Advanced Techniques for Modelling Maternal and Child Health in Africa

THE SPRINGER SERIES ON

DEMOGRAPHIC METHODS AND POPULATION ANALYSIS

Series Editor

KENNETH C. LAND

Duke University

In recent decades, there has been a rapid development of demographic models and methods and an explosive growth in the range of applications of population analysis. This series seeks to provide a publication outlet both for high-quality textual and expository books on modern techniques of demographic analysis and for works that present exemplary applications of such techniques to various aspects of population analysis.

Topics appropriate for the series include:

- General demographic methods
- Techniques of standardization
- Life table models and methods
- Multistate and multiregional life tables, analyses and projections
- Demographic aspects of biostatistics and epidemiology
- Stable population theory and its extensions
- Methods of indirect estimation
- Stochastic population models
- Event history analysis, duration analysis, and hazard regression models
- Demographic projection methods and population forecasts
- Techniques of applied demographic analysis, regional and local population estimates and projections
- Methods of estimation and projection for business and health care applications
- Methods and estimates for unique populations such as schools and students

Volumes in the series are of interest to researchers, professionals, and students in demography, sociology, economics, statistics, geography and regional science, public health and health care management, epidemiology, biostatistics, actuarial science, business, and related fields.

For further volumes:
http://www.springer.com/series/6449

Ngianga-Bakwin Kandala • Gebrenegus Ghilagaber
Editors

Advanced Techniques for Modelling Maternal and Child Health in Africa

Springer

Editors
Dr. Ngianga-Bakwin Kandala
Warwick Medical School
Division of Health Sciences
University of Warwick
Coventry, UK

Prof. Gebrenegus Ghilagaber
Department of Statistics
Stockholm University
Stockholm, Sweden

ISSN 1389-6784
ISBN 978-94-007-6777-5 ISBN 978-94-007-6778-2 (eBook)
DOI 10.1007/978-94-007-6778-2
Springer Dordrecht Heidelberg New York London

Library of Congress Control Number: 2013945174

Printed on acid-free paper

Springer is part of Springer Science+Business Media (www.springer.com)

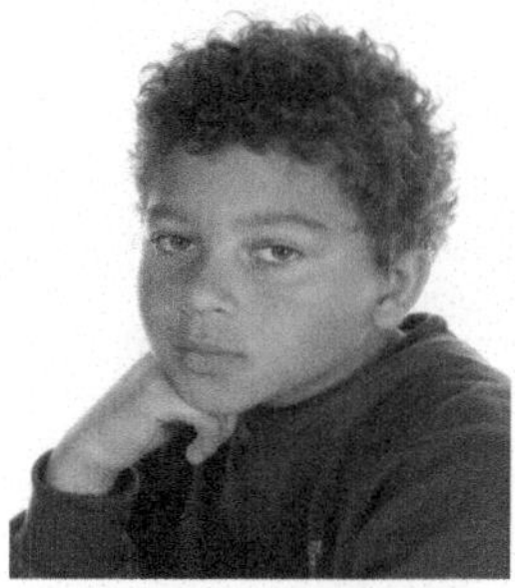

This book is firstly dedicated to the memory of my late son, Hendrick Kandala, who two months before his tragic death in London attended the 58th Congress of the International Statistical Institute (ISI) in Dublin, Ireland, August 21–26, 2011, and shared many wonderful things prior to his untimely death . . .

Then to my daughters, Catherine and Rose, God's blessings to me during good times and bad, whose unconditional and steadfast love has allowed me to get strength, and whom I will always love and cherish . . .

Summary

The estimation of levels, trends, and differentials in demographic and health outcomes in developing countries has, over the years, relied heavily on indirect methods that were devised to suit limited or deficient data. In recent decades, some worldwide surveys like the World Fertility Survey and its successor, the Demographic and Health Survey (DHS), have played an important role in filling the gap in the availability of survey data in developing countries. These surveys, conducted at enormous costs, are aimed at enabling investigators to make in-depth analyses that could guide policy intervention strategies. However, their utilization remains suboptimal, because optimal analyses of such data demand advanced statistical techniques.

Since the use of DHS data in developing countries, many developments in statistical modelling based on hierarchical models have been published, and our primary aim is to bring together the various methodological advances. Naturally, the choice of these recent developments reflects our own teaching and research interests.

We try to motivate and illustrate concepts with examples using real data from the DHS, and the data sets are available on http://www.measuredhs.com. We could not treat all recent developments in the area of health and survival in Africa in this book, and in such cases we point to references at the end of each chapter.

The book presents both theoretical contributions and empirical applications of such advanced techniques. We cover a range of new developments from both the classical and Bayesian approaches. In the Bayesian framework, Monte Carlo techniques, in particular MCMC, and their application to spatial and spatio-temporal data are covered. These include techniques such as geoadditive semi-parametric models that link individual health outcomes with area variables to account for spatial correlation; latent modelling that deals with the impact of spatial effects on latent, unobservable variables like "health status" or "frailty"; spatial modelling of multiple diseases that enables quantifying the correlation between relative risks of each disease as well as mapping of disease-specific residuals; and Bayesian structured geostatistical regression modelling that permits a joint estimation of the usual linear effects of categorical covariates, non-linear effects of continuous covariates and small-area district effects on health outcomes within a unified structured additive Bayesian framework.

Within the classical approach, we describe multilevel models which address issues of clustering within families and households; multiprocess models which account for interdependencies over life-course events and non-random utilization of health services; and flexible parametric alternatives to existing intensity models.

The techniques are illustrated mainly through modelling maternal and child health in the African context using data from the DHS in several countries in the continent. But the methods presented are universally applicable to other phenomena and geographical areas with similar data sets.

The book is coherently organized and clearly written so that readers can follow its contents without having to master the technical parts.

There are two parts to this book: (I) modelling child health and survival in Africa and (II) modelling maternal health and survival in Africa.

Part I covers recent developments in child health modelling techniques. We discuss the formulation of models using flexible geoadditive predictors accounting for the effects of different types of covariates. Such formulation embraces the usual famous regression models such as generalized additive models (GAM), generalized additive mixed models (GAMM), generalized geoadditive mixed models (GGAMM), and stepwise regression models, among others. We emphasize the modelling process and policy implications rather than explicit use of the techniques (which can be found in other textbooks).

Part II introduces modelling of maternal health outcomes. Readers are guided through these techniques with alternative software packages, such as WinBUGS and BayesX. Many of the applications of this part relate directly to the models discussed in Part I.

Although few authors worked on this text, it could not have been written without the support from various sources. We would particularly like to thank all participants of our session at the 57th Congress of the International Statistical Institute in Durban, South Africa, 2009, where the idea to write this book originated. We are also very grateful to the University of Aachen, Germany, for providing the environment and the financial support to run our subsequent workshop in 2010. In particular, we express our thanks to Professor Thomas Kraus, the head of the Institute of Occupational and Social Medicine, University of Aachen, who hosted and facilitated the workshop. Thanks to Professor Clifford Odimegwu of the University of Witwatersrand for valuable comments on earlier versions of this text. We also thank Professor Daniel Thorburn, Department of Statistics, Stockholm University, for reading parts of the manuscript and coming up with valuable comments. Our thanks also go to the anonymous reviewers from Springer who read and commented on the first draft of our manuscript. We also thank Diana Kandala for helping in copy-editing of the manuscript. Ngianga-Bakwin Kandala acknowledges the financial support he received from the British Council under the Development Partnership in Higher Education (DelPHE) scheme, Grant No. 788. Last, but by no means least, Gebrenegus Ghilagaber would like to thank his children Astér, Millen, and Simon for their unconditional love, patience, and understanding during the preparation of the book whose value may not have been clear to them at the time.

Contents

Contributors

Alfred A. Abiodun Department of Statistics, University of Ilorin, Ilorin, Nigeria

Samson Babatunde Adebayo Planning, Research and Statistics, National Agency for Food and Drug Administration and Control, Abuja, Nigeria

Diddy Antai Department of Public Health Sciences, Karolinska Institute, Stockholm, Sweden

Jennifer Anyanti Society for Family Health, Abuja, Nigeria

Bo Cai Department of Epidemiology and Biostatistics, University of South Carolina, Columbia, SC, USA

Woldeyesus Elisa Statistics and Evaluation Office, Asmara, Eritrea

Ezra Gayawan Department of Mathematical Sciences, Redeemer's University, Redemption City, Ogun State, Nigeria

Gebrenegus Ghilagaber Department of Statistics, Stockholm University, Stockholm, Sweden

***Stephen Obeng Gyimah** Department of Sociology, Queen's University, Kingston, Ontario, Canada

Ngianga-Bakwin Kandala Warwick Medical School, Division of Health Sciences, University of Warwick, Coventry, UK

KEMRI-University of Oxford-Welcome Trust Collaborative Programme, Nairobi, Kenya

Division of Epidemiology and Biostatistics, University of the Witwatersrand, Johannesburg, South Africa

Ngianga II Kandala (Shadrack) Division of Social Statistics, University of Southampton, Southampton, UK

Lawrence N. Kazembe Department of Statistics and Population Studies, University of Namibia, Windhoek, Namibia

Khaled Khatab Faculty of Health and Wellbeing, Centre for Health and Social Care Research, Sheffield Hallam University, Sheffield, UK

***Olaronke Ladipo** Society for Family Health, Abuja, Nigeria

Samuel O.M. Manda Biostatistics Unit, South African Medical Research Council, Pretoria, South Africa

Division of Epidemiology and Biostatistics, University of the Witwatersrand, Johannesburg, South Africa

Renate Meyer Department of Statistics, University of Auckland, Auckland, New Zealand

Benjamin A. Oyejola Department of Statistics, University of Ilorin, Ilorin, Nigeria

William Tigbe Division of Health Sciences, Warwick Medical School, University of Warwick, Coventry, UK

Waheed B. Yahya Department of Statistics, University of Ilorin, Ilorin, Nigeria

*Unfortunately, two contributors did not live long to see the end product of their efforts. **Stephen Obeng Gyimah** died on 11 May 2012 while **Olaronke Ladipo** died on 31 October 2012. Our thoughts will always be with their families, close friends and colleagues who are affected by their untimely death.

Chapter 1
Advanced Techniques for Modelling Maternal and Child Health in Africa

Samuel O.M. Manda, Ngianga-Bakwin Kandala, and Gebrenegus Ghilagaber

1.1 Introduction

More than ten million women die or experience adverse consequences during pregnancy and child birth each year (WHO 2005). Furthermore, nearly nine million children under the age of 5 years die each year, largely from preventable and treatable diseases (UNICEF 2010). The hardest hit countries by poor maternal health (defined as the health of mothers during pregnancy, childbirth, and in the postpartum period) and poor child health (defined as the health of children from birth through adolescence) are in the developing world. For example, even though the global estimates of maternal and child mortality rates in 2008 were at 260 per 100,000 and 60 per 1,000 live births, respectively, the rates ranged from 21 to 620 and 13 to 12, with the African region at the top of both ranges (WHO 2011).

Progress on maternal and child health has long been recognized as critical to fostering socio-economic development of a country. Thus, it was not surprising that improvements in maternal and child health (MCH) were two of the eight Millennium Development Goals (MDGs). In particular, MDG 4 targeted reducing under-five mortality rates by 67 % between 1990 and 2015, and MDG 5 set two targets: reducing maternal mortality ratio by 75 % and achieving universal access to reproductive health by 2015 (United Nations 2012). However, progress towards

S.O.M. Manda (✉)
Biostatistics Unit, South African Medical Research Council, Pretoria, South Africa
e-mail: Samuel.Manda@mrc.ac.za

N.-B. Kandala
Warwick Medical School, Division of Health Sciences, University of Warwick, Coventry, UK
e-mail: n-b.kandala@warwick.ac.uk

G. Ghilagaber
Department of Statistics, Stockholm University, SE-106 91 Stockholm, Sweden
e-mail: Gebre@stat.su.se

N.-B. Kandala and G. Ghilagaber (eds.), *Advanced Techniques for Modelling Maternal and Child Health in Africa*, The Springer Series on Demographic Methods and Population Analysis 34, DOI 10.1007/978-94-007-6778-2_1,

meeting these targets has been very slow in developing countries. For instance, the annual rate of under-five mortality decline is 2.1 %, which is below the target of 4.4 % per year. Furthermore, even though many pregnant women received at least one antenatal care visit with a skilled attendant, between 2000 and 2008, the prevalence of skilled attendance at birth in Africa was estimated at 46 %. The global estimate of this prevalence was put at 65 %, with a range of 46–96 % between the WHO regions (Friberg et al. 2010; WHO 2011).

In recognition of the slow progress towards MDGs 4 and 5 in Africa, major international bodies and funding agencies such as the United States Agency for International Development (USAID) and the World health Organization (WHO) have more than doubled their efforts at improving maternal and child health in the region (The Kaiser Family Foundation 2009; The PLoS Medicine Editors 2010). The interventions and programs that are mostly funded cover mitigating the adverse effects of HIV and malaria in pregnant women and their children. Support is also provided in the delivery of an evidence-based and cost-effective care for mothers and children. Individually, some governments have taken steps to improve maternal and child health. In South Africa, for instance, maternal and child health is one of the four health priority areas within the National Department of Health (Department of Health 2012).

Analyses of various data sources suggest that maternal and child health, for example maternal and child mortality have been declining in recent years in the sub-Saharan African (SSA) region. However, the levels of the decline vary considerably across the countries of the regions, with the wealthier and modernized regions having faster declines (UNICEF 2010; WHO 2011). But the data upon which these empirical evidences are based are inconsistent and their sources and quality vary between years and the countries. Thus, various governments and stakeholders have invested substantially into data collection and analysis for improved and reliable maternal and child health indicators.

Most of the empirical evidence upon which maternal and child health are assessed on to measure progress towards achieving targets sets under MDGs 4 and 5 are derived from the Demographic and Health Surveys (DHS) datasets. The DHS programme is funded by the USAID and is implemented by Macro International (a US based consultancy firm). The surveys provide nationally-representative data on population, health, HIV, and nutrition in over 90 developing countries. The data generated are used by various stakeholders for a wide range of monitoring and impact evaluation indicators in the areas of demographic and health in these countries. The DHS and its predecessor, the World Fertility Survey (WFS) have played important roles in filling the gap in the availability of MCH data in developing countries. The DHS datasets are available on http://www.measuredhs.com. Multiple Indicator Cluster Survey (MICS) and HIV/AIDS and Reproductive Health Survey are also increasingly used to provide comparative assessments of MCH outcomes. The samples drawn in these surveys mostly use stratified multistage cluster sampling designs, often with over-sampling of smaller domains such as urban areas or certain regions of a country.

Thus, any statistical analysis of data drawn from such complex surveys needs to account for the sampling design, in addition to account for data quality nonresponse, missing data, erroneous responses, and defective sampling frames. The importance of accounting for the sample design in regression modelling is widely acknowledged in the statistical literature (Binder 1983, 1992; Korn and Gruabard 1995, 1999; Pfeffermann 1993; Skinner et al. 1989). However, in many instances, these data are analyzed using statistical software designed for simple randomly sampled data. When such data are interrogated using statistical methods, the summary information used to inform public health policies regarding MCH can be misleading (Mathews et al. 1999). Whilst statistical methods exist to overcome this problem, these have not been extensively worked through in a coherent manner or packaged appropriately into a volume, which is why this volume fills that gap. These datasets, especially the DHS, include geographical information that could identify spatial patterns in MCH to target health policies. This new information must also be incorporated when analyses of such data are undertaken.

However, the utilization of a wealth of MCH data sources from high quality national representative samples in the Sub Saharan region Africa (SSA), collected at comparative enormous costs, remains sub-optimal because optimal analyses of such data demand advanced statistical techniques. These data when analyzed comprehensively using appropriate statistical methods for the robust evaluation of data in respect to the socio-economic, demographic, general and maternal and child health, can enable investigators to make in-depth assessments that could guide policy intervention strategies. Studies that utilized appropriate statistical modelling and analysis of MCH outcomes in the SSA region have increased recently (see for example, Gemperli et al. (2004); Kandala and Madise (2004); Kandala et al. (2006, 2007); Kazembe and Namangale (2007); Manda et al. (2012a, b) to name a few).

Our primary aim in this volume is to bring together these methodological advances to important applications in maternal and child health in Africa. Naturally, the choice of these recent developments reflects our own teaching and research interests. In order to make the volume widely read and accessible to the general practitioner and researchers who are routinely involved in the analyses of the MCH data; we have included motivating and illustrate concepts with examples using real data from the DHS and similar surveys. We could not treat all recent developments in the area of health and survival in Africa in this book, and in such cases, we point to references at the end of each chapter.

The volume presents both theoretical contributions and empirical applications of such recent and advanced techniques. We cover a range of new developments from both the classical and Bayesian approaches. Within the classical approach, we examine multilevel models that address the issue of clustering within families and households; multiprocess models that account for interdependencies over life-course events and non-random utilization of health services; and flexible parametric alternatives to existing intensity models.

On the other hand, within the Bayesian framework, Monte Carlo techniques, in particular Markov Chain Monte Carlo (MCMC) and their application to spatio-temporal data are covered. These include such techniques like geo-additive semi-parametric models that link individual health outcomes with area variables to account for spatial correlation; geo-additive latent modelling that deal with the impact of the spatial effects on the latent, unobservable health status or frailty; joint diseases mapping models that permit the quantification of common and specific risk profiles between diseases. Bayesian structured additive regression modelling that permits a joint estimation of the usual linear effects of categorical covariates, nonlinear effects of continuous covariates and small-area effects on health outcomes within a unified structured additive Bayesian framework.

Thus this volume presents wide theoretical and range of applications covering most aspects of the data structures arising from DHS and similar surveys. The techniques are illustrated through the modelling of maternal and child health in the African context using data from DHS in several countries in the continent, with a few example using Multiple Indicator Cluster Survey (MICS) and HIV/AIDS and Reproductive Health Survey. But, the methods presented are universally applicable to other phenomena and geographical areas with similar data sets.

1.2 Structure of the Volume

This volume is coherently organized and clearly written so that readers can follow its contents without having to master the technical parts. Apart from this Introductory Chapter and a Summary Chapter, it contains 14 chapters dedicated to case studies in maternal and child health in Africa; and for each a modern statistical method has been used to analyse the data. These 14 chapters are grouped into two parts: Part I contains eight case studies on child health and survival (2–9) and Part II contains six case studies on maternal health and survival (10–15). We emphasize the modelling process and policy implications, rather than explicit use of the techniques (which can be found in other textbooks).

Chapter 1 gives a general introduction of the volume. In Chap. 2 of the volume, Ghilagaber discusses multilevel modelling for clustered child survival data and the issue of selection bias in the utilization of maternal and child health services. He discusses the difficulties in assessing the impact of prenatal care and hospital delivery on child survival if the selection processes in the utilization of health facilities are not accounted for. These issues are addressed using data from three Africa countries: Egypt, Eritrea and Uganda. He constructs joint modelling of survival and selection processes, which he then estimated using likelihood based methods. Chapter 3 extends the ideas of multilevel modelling for child survival data to situation where the data are arranged in space. Ghilagaber and colleagues discuss the limitations of the independence assumptions by noting that neighbouring areas are more likely to have similar child survival experiences than children in areas far apart. Thus, they propose using spatial models to determine variations of childhood mortality between districts in Nigeria. The model proposed calls for time-varying as well as non-linear effects of some covariates on child survival by introducing smoothness structures for spatial and non-linear effects. These are estimated within a Bayesian perspective and fitted using the recently developed MCMC simulation techniques. The spatial modelling techniques in Chap. 3 are extended to Chap. 4, where Khatab examines the impact of socioeconomic and public health factors on childhood diseases and malnutrition by using latent or unobservable constructs. His Geo-additive latent variable modelling is exemplified using data on childhood disease and malnutrition in two African countries: Egypt and Nigeria.

In Chap. 5, Kazembe examines ecological associations between socio-economic inequalities and childhood health in Malawi. He constructs child health status using a number of combinations based on a child status on fever, diarrhoea, stunting and underweight to a multinomial response with five categories within a geoadditive spatial model. The empirical Bayesian method, using penalised likelihood estimation techniques, is used to fit the individual and spatially relevant fixed and random effects. In the analysis of time-to-event data Ghilagaber, in Chap. 6, shows that indirect standardization and loglinear regression models for count data are special cases of the well-known proportional hazards regression portrayed as belonging to distinct fields or as competing methodologies. He further shows that these seemingly different models can be synthesised in standard packages such as SPSS and SAS. These issues are illustrated by an empirical analysis of a data set on mortality experiences among Eritrean children. The spatial modelling techniques discussed in Chaps. 3 and 4 dealing with flexible Bayesian structured additive regression for joint estimation of trend, nonlinear effects of continuous covariates, geographical variations and fixed effects of categorical covariates is also adopted for Chap. 7 by Adebayo and Yahya. They analyse individual and ecological determinants of vaccination coverage in Nigeria. Chapter 8 discusses the modelling of both individual and ecological association with childhood survival in South Africa. Here, Manda introduces robust and flexible spatial distributions based on the double exponential model as opposed to the standard normal autoregressive model. He uses a mixture of spatial distributions to offer more flexibility and less restrictive form and shape of the spatial distribution assumed. Finally, Chap. 9 rounds off Part I of the book by discussing socio-demographic determinants of anaemia in children by Kandala (Shadrack), where he uses multilevel modelling to estimate the effects of predictors. The resulting models are estimated using restricted iterative generalized least squares (RIGLS) within MLwiN statistical package.

Part II starts off with Chap. 10, where Ghilagaber and co-authors discuss flexible family of parametric survival models to the analysis of birth interval data. The models are illustrated by an analysis of correlates of birth spacing in Eritrea, Ghana, and Kenya. Kandala in Chap. 11 discusses health threats posed by emerging burden of non-communicable diseases in the SSA region. He uses geostatistical modelling described in various chapters in Part I to analyse spatial variations of hypertension in South Africa. In Chap. 12, Manda and co-authors discuss modelling options for stratified survival data. They discuss unstratified and parametric stratified survival analyses and show the advantages of a non-parametric approach based on mixtures of triangular distributions to estimate baseline hazard rates. Within a Bayesian formulation via Markov chain Monte Carlo algorithm for posterior computation, they analyse determinants of timing of first childbirth in South Africa where the data are heavily stratified.

Adebayo and Gayawan discuss the issues regarding levels and trends of fertility in Nigeria. In particular, they consider number of children born to a woman and model its individual and spatial determinants using flexible geoadditive approaches, which as indicated earlier, permit non-linear or time-varying effects of covariates and the usual linear effects in a joint model. These are discussed in Chap. 13. In Chap. 14, Abiodun and colleagues use geostatistical models to investigate geographical variation of timing of sexual initiation in Nigerian youth and discuss the implications for HIV prevention. In Chap. 15, Kandala and coauthors extend the work in Chap. 11 to modelling geographic co-morbidity of four vascular diseases: high blood pressure, stroke, heart attack and high blood cholesterol in order to understand interactions and dynamics between chronic diseases. In particular, they use the shared component spatial models to estimate common and specific risk in the four vascular diseases. Finally, in Chap. 16 Ghilagaber ties up the findings of the volume by way of summary and direction for future research.

References

Binder, D. A. (1983). On the variance of the asymptotically normal estimators from complex surveys. *International Statistical Review, 51*, 279–292.

Binder, D. A. (1992). Fitting Cox's proportional hazards model from survey data. *Biometrika, 79*, 139–147.

Department of Health. (2012). *Maternal and child health*. http://www.doh.gov.za/list.php?type=Maternalandchildhealth. Accessed November 10, 2012.

Friberg, I. K., Kinney, M. V., Lawn, J. E., Kerber, K. J., Odubanjo, M. O., et al. (2010). Sub-Saharan Africa's mothers, newborns, and children: How many lives could be saved with targeted health interventions? *PLoS Medicine, 7*, e295.

Gemperli, A., Vounatsou, P., Kleinschmidt, I., et al. (2004). Spatial patterns of infant mortality in Mali: The effect of malaria endemicity. *American Journal of Epidemiology, 159*(1), 64–72.

Kandala, N.-B., & Madise, J. (2004). The spatial epidemiology of childhood diseases in Malawi and Zambia. *African Population Studies, 19*(3), 199–226.

Kandala, N.-B., Magadi, M. A., & Madise, N. J. (2006). An investigation of district spatial variations of childhood diarrhoea and fever in Malawi. *Social Science & Medicine, 62*(5), 1138–1152.

Kandala, N.-B., Ji, C., Stallard, N., et al. (2007). Spatial analysis of risk factors for childhood morbidity in Nigeria. *The American Journal of Tropical Medicine and Hygiene, 77*(4), 770–778.

Kazembe, L. N., & Namangale, J. J. (2007). A Bayesian multinomial model to analyse spatial patterns of childhood co-morbidity in Malawi. *European Journal of Epidemiology, 22*(8), 545–556.

Korn, E. L., & Graubard, B. I. (1995). Analysis of large health surveys: accounting for the sampling design. *Journal of the Royal Statistical Society A, 158*, 263–295.

Korn, E. L., & Graubard, B. I. (1999). *Analysis of large health surveys*. New York: Wiley.
Manda, S. O. M., Lombard, C. L., & Mosala, T. (2012a). Divergent spatial patterns in the prevalence of human immunodeficiency virus and syphilis in South African pregnant women. *Geospatial Health, 6*(2), 221–231.
Manda, S. O. M., Feltbower, R. G., & Gilthorpe, M. S. (2012b). A multivariate frailty model for multiple spatially dependent survival data. In Y.-K. Tu & D. C. Greenwood (Eds.), *Modern methods for epidemiology* (pp. 157–172). Dordrecht/New York: Springer.
Mathews, Z., Madise, N., & Stephenson, R. (1999). Regression modelling for complex survey data: An application to child nutritional status in four African Countries. *Proceedings of the Third African Population Conference, Durban, South Africa, 1,* 333–347.
Pfeffermann, D. (1993). The role of sampling weights when modelling survey data. *International Statistical Review, 61*, 317–337.
Skinner, C., Holt, D., & Smith, T. (1989). *Analysis of complex surveys*. New York: Wiley.
The Kaiser Family Foundation. (2009). *The U.S. and global maternal and child health. kaiser fast facts. Data Source: #7963*. http://www.kff.org/globalhealth/upload/7963.pdf. Accessed November 10, 2012.
The PLoS Medicine Editors. (2010). Maternal health: Time to deliver. *PLoS Medicine* 7(6), e1000300.
UNICEF. (2010). *ChildInfo: Monitoring the situation of children and woman*. Available at http://www.childinfo.org/mortality.html. Accessed November 10, 2012.
United Nations. (2012). *The millennium development goals report 2012*. New York: United Nations.
WHO. (2005). *The World health report 2005 – Make every mother and child count*. Geneva: World Health Organization. http://www.who.int/whr/2005/en. Accessed November 10, 2012.
WHO. (2011). *World health statistics 2011*. Geneva: WHO Press/World Health Organization.

Part I
Child Health and Survival

Chapter 2
Disentangling Selection and Causality in Assessing the Effects of Health Inputs on Child Survival: Evidence from East Africa

Gebrenegus Ghilagaber

2.1 Introduction

Many demographic data have a hierarchical or clustered structure. For example, the analysis of childhood mortality involves a natural hierarchy where children are grouped within mothers or families, and the latter, in turn, are grouped into communities. Children from the same parents tend to be more alike in their characteristics than children chosen at random from the population at large. To ignore this grouping risks overlooking the importance of group effects, and may render invalid many of the traditional statistical analysis techniques used for studying data relationships.

The present chapter addresses the relationship between childhood mortality on the one hand, and use of health care and other socioeconomic variables on the other, in three African countries – Egypt, Eritrea, and Uganda. In contrast to most previous works where the collection of children is assumed to be an independent random sample, we treat children with the same mother as correlated cases (level 1) within the same mother (level 2). This is consistent with the data collection where a nationally representative random sample of women is selected (National Statistics Office [Eritrea] and Macro International Inc 1995). Our formulation also enables us to allow for unobserved mother-specific heterogeneity in the models.

A second and important issue that is addressed in this chapter is that of selection bias. The public policy response to the problem of high childhood mortality in developing countries has primarily focused on encouraging prenatal care and institutional delivery. Since there are no randomized trials of standard prenatal care and hospital delivery, it is difficult to assess the impact of such health inputs on

G. Ghilagaber (✉)
Department of Statistics, Stockholm University, SE-106 91 Stockholm, Sweden
e-mail: Gebre@stat.su.se

N.-B. Kandala and G. Ghilagaber (eds.), *Advanced Techniques for Modelling Maternal and Child Health in Africa*, The Springer Series on Demographic Methods and Population Analysis 34, DOI 10.1007/978-94-007-6778-2_2,

survival chances without accounting for selection processes in the utilization of health facilities.

Generally, selection bias can arise when there is a systematic difference in characteristics between those who are selected for the study and those who are not. If these unobserved factors also influence the impacts of the studied subject, selection bias will occur. However, selection bias will only arise if these unobserved factors, which influence the selection, also influence the phenomena under investigation.

Two common types of selection are adverse selection and favorable selection. Suppose women who receive prenatal health care have a higher risk of losing their child than women who do not receive prenatal health care. It is possible that women who seek prenatal childcare in fact have characteristics that separate them from others. If such characteristics are such that they lead to poorer outcome of prenatal care than it really is, then the contribution of prenatal care may be underestimated due to adverse selection.

In contrast, favourable selection arises when the studied individuals have characteristics that lead to overestimation of the effects of a covariate on the phenomenon under investigation.

In the present chapter, we examine the effects of selection on estimates of the efficacy of prenatal care and hospital delivery (health inputs) by using multiprocess models developed and earlier used by Lillard and Panis (see, Lillard 1993; Panis and Lillard 1994; Lillard and Panis 2000).

2.2 Statistical Methods: Multilevel and Multiprocess Modeling

2.2.1 *A Piece-Wise Log-Linear Hazard Model with Heterogeneity*

A piece-wise log-linear hazards model of mortality is given by[1]:

$$\ln \lambda_{ij}(t) = \gamma T_{ij}(t) + \beta' X_{ij} + \varepsilon_i \tag{2.1}$$

where $\ln \lambda_{ij}(t)$ is the log-hazard of death at age t associated to child j of mother i. The baseline log-hazard $\gamma T_{ij}(t)$ is assumed to be piecewise linear in the child's age; X_{ij} represents regressors, and ε captures unobserved heterogeneity, at the mother level, that is associated with mortality, $\varepsilon \sim N\left(0, \sigma_\varepsilon^2\right)$. The regressors may be time-varying but all covariates used in this chapter are fixed. Regressors add to the log-hazard

[1]The presentation in this and the next sections follows largely that of Lillard and Panis (2000).

and thus shift the hazard proportionally. Time is written as an argument in $T_{ij}(t)$ to indicate that it varies continuously over the duration of an interval but the slope may vary between intervals.

This is a two-level piece-wise linear survival model with mothers as the level-2 units and children as repeated outcomes (level-1) within observations.

Conditional on the heterogeneity component ε, the likelihood of the hazard for child j from the ith mother is:

$$L_{ij}^{(M)}(\varepsilon) = \begin{cases} S_{ij}\left(t^{*},\varepsilon\right), & \textit{if the child is alive (censored) at time } t^{*} \\ S_{ij}\left(t^{l},\varepsilon\right) - S_{j}\left(t^{u},\varepsilon\right), & \textit{if the child died between at } t^{l} \textit{ and } t^{u} \end{cases} \tag{2.2}$$

where $S_{ij}(t,\varepsilon)$ is the survivor function at time t. In the absence of time-varying covariates,

$$S_j(t,\varepsilon) = \left[S_{0j}(t,\varepsilon)\right]^{\exp\left(\beta' X_j + \varepsilon\right)}, \tag{2.3}$$

where

$S_{0j}(t,\varepsilon)$ representing the baseline survivor function at time t., i.e., the survivor function based on the baseline duration dependency (or dependencies) only:

$$S_{0j}(t) = \exp\left\{-\int_{\tau=t_b}^{t} \lambda_{j0}(\tau)\,d\tau\right\},$$

where $\lambda_{j0}(t) = \gamma T_j(t)$ and t_b denotes the beginning of the hazard spell (interval).

Conditional on the heterogeneity, the likelihood contributions in (2.2) are independent. The joint likelihood of multiple hazard intervals in the presence of heterogeneity is thus found by the product of conditional likelihoods of individual hazard modules:

$$L^{(M)} = \prod_{j} L_j^{(M)} \tag{2.4}$$

The baseline duration pattern is the model's dependency on time without any covariates or heterogeneity. In the model above, it is represented by $\gamma T_{ij}(t)$. A constant baseline hazard (exponential model) may be achieved by defining a spline with intercept and without nodes, and fixing the slope coefficient to zero. A Gormpertz (linear) log-hazard may be specified by defining a spline without nodes, so that the slope is the Gompertz slope. A piecewise-constant hazard may be achieved by estimating regression coefficient on time-varying indicator variables. Piecewise-linear duration patterns are very attractive because they adjust to any pattern in the data (with sufficiently many nodes), and because linear combinations of piecewise-linear patterns are again piecewise-linear (Lillard and Panis 2000).

2.2.2 Multilevel Probit Models with Unobserved Heterogeneity

A Probit Model of Prenatal Care

We model the ith mother's decision to visit a prenatal care center (as opposed to no such visit at all) during pregnancy of the jth child as a binary probit model:

$$P_{ij}^{*} = \alpha' X_{ij} + \delta_i \tag{2.5}$$

where X are mother-specific explanatory variables ($X_{ij} = X_i$ for all children j of the same mother); and δ_i represents unobserved heterogeneity at the mother level that is associated with utilization of prenatal care. We assume that the heterogeneity component is distributed normally, $\delta \sim N\left(0, \sigma_{\delta}^{2}\right)$. Thus, the likelihood for a binary probit model is given by

$$L_j^{(P)} = \begin{cases} \Phi\left(-\alpha' X\right), & if\ P_j = 0 \\ 1 - \Phi\left(-\alpha' X\right), & if\ P_j = 1 \end{cases}, \tag{2.6}$$

where $\Phi(.)$ is the (cumulative) distribution function of the standard normal density:

$$\Phi(z) = \frac{1}{\sqrt{2\pi}} \int_{-\infty}^{z} \exp\left(-\frac{u^2}{2}\right) du \tag{2.7}$$

The Prenatal Care decision for child j is:

$$P_j = \begin{cases} 0, & if\ P_{ij}^{*} < 0\ (no\ prenatal\ care) \\ 1, & if\ P_{ij}^{*} \geq 0\ (prenatal\ care) \end{cases} \tag{2.8}$$

Conditional on the heterogeneity, the likelihood contributions in (2.6) are independent. The joint likelihood of multiple probit modules in the presence of heterogeneity is thus given by the product of conditional likelihoods of individual probit contributions:

$$L^{(P)} = \prod_{j} L_j^{(P)} \tag{2.9}$$

A Probit Model of Hospital Delivery

As with the prenatal care we model the decision to deliver in hospital (as opposed to home delivery) as a binary probit model:

$$H_{ij}^{*} = \phi' X_{ij} + \omega_i \tag{2.10}$$

where X are mother-specific explanatory variables, and ω represents unobserved heterogeneity at the mother level. We assume that the heterogeneity component is distributed normally, $\omega \sim N\left(0, \sigma_{\omega}^2\right)$.

The delivery decision for child j is:

$$H_j = \begin{cases} 0, & \textit{if } H_j^* < 0 \; (\textit{delivery at home}) \\ 1, & \textit{if } H_j^* \geq 0 \; (\textit{institutional delivery}) \end{cases} \tag{2.11}$$

The likelihood for a binary probit model (module) is then

$$L_j^{(H)} = \begin{cases} \Phi\left(-\phi' X\right), & \textit{if } H_j = 0 \\ 1 - \Phi\left(-\phi' X\right), & \textit{if } H_j = 1 \end{cases} \tag{2.12}$$

where $\Phi(.)$ is the distribution function of the standard normal density as given in (2.8).

Conditional on the heterogeneity, the likelihood contributions in (2.12) are independent. The joint likelihood of multiple probit modules in the presence of heterogeneity is thus given by the product of conditional likelihoods of individual probit modules:

$$L^{(H)} = \prod_j L_j^{(H)} \tag{2.13}$$

2.2.3 Multiprocess Models: Disentangling Selection and Causality

A Joint Model of Child Mortality and Prenatal Care

Suppose we estimated a hazard model of child mortality and found a significant evidence of unobserved mother-specific characteristics that affect children's survival. If the mothers themselves are aware of at least some of those characteristics, they may respond to this private knowledge. Suppose that those women who are at above-average risk of losing their baby decide to reduce the risks by visiting prenatal care centers. The result will, then, be that prenatal care centers get a disproportionately high-risk mix of babies. If ignored, this adverse selection will underestimate the beneficial effect of prenatal care on childhood mortality. Conversely, prenatal care centers may get disproportionately low-risk mix of babies. This happens when selection is favorable – that women with below-average risk of losing their babies have a higher propensity of visiting prenatal care centers. These may include more educated women who are more aware of the benefits of prenatal care and/or urban residents for whom access is relatively easier. In this later type of selection, ignoring the favorable selection will overestimate the effect of prenatal care. These problems prompt us to address the potential endogeneity of prenatal care and estimate a joint model of child mortality and prenatal care decisions.

The joint model consists of two sets of equations:

- A hazard of child mortality:

$$\ln \lambda_{ij}(t) = \gamma T_{ij}(t) + \beta' X_{ij} + \varepsilon_i \tag{2.14}$$

- A probit of prenatal care:

$$P_{ij}^* = \alpha' X_{ij} + \delta_i \tag{2.15}$$

The main issue addressed here is that we wish to allow for the possibility that unobserved mother-specific characteristics affect both child survival and prenatal care decisions, i.e., we wish to allow for correlation between ε and δ:

$$\begin{pmatrix} \varepsilon \\ \delta \end{pmatrix} \sim N\left[\begin{pmatrix} 0 \\ 0 \end{pmatrix}, \begin{pmatrix} \sigma_\varepsilon^2 & \\ \sigma_{\varepsilon\delta} & \sigma_\delta^2 \end{pmatrix}\right] \tag{2.16}$$

The bias due to selection effects is eliminated by making the source of the bias (the correlation) part of the model. In our present case, the effect of prenatal care on mortality may be biased because of non-random prenatal care decisions. We therefore estimate a joint or multiprocess (to borrow a word from Lillard and Panis 2000) model of child survival and the decision to visit a prenatal care center.

The joint likelihood of the continuous and probit outcomes may be separated into a continuous and a probit part:

$$L^{(MP)} = L_1^{(M)} L_2^{(P)} \tag{2.17}$$

where

$$L_1^{(M)} = \frac{1}{\sigma_\varepsilon \sqrt{2\pi}} \exp\left\{-\frac{(y - \beta' X)^2}{2\sigma_\varepsilon^2}\right\} \tag{2.18}$$

and

$$L_2^{(P)} = \begin{cases} \Phi\left(\dfrac{\mu_{\delta|\varepsilon} - \alpha' X}{\sigma_{\delta|\varepsilon}}\right), & \mathit{if}\ P = 0 \\ 1 - \Phi\left(\dfrac{\mu_{\delta|\varepsilon} - \alpha' X}{\sigma_{\delta|\varepsilon}}\right), & \mathit{if}\ P = 1 \end{cases} \tag{2.19}$$

where the distribution of $\delta|\varepsilon$ is such that:

$$\begin{pmatrix}\varepsilon\\ \delta\end{pmatrix} \sim N\left[\begin{pmatrix}0\\ 0\end{pmatrix}, \begin{pmatrix}\sigma_\varepsilon^2 & \\ \sigma_{\varepsilon\delta} & \sigma_\delta^2\end{pmatrix}\right] \tag{2.20}$$

so that

$$\delta|\varepsilon \sim N\left[\frac{\sigma_{\varepsilon\delta}}{\sigma_\varepsilon^2}(\ln\lambda - \beta' X),\ \sigma_\delta^2 - \frac{\sigma_{\varepsilon\delta}}{\sigma_\varepsilon^2}\right] \tag{2.21}$$

From (2.17), (2.18), (2.19), (2.20), and (2.21) we note that the probit residual δ is conditional on the realized value of ε and, hence, $L_2^{(P)}$ is conditional on $L_1^{(M)}$.

A Joint Model of Child Mortality and Hospital Delivery

By analogous argument to the above subsection we address the potential endogeneity of institutional delivery by estimating a joint model of child mortality and hospital delivery decisions.

- A hazard of child mortality:

$$\ln\ \lambda_{ij}(t) = \gamma T_{ij}(t) + \beta' X_{ij} + \varepsilon_i \tag{2.22}$$

- A probit of hospital delivery:

$$H_{ij}^* = \phi' X_{ij} + \omega_i \tag{2.23}$$

Again, the joint likelihood of the continuous and probit outcomes may be separated into a continuous and a probit part,

$$L^{(MH)} = L_1^{(M)} L_2^{(H)} \tag{2.24}$$

where $L_1^{(M)}$ is as defined in (2.18) and

$$L_2^{(H)} = \begin{cases} \Phi\left(\dfrac{\mu_{\omega|\varepsilon} - \alpha' X}{\sigma_{\omega|\varepsilon}}\right), & if\ H = 0 \\ 1 - \Phi\left(\dfrac{\mu_{\omega|\varepsilon} - \alpha' X}{\sigma_{\omega|\varepsilon}}\right), & if\ H = 1 \end{cases} \tag{2.26}$$

where the distribution of $\omega|\varepsilon$ is such that:

$$\begin{pmatrix}\varepsilon\\ \omega\end{pmatrix} \sim N\left[\begin{pmatrix}0\\ 0\end{pmatrix}, \begin{pmatrix}\sigma_\varepsilon^2 & \\ \sigma_{\varepsilon\omega} & \sigma_\omega^2\end{pmatrix}\right] \tag{2.27}$$

so that

$$\omega|\varepsilon \sim N\left[\frac{\sigma_{\varepsilon\omega}}{\sigma_{\varepsilon}^{2}}\left(\ln\lambda - \phi' X\right),\ \sigma_{\omega}^{2} - \frac{\sigma_{\varepsilon\omega}}{\sigma_{\varepsilon}^{2}}\right] \tag{2.28}$$

We now wish to investigate whether unobserved characteristics at the mother level that affect the prenatal care decision are correlated with those that affect the decision to deliver in hospital. If these characteristics are correlated and the correlation is not accounted for, the effects of prenatal care and hospital deliveries on child mortality may be incorrect because these two effects may compete with each other or reinforce each other depending on the direction of the correlation.

The next step is, therefore, to estimate the hazard of child mortality jointly with both prenatal care and hospital delivery in order to control for the correlation between unobserved characteristics that affect these two health care decisions.

A Joint Model of Child Mortality, Prenatal Care, and Hospital Delivery

The effect of prenatal care and hospital delivery on mortality may be biased because of non-random prenatal care and hospital delivery decisions. More importantly, these effects may be biased because of a disproportionately high number of hospital deliveries with mothers who have visited a prenatal care center. We, therefore, model prenatal care and hospital delivery decisions jointly with the hazard of mortality.

The three-process joint model consists of three sets of equations:

- A hazard of child mortality:

$$\ln\ \lambda_{ij}(t) = \gamma T_{ij}(t) + \beta' X_{ij} + \varepsilon_i \tag{2.29}$$

- A probit of prenatal care:

$$P_{ij}^{*} = \alpha' X_{ij} + \delta_i \tag{2.30}$$

- A probit of hospital delivery:

$$H_{ij}^{*} = \phi' X_{ij} + \omega_i \tag{2.31}$$

The key issue here is that we wish to allow for the possibility that unobserved mother-specific characteristics affect all three dimensions: child survival, prenatal care, and hospital delivery decisions. In other words, the mother-specific heterogeneities in the three models ($\varepsilon, \delta\ and\ \omega$) are allowed to be pairwise correlated:

$$\begin{pmatrix}\varepsilon\\ \delta\\ \omega\end{pmatrix} \sim N\left[\begin{pmatrix}0\\0\\0\end{pmatrix},\begin{pmatrix}\sigma_{\varepsilon}^{2} & & \\ \sigma_{\varepsilon\delta} & \sigma_{\delta}^{2} & \\ \sigma_{\varepsilon\omega} & \sigma_{\delta\omega} & \sigma_{\omega}^{2}\end{pmatrix}\right]$$

The joint likelihood in the three process model is given as a product of the three likelihoods in (2.18), (2.19), and (2.26).

2.3 Data and Correlates of Childhood Mortality in Egypt, Eritrea, and Uganda

2.3.1 Data Sources

Egypt

The 1995 Egypt Demographic and Health Survey is the third survey in a series of Demographic and Health surveys that have been carried out in Egypt. The survey is a nationally-representative survey of 14,779 ever married women aged 15–49. These women gave birth to a total of 56,681 children but information on antenatal care visits and assistance, etc. is available only for children born within 5 years before the survey. For the purpose of this chapter, therefore, we concentrate on these 12,051 children from 8,008 mothers. For comparison purposes we also use a subset of 7,483 children from 6,140 mothers who were born within 3 years before the survey. Details concerning the 1995 Egyptian Demographic and Health Survey is documented in El-Zanaty et al. (1996).

Eritrea

The data used for illustration in the present section come the 1995 Demographic and Health Surveys (DHS) in the three countries.

The Eritrean Demographic and Health Survey (EDHS) is a nationally-representative survey of 5,054 women age 15–49 and 1,114 men age 15–59. It is the first survey ever undertaken by the National Statistics Office (NSO) of the Department of Macro Policy and International Economic Cooperation, Office of the President. It was implemented through the worldwide Demographic and Health Surveys (DHS) program of Macro International Inc.

One of the main objectives of the EDHS was to collect reliable data on maternal and child health indicators among children in early ages of their life. These include, among others, antenatal care visits and assistance at delivery. While the 5,054 women had a total of 14,268 children, information on antenatal care visits and assistance, etc. is available only for children born within 3 years before the survey. After deleting children with incomplete information on important factors we were left with 2,284 children belonging to 1,969 mothers. The maximum number of children per women was 3.

More details concerning the EDHS sample design, estimations of sampling errors for selected variables as well as summary tabulations are provided in National

Statistics Office (Eritrea), and Macro International Inc. (1995). In the present illustration we use the 1,969 mothers as experimental units and treat the 2,284 children as levels nested within these 1,969 mothers.

Uganda

The 1995 Uganda Demographic and Health Survey is a second survey in a series of Demographic and Health surveys that have been carried out in that country. It is a nationally-representative survey of 7,070 women age 15–49. By the survey time these women had a total of 22,752 children but the usable records for the purpose of this chapter are the 5,677 children from 3,988 mothers who were born within 4 years before the survey and a subset of it – the 4,533 children from 3,670 women who were born within 3 years before the survey. Tables of preliminary results and other details on the 1,995 Uganda Demographic and Health Survey may be found in Statistics Department [Uganda] and Macro International Inc. (1996).

2.3.2 Correlates of Child Mortality

The dependent variable is the log-hazard (logarithm of the rate at which the event of death occurs). The time variable (duration) measures the number of months from birth to death or the survey date, whichever comes first. Time varies between 0 and 35 months. The period between 0 and 35 months was partitioned into four: (0, 1), (1, 6), (6, 12), and (12, 35). The slope of the log-hazard was assumed to be constant within each interval but may vary between intervals. Additional models with time ranging between 0 and 47 months (in Uganda) and between 0 and 59 months (in Egypt) were also fit. In these models additional intervals for the time variable were used. These were (12, 24) in the case of Uganda and (12, 24), and (24, 36) in the case of Egypt.

Three mother-specific and five child-specific variables were used as explanatory variables.

The mother-specific variables are:

X_1 – Mother's Age-group at survey time (15–19, 20–24, 25–29, ..., 45–49).
X_2 – Mother's Level of Education (None, Primary, Secondary or higher).
X_3 – Residence (Urban, Rural).

The child-specific variables are:

X_4 – Preceding birth interval (First born, <18, 18–29, 30–47, 48+ months).
X_5 – Prenatal Care during pregnancy (None, Some prenatal care).
X_6 – Place of delivery of index child (Home, Hospital or clinic).
X_7 – Sex of index child (Girl, Boy).
X_8 – Multiplicity of index child (Single birth, One of multiple births).

The first level of each covariate was used as baseline (reference) level and, thus, no estimates are reported for these levels.

These variables are among those considered to be correlated with childhood mortality in previous analyses of the same data set (for the Eritrean data) or other data sets. However, because our main aim is of methodological nature, we have not strived to include all relevant covariates of mortality suggested in the literature or discuss the theoretical expectations of the effects of the covariates included in the analysis.

2.4 Results

2.4.1 Covariates Effects

The results of fitting the various models described in Sect. 2.2 to data on Egypt, Eritrea, and Uganda, are shown in Tables 2.1, 2.2, and 2.3, respectively. The five columns of results refer to the following situations:

- Model 1 refers to the multilevel piecewise log-linear hazards model in (2.1) but without heterogeneity term.
- Model 2 refers to the multilevel piecewise log-linear hazards model in (2.1) with mother-specific heterogeneity.
- Model 3 refers to the multilevel multiprocess model where (2.14) and (2.15) – that is a hazard model of child mortality and a probit model of prenatal care – are estimated simultaneously; we allow for mother-specific unobserved heterogeneity in both models; and allow these two heterogeneity terms to correlate.
- Model 4 refers to the multilevel multiprocess model where (2.22) and (2.23) – that is a hazard model of child mortality and a probit model of hospital delivery –

Table 2.1 Estimates of effects of prenatal care and hospital delivery on log-hazards of mortality (M) in various models: **Egypt (1995)**

Parameters	Model 1 (No Hetro)	Model 2 (Hetro)	Model 3 (M and P)	Model 4 (M and H)	Model 5 (M, P & H)
β_P	−0.3493*	−0.3959*	−1.4141*	−0.4037*	−1.2112*
β_H	0.0748	0.0945	0.0800	−0.6066*	−0.5283*
σ_ε	–	0.7393*	0.9082*	0.7408*	0.8469*
σ_δ	–	–	2.2458*	–	2.6563*
$\rho_{\varepsilon\delta}$	–	–	0.7531*	–	0.6314*
σ_ω	–	–	–	2.6997*	2.2649*
$\rho_{\varepsilon\omega}$	–	–	–	0.6182*	0.7741*
$\rho_{\delta\omega}$	–	–	–	–	0.4786*

*Estimate significant at 10 % significance level

Table 2.2 Estimates of effects of prenatal care and hospital delivery on log-hazards of mortality (M) in various models: **Eritrea (1995)**

Parameters	Model 1 (No Hetro)	Model 2 (Hetro)	Model 3 (M and P)	Model 4 (M and H)	Model 5 (M, P & H)
β_P	−0.4624*	−0.4928**	0.4632	−0.5038*	0.4432
β_H	−0.1142	−0.1107	−0.0920	−0.7188	0.1190
σ_ε	–	1.2488***	1.3324***	1.2367***	1.3165***
σ_δ	–	–	1.3193***	–	1.2913***
$\rho_{\varepsilon\delta}$	–	–	−0.5265*	–	−0.5412*
σ_ω	–	–	–	1.9301***	1.7889***
$\rho_{\varepsilon\omega}$	–	–	–	0.3138**	−0.2285
$\rho_{\delta\omega}$	–	–	–	–	0.6233***

*Estimate significant at 10 % level; **Estimate significant at 5 % level; ***Estimate significant at 1 % level

Table 2.3 Estimates of effects of prenatal care and hospital delivery on log-hazards of mortality (M) in various models: **Uganda (1995)**

Parameters	Model 1 (No Hetro)	Model 2 (Hetro)	Model 3 (M and P)	Model 4 (M and H)	Model 5 (M, P & H)
β_P	−0.4163*	−0.4280*	−0.1284	−0.4258*	−0.1713
β_H	−0.2945*	−0.2996*	−0.2942*	0.0271	−0.0211
σ_ε	–	0.5118*	0.4417**	0.5180*	0.4899*
σ_δ	–	–	1.9376*	–	2.0197*
$\rho_{\varepsilon\delta}$	–	–	−0.3654***	–	−0.4036***
σ_ω	–	–	–	2.0799*	1.8867*
$\rho_{\varepsilon\omega}$	–	–	–	−0.4099*	−0.3525**
$\rho_{\delta\omega}$	–	–	–	–	0.4625*

*Estimate significant at 10 % level; **Estimate significant at 5 % level; ***Estimate significant at 1 % level

are estimated simultaneously; we allow for mother-specific unobserved heterogeneity in both models; and allow these two heterogeneity terms to correlate.

- Model 5 refers to the multilevel multiprocess model where the three Eqs. (2.29), (2.30), and (2.31) – that is a hazard model of child mortality and two probit models for hospital delivery and prenatal care, respectively, – are estimated simultaneously; we allow for mother-specific unobserved heterogeneity in all three models, and allow for pairwise correlation between these three heterogeneity terms.

We have reported results related to hazard models alone and left out those from probit models. Further, only estimates of Prenatal care and Hospital delivery are presented in the Tables while estimates of the other background variables are suppressed.

We can, however, mention that, in the Egyptian case for instance, children from older cohort of mothers (aged 35 years or above at the time of the survey) had higher mortality risks than children from the very youngest cohort (15–19 years at survey time). Further, children of mothers with higher education (secondary or above level) had lower mortality; that 2nd and higher order births with short preceding birth intervals (< 18 months) had higher risks than first born children, while those born after long interval (at least 30 months) had significantly lower risks. The results for Eritrea and Uganda, in terms of the unreported covariate effects, were not much different.

2.4.2 Selection Bias in Prenatal Care Utilization

Again, beginning with Egypt (Table 2.1), a comparison of Models 2 and 3 shows that while both models show a significant beneficial effect of prenatal care on child mortality hazard, the magnitude is underestimated in the separate specification (from −1.4141 to −0.3959). This, again, is due to the positive correlation (0.7531) between the unobserved mother-specific characteristics that affect childhood mortality risks and the decision to visit a prenatal care during pregnancy. Thus, we can say that there is also adverse selection into prenatal care, and failure to account for this selectivity severely underestimates the magnitude of the beneficial effect of prenatal care.

The effect of selection in prenatal care is in the opposite direction in Eritrea. While separate specification (Model 2) shows a marginally significant beneficial effect of prenatal care (−0.4928), joint modeling (Model 3.) shows a positive but insignificant effect (0.4632). The correlation between the unobserved mother-specific characteristics that affect childhood mortality risks and the prenatal care is negative (−0.5265) and it is this negative correlation that pushed the effect of prenatal care far to the left of zero. In any case, we note that there is a mild favorable selection to prenatal care in Eritrea.

In the case of Uganda the selection bias is in the same direction as in Eritrea but it is stronger. The relatively weak and negative correlation (−0.3654) inflates the effect of prenatal care from an insignificant value (−0.1284) to a strongly significant effect (−0.4280) if this favorable selection is not accounted for.

2.4.3 Selection Bias in Hospital Delivery

Beginning with Egypt (Table 2.1), while the separate specification (Model 2) shows an insignificant and positive effect of hospital delivery on child mortality hazard (0.0748), joint estimation (Model 4) reveals a highly significant and strong negative effect (−0.6066). As stated in Lillard and Panis (2000), the mechanical reason lies in the positive correlation (0.6182) between the unobserved mother-specific characteristics that affect childhood mortality risks and the decision to delivery a child in hospital. An ignored positive correlation biases parameter estimates in positive direction, i.e., toward zero in the present case. Substantively, women with above-average risks of losing a baby ($\varepsilon > 0$) also tend to have above-average propensities to deliver in a hospital ($\omega > 0$); and vice versa. In other words, there is adverse selection into hospital delivery, and failure to account for this selectivity severely underestimates the beneficial effect of hospital delivery.

The effect of selection bias is in the same direction in Eritrea as well (Table 2.2) but the effect is milder in the case of Eritrea than in Egypt. While the estimate changes from −0.1107 to −0.7188, it is insignificant in both Models 2 and 4. This is due to the relatively weaker correlation (0.3138) between the unobserved mother-specific characteristics that affect childhood mortality risks and the decision to delivery a child in hospital, in the case of Eritrea.

A different picture is depicted in the case of Uganda (Table 2.3). To begin with, the correlation between the unobserved mother-specific characteristics that affect childhood mortality risks and the decision to deliver a child in hospital is negative (−0.4099) in the case of Uganda.

This implies that, women with above-average risks of losing a baby ($\varepsilon > 0$) tend to have below-average propensities to deliver in a hospital ($\omega < 0$); and vice versa. Thus, the effect of hospital delivery on child mortality shifts from a highly significant beneficial effect (−0.2996) to an insignificant effect (0.0271). In other words, there is favorable selection into hospital delivery in Uganda, and failure to account for this selectivity severely overestimates the effect of hospital care.

2.4.4 Correlation Between Prenatal Care Utilization and Hospital Delivery

The results in the above subsections indicated that there is significant correlation between the mother-specific unobserved heterogeneities in the hazard and probit models and that failure to account for such correlation would bias the parameter estimates of the effects of prenatal care and hospital delivery.

An important question that still remains to be answered is as to whether the two decisions (prenatal care and hospital delivery) are also correlated. It is quite likely that mothers who visited prenatal care centers during pregnancy would have a higher propensity to deliver their child in hospital than mothers who never did so. The result will, then, be that delivery centers get a disproportionately high proportion of babies whose mothers have visited prenatal care centers during pregnancy. If ignored, it would be difficult to distinguish between the relative strengths of the effects of prenatal care and hospital delivery on child mortality when both effects are considered together.

We therefore address the potential endogeneity of both decisions and estimate a joint (three-process) model of child mortality, prenatal care, and hospital delivery decisions.

The results from such a three-process models are shown in the last column (Model 5) of Tables 2.1, 2.2, and 2.3. In all three tables we see, as expected, that there is a highly significant positive correlation between the decisions of visiting prenatal care during pregnancy and delivering the child in hospital. How does this affect the relative magnitudes of the effects of these two endogenous factors on the risk of childhood mortality?

In the case of Egypt Table 2.1 we note that failure to account for this positive correlation raises the magnitude of effect of both factors – from −1.2112 (Model 5) to −1.4141 (Model 3.) for prenatal care, and from −0.5283 (Model 5) to −0.6066 (Model 4) for hospital delivery.

The same is true for Eritrea Table 2.2 – from 0.4432 (Model 5) to 0.4632 (Model 3.) for prenatal care, and from 0.1190 (Model 5) to −0.7188 (Model 4) for hospital delivery.

In Uganda Table 2.3 the changes are from −0.1713 (Model 5) to −0.1284 (Model 3.) for prenatal care, and from −0.0211 (Model 5) to 0.0271 (Model 4) for hospital delivery.

2.4.5 Comparison of the Standard Model and the Multiprocess Model with Unobserved Heterogeneity and Correlated Health Input Variables

As a final remark in this section, it may be worth examining what happens to the effects of prenatal care and hospital delivery on the log-hazard of childhood mortality as we move from the standard model (Model 1) to the final model (Model 5). The changes in estimates of such effects may be examined by comparing the estimates in columns 1 and 5 of Tables 2.1, 2.2, and 2.3.

The results for Egypt Table 2.1 show that while the standard model reports a significant beneficial effect of prenatal care (−0.3493) but no effect of hospital delivery (0.0748), the final model, where selection and correlation are accounted for, shows that both factors have significant beneficial effects (−1.2112 and −0.5283, respectively). Thus, it seems that at least part of the effect of hospital delivery was transferred to that of prenatal care in the standard model, which does not account for the correlation between these two factors.

The Eritrean case Table 2.2 shows to the contrary. While the true picture is that the two health inputs have no beneficial effects (0.4432 and 0.1190, respectively for prenatal care and hospital delivery), failure to account for selection bias into these two processes and the correlation between them would lead to concluding that one of them (prenatal care) has strong beneficial effect (−0.4624) while the other (hospital care) has no effect at all (−0.1142).

Ugandan results Table 2.3 show another interesting case. The right picture (Model 5) is that none of these two health inputs has any beneficial effect on childhood mortality (−0.1713 and −0.0211, respectively for prenatal care and hospital delivery). If one ignores selection biases and the correlation between the two health inputs, however, one would be led to the erroneous conclusion that the two health inputs have highly significant beneficial effects in reducing childhood mortality (−0.4163 and −0.2945, respectively).

Are these changes statistically significant? This question may be answered by comparing the differences in log-likelihoods in the models under consideration because the models are nested within the next higher model.

It may also be of interest to examine the effects of unobserved heterogeneity, selection bias, and correlation between health input variables, affects the effects of the exogenous variables Education and Residence. A priori, one would suspect that these two variables are correlated with the health input variables (prenatal care and hospital delivery) because we expect the more educated women and those in urban areas would have a higher propensity to use health care facilities.

The results (details not shown here) show that as long as Prenatal Care is treated as exogenous variable, Education (at higher level) continues to have beneficial effects in reducing childhood mortality in the Egyptian data set (with estimates −0.4188, −0.4429, and −0.2279, respectively in Models 1, 2, and 4). Once we treat Prenatal Care as endogenous variable (Model 3) and/or account for its correlation with Hospital Delivery (Model 5), however, the beneficial effect of Education fades away (the estimate reduces to −0.0916 and 0.0180, respectively, in Models 3 and 5). One would, thus, be tempted to suspect that the effects of Education, at least in Egypt work, via higher propensity of educated women to make use of prenatal care centers. But we also need to reconcile this suspicion with our earlier results of adverse selection into prenatal care. The effect of Residence is more blurred though there is marginal evidence that the estimate shifts from insignificant difference towards rural advantages in childhood mortality when proper care is taken of selection effects.

The opposite is true in Eritrea. Results from model 1, 2 and 4 show that there is no effect of education on the hazard of childhood mortality. Once Prenatal Care is treated at endogenous variable and/or its correlation with Hospital Delivery is accounted for, it turns out that Education (now at primary level) has a strong beneficial effect in reducing the risk of childhood mortality. We already know that selection into prenatal care is favorable in Eritrea prompting that it is the more educated women who benefit from such services. Thus, accounting for such favorable selection brings to the surface the true and beneficial effect of education on childhood mortality risks. The effect of Residence is also interesting in the case of Eritrea. The standard model (Model 1) shows that Rural areas have significantly lower risks of childhood mortality than urban areas. In Models 3 and 5, however, it is shown that there are no differential mortality risks by mother's place of residence. We also know that we have favorable selection into prenatal care and that we suspect this would be so due to the fact that urban residents benefit more from prenatal care centers than their rural counterparts. Thus, failure to account for this selection would have underestimated the urban advantage.

Uganda provides another interesting result. Here, there is relatively weaker impact of our procedure on the effects of Education and Residence. If any, it is when we account for Hospital Delivery that the effects of Education are strengthened. It may be noted that there is a stronger correlation between the heterogeneity terms of Hospital Delivery and Mortality in Uganda than in Egypt and Eritrea. On the other hand, there is a weaker correlation between the heterogeneity terms of Prenatal Care and Mortality in Uganda than in Egypt and Eritrea.

The effects of accounting for selection biases and correlation between health input variables are relatively minor on the other exogenous variables (Interval, Sex, and Multiplicity) that we don't give much space to discuss them.

2.5 Summary and Concluding Remarks

For the last two decades Demographic and Health Surveys have been collected to provide information on family planning, maternal and child health, child survival, and reproductive health in Africa, Asia, the Near East, Latin America, and the Caribbean. The availability of such surveys has helped to shift the focus of investigations from indirect methods of estimation of summary measures to the use modern analytic methods in order to examine correlates of demographic behavior and their policy implications.

The surveys have been collected hierarchically at the family, household, and community levels. However, not many analysts seem to be aware of this nature of the data. The data in the surveys are collected by interviewing a nationally representative sample of women (and men in some cases). These women are independent observations once we account for their communities. Thus, in the analysis of marriage behavior, using these women as experimental units is a correct procedure.

In the analysis of childhood mortality, however, the situation is different. To analyze childhood mortality the original women data is converted to child data. In so doing a number of children are nested within the same woman (mother) and the data on children no longer consists of independent (random) observations unless we select just one child, say of a given birth order, from each mother. Children of the same mother are more alike than children selected at random from the population and analytical methods must pay due attention to this nature of the data.

Other issues of concern in the analysis of Demographic and Health Surveys Data include accounting for correlation structure among various determinants (such as that between death of previous child and preceding birth interval) and, more importantly, selection biases in the utilization of health facilities.

The present chapter attempts to address some of above issues through analyses of childhood mortality in three African countries – Egypt, Eritrea, and Uganda based on their 1995 DHS data.

In contrast to previous approaches where children are used as independent experimental units, we have treated children of the same mother as correlated cases (multilevels) within the same experimental unit (mother). We have also allowed for mother-specific unobserved heterogeneity at the mother level. Further, we have paid due account to selection into health care utilization by treating health care variables like prenatal care and hospital delivery as endogenous variables and modeling them simultaneously with the hazard of mortality.

Our results show that there are significant mother-level heterogeneities in the three countries. More interestingly, we have demonstrated that while there are selection biases of health care utilization in all three countries, their effects and, hence, policy implications are different. In one of the countries (Egypt) we have shown that there is adverse selection bias and failure to account for this selection underestimates the beneficial effects of health care inputs. In the other two countries (Eritrea and Uganda) the selection is that of favorable selection and failure to account for it overstates the effect of health inputs.

We have also accounted for the possible correlation between the various health input variables and demonstrated that failure to account for such correlation would benefit one of the variables at the expense of the other. Further, we have demonstrated how the effects of exogenous variables like education and residence may be under/over-estimated if proper care is not taken to address selection into health care utilization.

References

El-Zanaty, F., Hussein, E. M., Shawky, G. A., Way, A. A., & Kishor, S. (1996). *Egypt demographic and health survey 1995*. Calverton: National Population Council [Egypt] & Macro International Inc.

Lillard, L. A. (1993). Simultaneous equations for hazards: Marital duration & fertility timing. *Journal of Econometrics, 56*, 189–217.

Lillard, L. A., & Panis, C. W. A. (2000). aML multilevel multiprocess statistical software, Release 1.0. EconWare, Los Angeles.

National Statistics Office [Eritrea], & Macro International Inc. (1995). Eritrea demographic and health survey 1995. Calverton: National Statistics Office [Eritrea] & Macro International Inc.

Panis, C. W. A., & Lillard, L. (1994). Health inputs and child mortality: Malaysia. *Journal of Health Economics, 13*, 455–489.

Statistics Department [Uganda], & Macro International Inc. (1996). Uganda demographic and health survey 1995. Calverton: Statistics Department [Uganda] & Macro International Inc.

Chapter 3
Modeling Spatial Effects on Childhood Mortality Via Geo-additive Bayesian Discrete-Time Survival Model: A Case Study from Nigeria

Gebrenegus Ghilagaber, Diddy Antai, and Ngianga-Bakwin Kandala

3.1 Introduction

Childhood mortality is an important indicator of overall health and development in a country. It is the result of a complex interplay of determinants at many levels, and as such several studies have recognized that, for instance, maternal (Caldwell 1979; Cleland and van Ginneken 1988), socio-economic (Castro-Leal et al. 1999; Wagstaff 2001), and environmental (Wolfe and Behrman 1982; Lee et al. 1997) factors are important determinants of childhood mortality. However, only a few studies have incorporated environmental factors that are spatial in nature and derived from geographic databases, such as distances from households or communities (Watson et al. 1997).

While the commonly used approaches, such as correlation coefficients and regression analysis may produce statistical outcomes and measures of association, which are limited to a particular location, these relationships cannot be readily generalized for other locations within a country. In order to determine that the observed social phenomena are not distributed in a spatially random manner,

G. Ghilagaber (✉)
Department of Statistics, Stockholm University, SE-106 91 Stockholm, Sweden
e-mail: Gebre@stat.su.se

D. Antai
Department of Public Health Sciences, Karolinska Institute, Stockholm, Sweden

N.-B. Kandala
Warwick Medical School, Division of Health Sciences, University of Warwick, Coventry, UK
e-mail: n-b.kandala@warwick.ac.uk

N.-B. Kandala and G. Ghilagaber (eds.), *Advanced Techniques for Modelling Maternal and Child Health in Africa*, The Springer Series on Demographic Methods and Population Analysis 34, DOI 10.1007/978-94-007-6778-2_3,

spatial analysis is employed. Spatial analysis could be defined as a quantitative data analysis, which focuses on the role of space and relies explicitly on spatial variables in order to explain or predict the phenomenon under investigation (Cressie 1993; Chou 1997). It tests theories that stress that the location of an individual influences social attitudes and behaviour, and that observed social phenomena are not distributed in a spatially random fashion (Weeks 2004). Studies of childhood mortality in developing countries using aggregated data and methodologies that ignore spatial dimensions run the risk of explaining very little of the variations in mortality rates as well as masking spatial variations. For instance, results of the 2003 Nigeria Demographic and Health Survey (NDHS), disaggregated by geopolitical zones, shows that the infant mortality rate (IMR) for the period 10–14 years preceding the 2003 NDHS (1989–1993) at the national level was 113 per 1,000 live-births, while the corresponding IMR for the then four geopolitical zones was North East (129/1,000), North West (136/1,000), and South East (74/1,000), South West (81/1,000) (NPC 2004).

Crude under-five mortality rates stratified by districts (states) are displayed in Table 3.1, and reveal wide variations between districts within the same geopolitical region, information that would otherwise be "hidden" in the overall picture of crude mortality rate for that region or states had spatial analysis not been carried out, thereby exemplifying the significance of spatial analysis.

This chapter is intended to account simultaneously for spatial and time-varying effects on childhood mortality by employing a geo-additive Bayesian model with dynamic and spatial extensions of discrete-time survival models in estimating temporal and spatial variation in the determinants of childhood mortality, as well as any associations between risk factors and childhood mortality in the presence of spatial correlation. To ignore this correlation would mean an underestimation of the variance of the effects of risk factors (Weeks 2004). The impact of some determinant factors of child survival is allowed to vary over time, as well as allowing for non-linear effects of some covariates on child survival. This model introduces appropriate smoothness priors for spatial and non-linear effects, as well as Markov chain Monte Carlo simulation techniques (Gelfand and Smith 1990; Smith and Roberts 1993), used to estimate the model parameters. The models are subsequently used to examine spatial variation in childhood mortality rates in Nigeria, and explore district-level clustering of mortality rates across both space and time (Fig. 3.1). This chapter will however be limited to the older 31 states (i.e. states created before 1996) due to lack of spatial data including the last five states. Figure 3.1 displays spatial distribution of mortality rates (per 1,000) across these states/districts for crude neonatal mortality (panel b); crude peri-natal mortality (panel c); crude infant mortality (panel d); crude child mortality (panel e); and crude under-five mortality (panel f).

Table 3.1 Under-five mortality rates (per 1,000) by older states (districts) in Nigeria for 0–4 years prior to the survey (1999–2003)

Region	No.	District	Mortality rate (per 1,000)
North Central		**All**	**172**
	1	Plateau	65[a]
	2	Benue	112[a]
	3	Kogi	131
	4	Kwara	96[a]
	5	Niger	202
	6	Abuja (FCT)	123[a]
North East		**All**	**270**
	7	Taraba	132[a]
	8	Adamawa	270[a]
	9	Borno	262
	10	Bauchi	278[a]
	11	Yobe	299
North West		**All**	**264**
	12	Jigawa	263[a]
	13	Kano	266
	14	Kebbi	240
	15	Kaduna	221
	16	Katsina	222
	17	Sokoto	304[a]
South East		**All**	**92**
	18	Anambra	54[a]
	19	Enugu	192
	20	Abia	126
	21	Imo	98[a]
South South		**All**	**187**
	22	Cross River	136[a]
	23	Akwa Ibom	154[a]
	24	Rivers	242[a]
	25	Delta	117[a]
	26	Edo	134[a]
South West		**All**	**101**
	27	Lagos	101
	28	Oyo	52
	29	Osun	86[a]
	30	Ogun	124
	31	Ondo	118[a]

[a]Imputed rates, which correspond to Harmonic means of neighbouring states whenever available

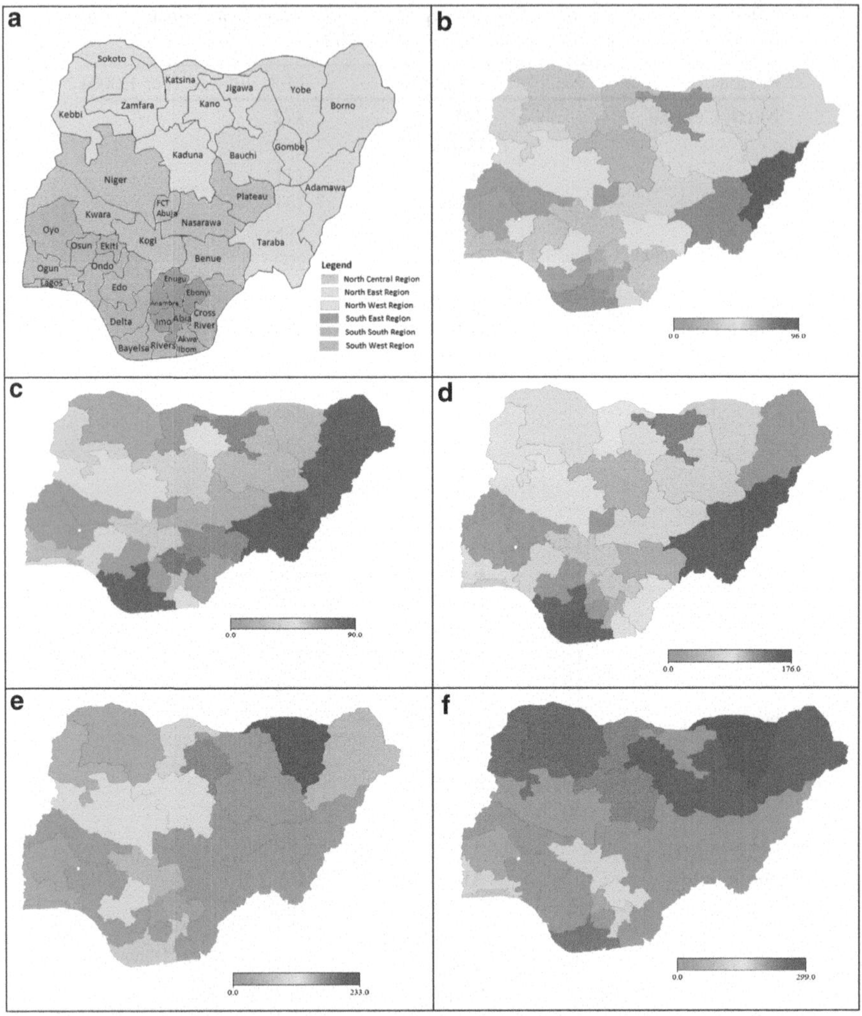

Fig. 3.1 Map of Nigeria (**a**) and spatial distribution of mortality rates across the 36 states/districts (**b–f**), in Nigeria 1999-2003 (Source: Table 3.1)

3.2 Study Area and Study Population

Nigeria, with a 2006 population of 140 million people, is the most populous country in Africa (Onuah 2006). It is also the tenth largest country by population in the world. The country lies on the west coast of Africa between 4° and 14° North latitude and 2° and 15° East longitude, and is bordered by Benin, Niger, Chad, Cameroon, and the Gulf of Guinea. It has a landmass extending over 923,768 km^2 and is located on the eastern terminus of the bulge of West Africa (Population

Resource Centre 2000). With an average density of approximately 124 persons per square kilometer (Ali-Akpajiak and Pyke 2003) Nigeria is one of the most densely populated countries in the world. The spatial distribution of the population is uneven, with some areas of the country sparsely inhabited while other areas are densely populated. With the exception of Lagos, which has the highest population density in the country, the South East of Nigeria has the highest densities. Sixty four percent of the population is concentrated in the rural areas (Ali-Akpajiak and Pyke 2003). Nigeria is made up of 36 states (districts) and a Federal Capital Territory at Abuja. The 36 states are grouped into six geopolitical zones (regions). The mean temperature ranges between 25 °C and 40 °C, and rainfall ranges between 2,650 mm in the Southeast and less than 600 mm in some parts of northern Nigeria that lies mainly in the Sahara desert. These climatic differences give rise to both vegetational differences ranging from mangrove swamp forest in the Niger delta and Sahel grassland in the North, and different soil conditions. This results in a variation in agricultural produce and natural resources in the different parts of Nigeria. A map of Nigeria indicating the geographical location of the states (districts) is shown in Fig. 3.1.

3.3 Geo-Additive Bayesian Discrete-Time Survival Model

3.3.1 The Basic Model

Let T denote a discrete survival time, where $t \in \{1, \ldots, q+1\}$ represents the t th month after birth and let $x_i = (x_1, \ldots, x_t)$ denote the history of a covariate up to month t. The discrete-time conditional probability of death at month t is then given by

$$\lambda(t, x_i) = pr(T = t \mid T \geq t, x_i), \quad t = 1, \ldots, q. \tag{3.1}$$

Survival information on each child is recorded by (t_i, δ_i), $i \in \{1, \ldots, N\}$, where $t_i \in \{1, \ldots, 60\}$ is the child's observed survival time in months, and δ_i is a survival indicator with $\delta_i = 1$ if child i died, and $\delta_i = 0$ if it is still alive. Therefore for $\delta_i = 1$, t_i is the age (in months) of the child at death, and for $\delta_i = 0$, t_i is the current age of the child (in months) at the time of interview.

The assumption is non-informative censoring as applied by Lagakos (see Lagakos 1979), so that the risk set R_t includes all individuals who are censored in interval ending in t. A binary event indicator is then defined as:

$$y_{it}\{i \in R_t,\ t = 1, \ldots, t_i\}$$
$$y_{it} = \{1 \ \text{if}\ t = t_i \ \text{and}\ \delta_i = 1$$
$$\{0 \quad \text{otherwise}, \tag{3.2}$$

The event of death of individual i could then be considered as a sequence of binary "outcomes" – dying at age t ($y_{it} = 1$) or in the case of survival beyond age t ($y_{it} = 0$). Such formulation yields a sequence of 0 s and 1 s indicating survival histories of each child at the various time points.

3.3.2 *Incorporation of Fixed-, Time-Varying and Spatial-Effects*

Parallel with the sequence of 0 s and 1 s, the values of relevant explanatory variables $x_{it} = (x_{i1}, \ldots, x_{it})$, $i = 1, 2, \ldots$ could be recorded. These variables may be fixed over time, for example sex, place of residence; or may vary over time, for example breastfeeding of a child, at time t.

The indicator y_{it} could be linked to the covariates x_{it} by an appropriate link function for binary response model such as probit, logit or multinomial link function, and a predictor η_{it} (x_{it}). Assuming that y_{it} has a binomial distribution and using a probit link function for $i \in Rt$, the probability of death for a child i is denoted by:

$$\Phi(\eta_{it}) = \mathrm{pr}\,(y_{it} = 1|x_{it}). \tag{3.3}$$

The usual form of the predictor is

$$\eta_{it} = f_0\,(t) + x_{it}\,\beta \tag{3.4}$$

where the baseline effect f_0 (t), $t = 1, 2, \ldots$ is an unknown, usually non linear, function of t to be estimated from data and β is the vector of fixed covariate effects. In parametric framework, the baseline hazard is often modelled by a few dummy variables, which divide the time-axis into a number of relatively small segments or by some low-order polynomial. In practice however, it is difficult to correctly specify such parametric functional forms for the baseline effects in advance. Non-parametric modelling based on some qualitative smoothness restrictions offers a more flexible framework to explore unknown patterns of the baseline.

Restriction to fixed effects alone might not be adequate in most cases, due to the covariates whose value may vary over time. The predictor in (3.4) is subsequently extended to a more flexible semi-parametric model, which could accommodate time-varying effects. On further inclusion of another expression to represent spatial effects, this semi-parametric predictor is given by

$$\eta_{it} = f_0(t) + f_1(X) + f(t)X_{it} + f_{spat}(s_i) + X_{it}\,\beta. \tag{3.5}$$

Here, $f_0(t)$ is the baseline function of time, and f_1 is a nonlinear effect of metrical covariate X. The effects, f (t), of the covariates in X_{it} are time-varying, while X_{it} comprises fixed covariates whose effect is represented by the parameter vector β; and f_{spat} is the non-linear spatial component of, for instance, district s ($s = 1, \ldots, S$), where the child lives. The spatial effects f_{spat} (s_i) may be further split-up into spatially correlated (structured) and uncorrelated (unstructured) effects of the form f_{str} $(s_i) + f_{unstr}$ (s_i). The fundamental reason behind this is that a spatial effect is a surrogate of many unobserved influencing factors, some of which may obey a strong spatial structure while others may only be present locally. The analyses in this chapter are based on (3.4) and (3.5), and would be subsequently referred to as "constant fixed effects model" and "geo-additive model" respectively.

3.3.3 The Estimation Process

The functions f_0, f_1, and f are smooth over by second-order random walk priors using the MCMC techniques implemented in *BayesX* (Fahrmeir and Lang 2001a, b; Brezger et al. 2002).

Let $f = \{f(1), \ldots, f(m), m \leq n\}$ be a vector of corresponding function evaluations at the observed values of x. The general form of the prior for f would be:

$$\mathrm{f}|\tau^2 \ \alpha \exp\left(-1/2\tau^2(\mathrm{f}_2\ \mathrm{f}/\mathrm{Kf})\right) \tag{3.6}$$

where K is a penalty matrix that penalizes too abrupt jumps between neighbouring parameters. In most cases, K is rank deficient, therefore the prior for f is improper.

Traditionally, the smoothing parameter is equivalent to the variance parameter τ^2, which controls the trade-off between flexibility and smoothness. A highly dispersed but proper hyperprior is assigned to τ^2 so as to estimate the smoothness parameter simultaneously with f. A proper prior for τ^2 is required in order to obtain a proper posterior for f (Hobart and Casella 1996). In the event of the selection of an Inverse Gamma distribution with hyper-parameters a and b, ($\tau^2 \sim \mathrm{IG}$ (a, b)), a first- and second-order random walk priors for f would be defined respectively by:

$$\mathrm{f(t) = f(t-1) + u(t), \ and \ f(t) = 2f(t-1) - f(t-2) + u(t),} \tag{3.7}$$

with Gaussian errors $u(t) \sim N$ $(0;\tau^2)$ and diffuse priors $f(1)$ α const, or $f(1)$ and $f(2)$ α const, as initial values. A first order random walk penalizes abrupt jumps $f(t) - f(t-1)$ between successive states, and a second order random walk penalizes deviations from the linear trend $2f(t-1) - f(t-2)$. The trade-off between flexibility and smoothness of f is controlled by the variance parameter τ^2. This chapter adopts the approach of estimating the variance parameter and the smoothing function simultaneously; this is achieved by introducing an additional hyperprior for τ^2 at a further stage of the hierarchy. A highly dispersed but proper Inverse Gamma prior, p $(\tau^2) \sim \mathrm{IG}$ $(a; b)$ is chosen, with $a = 1$ and $b = 0.005$. Similarly, a highly dispersed Inverse Gamma prior is defined for the overall variance σ^2.

For the spatially correlated or structured effect, f_{str} (s), $s=1,\ldots,S$, Marked random field priors common in spatial statistics are chosen (Besag et al. 1991) of the form

$$\mathrm{f_{str}(s)|\,f_{str}(r),\ r \neq s,\ \tau^2{}_{str}} \sim \mathrm{N}\left(\sum \mathrm{f_{str}(r)/\,Ns,\ \tau^2{}_{str}/Ns}\right)$$
$$r\epsilon\partial s \tag{3.8}$$

where N_s is the number of adjacent regions, and $r\ c\ \partial s$ indicates that region r is a 'neighbour' of region s. Therefore the conditional mean of f_{str} (s) is an unweighted average of function valuations for neighbouring regions. In addition, the variance parameter $\tau^2{}_{str}$ controls the degree of smoothness.

For a spatially uncorrelated (unstructured) effect, f_{unstr}, $s=1,\ \ldots,S$, common assumptions are that the parameters f_{unstr} (s), are i.i.d. Gaussian:

$$f_{unstr}(s)|\tau^2{}_{unstr} \sim N(0,\ \tau^2{}_{unstr}). \tag{3.9}$$

Variance or smoothness parameters $\tau^2{}_j$, $j=$ str, unstr, are also considered as unknown in a fully Bayesian analysis, and are therefore estimated simultaneously with the corresponding unknown functions f_j. As such, hyperpriors are assigned to them in a second stage of the hierarchy by highly dispersed Inverse Gamma distributions $p\ (\tau^2{}_j) \sim \mathrm{IG}\ (a_j,\ b_j)$ with known hyperparameters a_j and b_j.

Standard choices for the hyperparameters are $a=1$ and $b=0.005$ or $a=b=0.001$. The results of the illustration in this chapter are however not sensitive to the choice of a and b, and the later choice is close to Jeffrey's non-informative prior. Fully Bayesian inference is based on the posterior distribution of model parameter, which is not a known form. As such, MCMC sampling from full conditionals for nonlinear effects, spatial effects, fixed effects and smoothing parameters is used for posterior analysis. For the nonlinear and spatial effects, the sampling scheme of Iterative Weighted Least Squares (IWLS) implemented in BayesX (see Brezger et al. 2002) is applied. This is an alternative to the general Metropolis–Hastings algorithms based on conditional prior proposals, suggested first by Knorr-Held (1999) in the context of state space models as an extension to Gamerman (1997), and given in more detail in Knorr-Held and Rue (2002).

An essential task in the model-building process is the comparison of a set of plausible models, for instance, rating the impact of covariates and assessing whether their effects are time-varying or not; or comparing geo-additive models with simpler parametric alternatives. The measure of complexity and fit suggested by Spiegelhalter et al. (2002) is adopted in this chapter for comparison, and the model that takes all relevant structure into account while remaining parsimonious is selected.

The *Deviance Information Criteria* (DIC), which may be used for model comparison, is defined as

$$\overline{\mathrm{DIC}}(\mathrm{M}) = \mathrm{D(M)} + \mathrm{pD}. \tag{3.10}$$

Therefore, the posterior mean of the deviance $\overline{D}(M)$ is penalized by the effective number of model parameters pD. Models could be validated by analyzing the DIC, which is smaller in models with covariates of high explanatory value.

3.3.4 Advantages of the Bayesian Geo-additive Model

There are several potential advantages of the Bayesian geo-additive model described above over the more conventional approaches such as, discrete-time Cox models with time-varying covariates and fixed or random districts effects, or the standard 2-level multilevel modelling with unstructured spatial effects (Goldstein 1999). In the conventional models, it is assumed that the random components at the contextual level (district in this case) are mutually independent. In practice however, these approaches specify correlated random residuals (see Langford et al. 1999), which is contrary to the assumption. Furthermore, Borgoni and Billari (2003) point out that the independence assumption has an inherent problem of inconsistency. They argue that if the location of the event matters, it is only logical to assume that areas close to each other are more similar than areas that are far apart. In addition, treating groups (in this case, districts) as independent is unrealistic and may lead to poor estimates of the standard errors. As Rabe-Heskesth and Everitt (2000) stipulate, standard errors for between-district factors are likely to be underestimated as a result of observations from the same districts being treated as independent, and thereby increasing the apparent sample size. In contrast, standard errors for within-district factors are likely to be overestimated (see also Bolstad and Manda 2001). Demographic and Health Survey data on the other hand are based on the random sampling of districts that introduces a structured component, which allows for the borrowing of strength from neighbors in order to cope with the posterior uncertainty of the district effect and obtain estimates for areas that may have inadequate sample sizes or are not represented in the sample. In order to highlight the advantages of the Bayesian geo-additive model approach used in this chapter, and examine the potential bias incurred when ignoring the dependence between aggregated spatial areas, several models shall be fitted with, and without the structured and random components, as seen in the illustration below.

3.4 Illustration: Spatial Modelling of Under-Five Mortality in Nigeria

3.4.1 Data Set

Data from the 2003 Nigeria Demographic and Health Survey (NDHS) was used in this chapter. The sample included 7,620 women aged 15–49 years, and all men aged 15–59 in a sub-sample of one-third (i.e. 2,346) of the households. The data contains

6,029 children born within 5 years prior to the survey, which came from 3,725 mothers who contributed between 1 child and 6 children. Technical details of the survey have been reported in the official 2003 NDHS report (NPC 2004). From the data collected, a retrospective child file consisting of all children born to the sample women was generated, of these, 1,559 children died before their fifth birthday. Each live birth and each subsequent child health outcome contains information on the household and each parent, thereby constituting the basic analytic sample.

The response variable used in this chapter is:

$$y_{\mathrm{it}} = \begin{cases} 1: & \text{if child } i \text{ dies in month } t \\ 0: & \text{if child } i \text{ survives beyond time } t, \end{cases} \tag{3.11}$$

3.4.2 *Specification and Measurement of Variables*

On the basis of previous studies, a selection of theoretically relevant variables was chosen as covariates of childhood mortality, and these include: *mab*, mother's age at birth of the child (in years) – nonlinear; *dobt*, duration of breastfeeding – time-dependent; *dist*, district (state) in Nigeria – spatial covariate; *X*, vector of categorical covariates, such as: sex of the child (male or female), asset index (low, middle or higher income household), place of residence (urban or rural), mother's educational level (no education, primary, secondary of higher), place of delivery (hospital or home/other), preceding birth interval long birth interval [$\geq$24 months], or short birth interval [<24 months], antenatal visits during pregnancy (at least one visit, or none), marital status of mother (single or married), and district level mortality rate per 1,000 (at least 6 children, or at less than six children per woman).

The last levels of each covariate were selected as reference or baseline levels; descriptive statistics of covariates used in the analysis are shown in Table 3.2. Available statistics suggest that child mortality levels in Nigeria exhibit wide geographic disparities (NPC 2000, 2004), with the northern regions and rural areas generally having higher childhood mortality rates compared to the southern regions and urban areas respectively. While the focus of previous studies in Nigeria have mainly been on effect of individual and household factors in explaining childhood mortality differences in the country, they have largely neglected the impact of small area variations and community-level variables (see Iyun 1992; Adetunji 1994; Folasade 2000; NPC 2004).

The aim of this present chapter is to highlight the regional- and district-level variations in under-five mortality in Nigeria, while improving current knowledge of district-level socio-economic and demographic determinants (thereby warranting the inclusion of a geographic location [districts] covariate). It is also intended to assist policy makers in evaluating and designing programme strategies needed to improve child health services, and reduce childhood mortality levels in Nigeria.

Table 3.2 Descriptive statistics of covariates used in the analysis, Nigeria Demographic and Health Survey, 2003

Variables	Frequency (%)	Coding
Place of residence:		
Urban	2,118 (35 %)	1
Rural	3,911 (65 %)	Reference category
Sex of the child:		
Male	3,062 (51 %)	1
Female	2,967 (49 %)	Reference category
Preceding birth interval:		
Long birth interval [25+ months]	3,266 (58 %)	1
Short birth interval [<25 months]	2,326 (42 %)	Reference category
Mother's current age (in years):		
Less than 20 years	264 (4 %)	1
20–35 years	5,765 (96 %)	Reference category
Antenatal visits during pregnancy:		
At least one visit	2,337 (64 %)	1
No antenatal visit	1,339 (36 %)	Reference category
Place of delivery:		
Hospital	2,094 (35 %)	1
Home/other	3,878 (65 %)	Reference category
Asset index [economic status of the household]:		
1st quintile	970 (16 %)	1
2nd quintile	2,332 (39 %)	2
3rd quintile	1,322 (22 %)	3
4th quintile	1,405 (23 %)	Reference category
Mother's educational level:		
No education	3,033 (50 %)	1
Primary, secondary of higher	2,966 (50 %)	Reference category
Partner's educational level:		
No education	2,343 (40 %)	1
Primary, secondary of higher	3,501 (60 %)	Reference category
Marital status of mother:		
Single	483 (8 %)	1
Married	5,546 (92 %)	Reference category
Household size:		
Large size	1,724 (29 %)	1
Medium size	2,927 (48 %)	2
Small size	1,378 (23 %)	Reference category

3.4.3 Statistical Method

An analysis and comparison of simpler parametric probit models, and probit models with dynamic effects, $pr\,(y_{it} = 1|x_{it}) = \Phi\,(\eta_{it})$, was made for the probability of dying in month t, i.e. the conditional probability of a child dying, given the child's age in months, the district where the child lived before death, and covariates in X above, is modeled with the following predictors:

$$M1 : \eta_{\text{it}} = f_0(t) + X_{\text{it}}\beta$$

$$M2 : \eta_{\text{it}} = f_0(t) + f_1(\text{mab}) + f(t)X_{\text{it}} + f_{\text{unstr}}(\text{dist}) + f_{\text{str}}(\text{dist}) + X_{\text{it}}\beta$$

The fixed effects in model $M1$ include all covariates described above with constant fixed effects. Mother's age at birth was split into three categories as shown in Table 3.2, and duration of breastfeeding was included as dichotomous (0, 1) variable. Model $M2$ will be superior to model $M1$ because Model $M2$ accounts for the unobserved heterogeneity that might exist in the data, all of which cannot be captured by the covariates (see Madise et al. 1999).

The effects of f_0 (t), f_1 and $f(t)$ are estimated using second-order random walk prior, and Markov random field priors for f_{str} (s). The analysis was carried out using BayesX-version 0.9 (Brezger et al. 2002), a software for Bayesian inference based on Markov Chain Monte Carlo simulation techniques. The sensitivity of the effects to choice of different priors for the non-linear effects (P-splines) and the choice of the hyperparameter values a and b are investigated.

Previous studies, for example, Berger et al. (2002), have shown that breastfeeding is an important factor. In order to assess its effect, a time-varying indicator variable (see Kandala 2002), that takes the value 1 in the months a child is breastfed, and 0 otherwise, is generated. In addition, temporal and spatial variations in the determinants of child mortality are also assessed. Common choices for discrete survival models are the grouped Cox model and probit or logit models. For this chapter, probit model for discrete survival data is used because binary response models (3.3) can be written equivalently in terms of latent Gaussian utilities, which lead to very efficient estimation algorithms. In addition, since survival time in the DHS data set is recorded in months and the longest observation time for this study is limited to 60 months, the data naturally contain a high amount of tied events. A constant hazard within each month is assumed.

At the exploratory stage, a probit model with constant covariate effects ($M1$) for the effects of breastfeeding and mother's age are fitted with a view to compare them to the dynamic probit models ($M2$).

3.5 Results

3.5.1 Fixed Effects

The estimates of posterior odds ratio of the fixed effect parameters for under-five mortality in Nigeria (Model 2) together with their standard errors and quantiles are presented in Table 3.3. Results indicate that children living in urban areas at

Table 3.3 Posterior Odds ratio of the fixed effect parameters for under-five mortality in Nigeria (Model 2)

Variable	Odds ration (OR)	2.5 % quantile	97.5 % quantile
Place of residence			
Urban	0.54*	(0.38;	0.83)
Rural	1		
Sex of the child			
Male	1.08	(0.83;	1.40)
Female	1		
Preceding birth interval			
<25 months	1		
25+ months	0.71*	(0.55;	0.94)
Antenatal visits during pregnancy			
At least one visit	0.57*	(0.40 ;	0.77)
No visit	1		
Place of delivery			
Home or other	1		
Hospital	0.95	(0.68;	1.40)
Asset index			
1st quintile	1		
2nd quintile	0.86	(0.55;	1.23)
3rd quintile	1.09	(0.78;	1.54)
4th quintile	0.93	(0.64;	1.37)
Mother's educational level			
No education	1.51*	(1.06;	2.25)
Primary, secondary, or higher	1		
Partner's educational level			
No education	0.76	(0.54;	1.20)
Primary, secondary, or higher	1		
Marital status of mother			
Single	1.27	(0.66;	2.47)
Married	1		
Household size			
Small size	1		
Medium size	0.99	(0.67;	1.68)
Large size	0.96	(0.64;	1.51)

*Estimate significant at 5% level. This is also indicated by the corresponding 95% confidence interval (which doesn't include 1)

lower risk of dying than children living in rural areas (posterior odds ratio 0.54), with positive corresponding 2.5 %- and 97.5 % quantiles indicating that the effect is statistically significant. Boys are only slightly at higher risk of dying than girls (posterior odds ratio 1.08), and the corresponding 2.5 %- and 97.5 % quantiles are both positive. The results also show that a short birth interval significantly reduces a child's chances of survival, as children with birth interval 25+ months were at lower risk of dying compared to those < 25 months (posterior odds ratio 0.71), the effect being statistically significant. In comparison to children whose mothers had no antenatal visits during pregnancy, children whose mothers had at least one antenatal visit were at lower risk of dying; the effect being statistically significant.

Children delivered in hospitals were at slightly lower risk of dying compared to children born at home or elsewhere (posterior odds ratio 0.95). Findings also indicate that child survival is associated with economic status of the household; while children living in households within the 2nd and 4th quintiles were significantly at lower risks of dying compared to those in the 1st quintile (richest households), those living in households within the 3rd quintile had a slightly higher risk of dying (posterior odds ratio 1.09) compared to those in the 1st quintile. Mothers' education, was associated with child survival and works in the expected direction (with children of uneducated mothers having 50 % higher risk). Partner's education, on the other hand, was insignificant.

Children of single mothers were at higher risk of dying (posterior odds ratio 1.27) compared to children whose mothers were married; both quantiles were positive, and therefore the relationship was significant. Remarkably, the larger the household size, the lower the risk of the children dying. Children living in medium-size households (posterior odds ratio 0.99), and those living in large-size households (posterior odds ratio 0.96), were at lower risk of dying compared to children living in small-size households; both relationships had positive quantiles and were therefore significant.

3.5.2 Baseline Effects

The estimated nonlinear effect of child's age (baseline time) and the time-varying effects, modelled and fitted through Bayesian P-splines are shown in Fig. 3.2. The posterior means are presented within 80–95 % credible intervals, and show that starting from a comparably high level in the first month, the baseline effect remains more or less constant until 25–26, and 40–41 months, where they peak. These observed peaks are likely to be caused by a "heaping" effect from the large number of deaths reported at these times (probably resulting from incorrect reporting of large number of deaths at these ages).

3.5.3 Time-Varying Effects

Figure 3.3 displays the time-varying effect of breastfeeding in Nigeria, and indicates that breastfeeding is on average associated with lower risk of mortality within the first 16–18 months using 80–95 % credible intervals. However, given the wide range of the 80–95 % credible region at the end of the observation period (most likely due to fewer numbers of cases), the results beyond 18 months should be interpreted with caution.

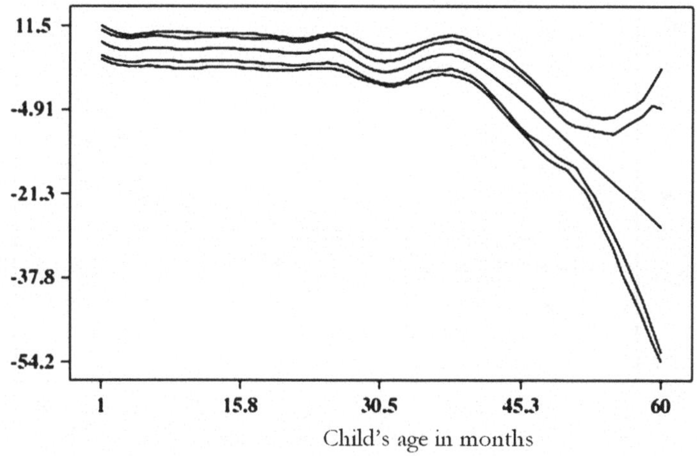

Fig. 3.2 Estimated nonlinear effect of baseline time. Shown is the posterior mean within 80–95 % credible intervals

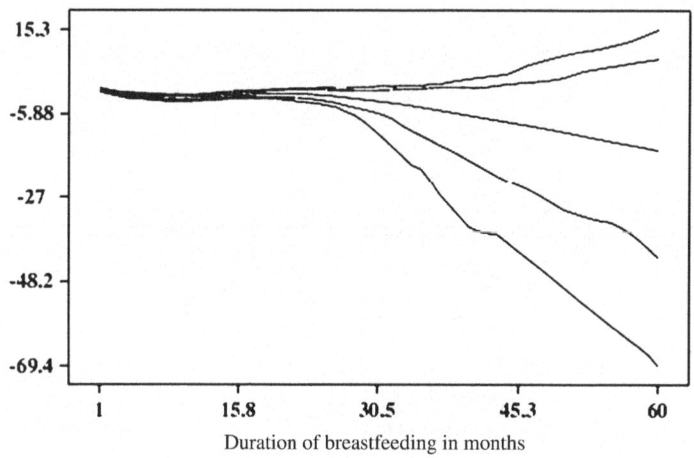

Fig. 3.3 Estimated nonlinear effect of time-varying effect of breastfeeding. Shown is the posterior mean within 80–95 % credible intervals

3.5.4 Nonlinear Effects

Figure 3.4 shows the non-linear or time-varying effect of mother's age at birth of the child. Children with younger mothers (<20 years) and older mothers (>35 years) have higher (but statistically insignificant) risk of dying compared to children of mothers within the middle age group (22–34 years). Figure 3.4 also shows that children of mothers 42–48 years are even at higher risk of dying compared to children of mothers <20 years.

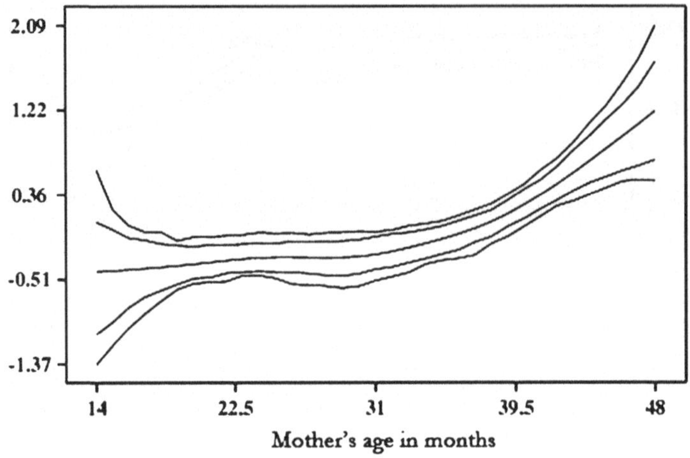

Fig. 3.4 Estimated nonlinear effect of mother's age at child's birth. Shown is the posterior mean within 80–95 % credible intervals

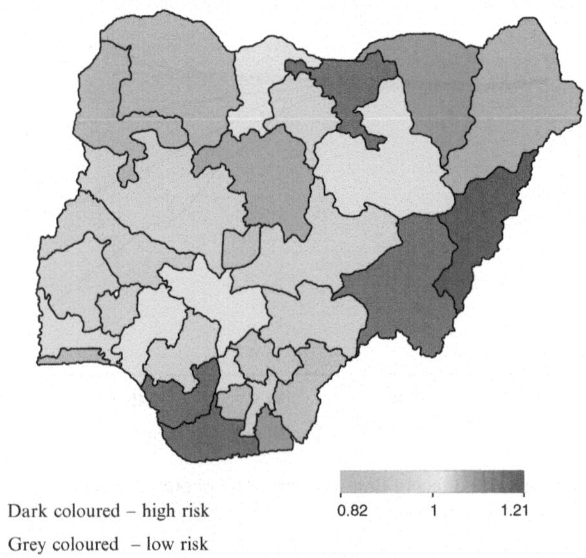

Fig. 3.5 Estimated odd ratio of total residual spatial states effects for under-five mortality in Nigeria. *Dark* coloured – high risk. *Grey* coloured – low risk

3.5.5 *Spatial Effects*

Posterior means of the estimated residual spatial states effects on under-five mortality in Nigeria are presented in Fig. 3.5. This map shows a strong spatial pattern, which suggests that survival chances of children under-5 years of age are highest within the North Western (Sokoto, and Kebbi) and South Western (Lagos) regions compared to the other regions. On the other hand, the survival chances of children under-5 years are lowest among children from Jigawa, Taraba, Delta, Rivers and Adamawa states compared to the children from the rest of the states. A comparison between the under-five mortality rates (Table 3.1) and the estimated odds ratio (Fig. 3.5) reveals the emergence of a clear spatial pattern of under-five mortality risk with the residual effects in Fig. 3.5. Therefore, failure to take into consideration the posterior uncertainty in the spatial location (states or districts) would invariably lead to an overestimation of the precision in predicting childhood mortality risks in unsampled districts. The spatial effects could therefore be interpreted as representing the cumulative effect of unidentified or unmeasured additional covariates that may reflect impacts of environmental and socio-cultural factors.

3.6 Discussion and Conclusion

After controlling for the spatial dependence in the data, almost all the covariates associated with under-five mortality in the fixed part of the model were found to have effects in the expected directions. A remarkable finding however, is that children in larger households are at slightly lesser risk of dying compared to children in small households; this may not be unconnected with factors that might contribute to a household's propensity to experience childhood deaths such as the burden of child ill-health and mortality being borne by only a small fraction of all households (Madise and Diamond 1995); household income (Vella et al. 1992); maternal education (Cleland and van Ginneken 1988); physical access to care (Kuate Defo 1996); and rural as opposes to urban setting (Sastry 1997).

The time-varying effects of breastfeeding emphasize the importance of breastfeeding, which is widely believed to be the most beneficial source of infant nutrition for the attainment of health and well-being of the infant (Weimer 2001). Results of this study show a lowered risk of mortality associated with breastfeeding within the first 16–18 months. However, results at the end of the observation period do not provide reliable information on the dynamic effect of breastfeeding (due to few cases), and should therefore be interpreted with caution. Results of the nonlinear effect of mother's age at the birth of the child are in the expected direction, emphasizing the risk associated with younger mother (also seen in Alam 2000) and late childbirth (see Hobcraft et al. 1985), especially the higher risk associated with children of women aged 42–48 years.

The estimated residual spatial effects for under-five mortality in Fig. 3.5 show clear differences between the significantly better survival chances of children in the North West (Sokoto, and Kebbi) and South West (Lagos) regions compared to the North East (Adamawa, Taraba, Yobe, Borno), South South (Delta, Rivers, Akwa Ibom) and South East (Enugu) regions. These state patterns are similar to analysis of poverty in Nigeria in which the Northeast zone had the highest poverty incidence with 67.3 %, followed by the Northwest with 63.9 %; the South South zone had the highest poverty rates (55 %) among the southern states, while the lowest poverty rates were recorded in the South East at 34.2 %, followed by Southwest with 43.0 % (National Bureau of Statistics 2005).

While some of these effects have been shown using traditional parametric methods, using Bayesian geo-additive models uniquely shows subtle differences when analysing for small-area spatial effects. Though the spatial effects do not show causality, careful interpretation could identify latent and unobserved factors that directly influence mortality rates. This geographic semi-parametric approach therefore appears to be able to discern subtle influences of the determinants, and identifies district-level clustering of under-five mortality.

The variation in the probability of childhood survival in Nigeria is spatially structured. This implies that adjusted mortality risks are similar among neighbouring states or districts, which may partly be explained by general health care practices, similar prevalence of common childhood diseases, and the residual spatial variation induced by variation in unmeasured district-specific characteristics (which any standard 2-level model with unstructured spatial effects assuming independence among districts would yield estimated that lead to incorrect conclusions).

References

Adetunji, J. A. (1994). Infant mortality in Nigeria: Effects of place of birth, mother's education and region of residence. *Journal of Biosocial Science, 26*(4), 469–477.

Alam, N. (2000). Teenage motherhood and infant mortality in Bangladesh: Maternal age-dependent effect of party one. *Journal of Biosocial Science, 32*, 229–236.

Ali-Akpajiak, S. C. A., & Pyke, T. (2003). *Measuring poverty in Nigeria*. Oxfam: Oxfam Working Papers. http://www.oxfam.org.uk/what_we_do/resources/wp_poverty_nigeria.htm

Berger, U., Fahrmeir, L., & Klasen, S. (2002). Dynamic modelling of child mortality in developing countries: Application for Zambia. *Sonderforschungsbereich 386* (Discussion Paper 299). University of Munich, Germany.

Besag, J., York, Y., & Mollie, A. (1991). Bayesian image restoration with two applications in spatial statistics. *Annual Institute of Statistical Mathematics, 43*, 1–59.

Bolstad, W. M., & Manda, S. O. (2001). Investigating child mortality in Malawi using family and community random effects: A Bayesian analysis. *Journal of the American Statistical Association, 96*(453), 12–19.

Borgoni, R., & Billardi, F. C. (2003). Bayesian spatial analysis of demographic survey data: An application to contraceptive use at first sexual intercourse. *Demographic Research, 83*, 61–92.

Brezger, A., Kneib, T., & Lang, S. (2002). *BayesX-software for Bayesian inference based on Markov chain Monte Carlo simulation techniques*. http://www.stat.uni-muenchen.de/~lang/

Caldwell, J. C. (1979). Education as a factor in mortality decline an examination of Nigerian data. *Population Studies, 33*(3), 395–413.

Castro-Leal, F., Dayton, J., Demery, L., & Mehra, K. (1999). Public social spending in Africa: Do the poor benefit? *World Bank Research Observer, 14*, 49–72.

Chou, Y.-H. (1997). *Exploring spatial analysis in geographic information systems*. Santa Fe: OnWard Press.

Cleland, J. G., & van Ginneken, J. K. (1988). Maternal education and child survival in developing countries: The search for pathways of influence. *Social Science & Medicine, 27*(12), 1357–1368.

Cressie, N. A. C. (1993). *Statistics for spatial data* (Rev. ed.). New York: Wiley.

Fahrmeir, L., & Lang, S. (2001a). Bayesian Inference for generalized additive mixed models based on Markov random field priors. *Applied Statistics (JRSS C), 50*, 201–220.

Fahrmeir, L., & Lang, S. (2001b). Bayesian semi-parametric regression analysis of multicategorical time-space data. *Annual Institute of Statistical Mathematics, 53*, 11–30.

Folasade, I. B. (2000). Environmental factors, situation of women and child mortality in southwestern Nigeria. *Social Science & Medicine, 51*(10), 1473–1489.

Gamerman, D. (1997). Efficient sampling from the posterior distribution in generalized linear mixed models. *Statistics and Computing, 7*, 57–68.

Gelfand, A. E., & Smith, A. F. R. (1990). Sampling-based approaches to calculating marginal densities. *Journal of the American Statistical Association, 85*, 398–409.

Goldstein, H. (1999, April). *Multilevel statistical models*. London: Institute of Education, Multilevel Models Project. http://www.soziologie.uni-halle.de/langer/multilevel/books/goldstein.pdf

Hobart, J., & Casella, G. (1996). The effect of improper priors on Gibbs sampling in hierarchical linear mixed models. *Journal of the American Statistical Association, 91*, 1461–1473.

Hobcraft, J. N., McDonald, J. W., & Rutstein, S. O. (1985). Demographic determinants of infant and early child mortality: A comparative analysis. *Population Studies, 39*(3), 363–385.

Iyun, B. F. (1992). Women's status and childhood mortality in two contrasting areas in southwestern Nigeria: A preliminary analysis. *GeoJournal, 26*(1), 43–52.

Kandala, N.-B. (2002). Spatial modelling of socio-economic and demographic determinants of childhood undernutrition and mortality in Africa. Ph. D. Thesis, University of Munich, Shaker Verlag.

Knorr-Held, L. (1999). Conditional prior proposals in dynamic models. *Scandinavian Journal of Statistics, 26*, 129–144.

Knorr-Held, L., & Rue, H. (2002). On block updating in Markov random field models for disease mapping. *Scandinavian Journal of Statistics, 29*, 597–614.

Kuate Defo, B. (1996). Areal and socioeconomic differentials in infant and child mortality in Cameroon. *Social Science & Medicine, 42*, 399–420.

Lagakos, S. W. (1979). General right censoring and its impact on the analysis of survival data. *Biometrics, 35*, 139–156.

Langford, I. H., Leyland, A. H., Rabash, J., & Goldstein, H. (1999). Multilevel modeling of the geographical distributions of diseases. *Journal of Royal Statistical Society, Series A (Applied Statistics), 48*, 253–268.

Lee, L.-F., Rosenzweig, M., & Pitt, M. (1997). The effects of improved nutrition, sanitation and water quality on child health in high-mortality populations. *Journal of Econometrics, 77*, 209–235.

Madise, N. J., & Diamond, I. (1995). Determinants of infant mortality in Malawi: An analysis to control for death clustering within families. *Journal of Biosocial Science, 27*, 95–106.

Madise, N. J., Matthews, Z., & Margetts, B. (1999). Heterogeneity of child nutritional status between households: A comparison of six sub-Saharan African countries. *Population Studies, 53*, 331–343.

National Bureau of Statistics (NBS). (2005). *Poverty profile for Nigeria report (1980–1996)*. Federal Republic of Nigeria.

National Population Commission (NPC) [Nigeria]. (2000). *Nigeria demographic and health survey 1999*. Calverton: National Population Commission and ORC/Macro.

National Population Commission (NPC) [Nigeria]. (2004). *Nigeria demographic and health survey 2003*. Calverton: National Population Commission and ORC/Macro.

Onuah, F. (2006, Dec 30). Nigeria gives census result, avoids risky details. *Reuters*. http://za.today.reuters.com. Accessed 30 March 2007

Population Resource Centre. Nigeria Demographic Profile. (2000). Accessed at: http://www.prcdc.org/summaries/nigeria/nigeria.html

Rabe-Heskesth, S., & Everitt, B. (2000). *A handbook of statistical analysis using Stata* (2nd ed.). Boca Raton: Chapman and Hall/CRC.

Sastry, N. (1997). What explains rural-urban differentials in child mortality in Brazil? *Social Science & Medicine, 44*, 989–1002.

Smith, A. F. M., & Roberts, G. O. (1993). Bayesian computation via the Gibbs sampler and related Markov chain Monte Carlo methods. *Journal of the Royal Statistical Society (B), 55*, 3–23.

Spiegelhalter, D., Best, N., Carlin, B., & Van der Line, A. (2002). Bayesian measures of models complexity and fit. *Journal of the Royal Statistical Society Series B, 64*, 1–34.

Vella, V., Tomkins, A., Nidku, J., & Marshall, T. (1992). Determinants of child mortality in South-West Uganda. *Journal of Biosocial Science, 24*, 103–112.

Wagstaff, A. (2001). *Poverty and health*. Geneva: Commission on Macroeconomics and Health working paper series. Washington, DC: The World Bank.

Watson, R. T., Zinyowera, M. C., & Moss, R. H. (Eds.). (1997). *The regional impacts of climate change: An assessment of vulnerability. A special report of the intergovernmental panel on climate change, Working Group II*. Cambridge: Cambridge University Press.

Weeks, J. R. (2004). The role of spatial analysis in demographic research. In M. F. Goodchild & D. G. Janelle (Eds.), *Spatially integrated social science*. Oxford: Oxford University Press.

Weimer, J. P. (2001). *The economic benefits of breastfeeding: A review and analysis*. (Food and Rural Food Assistance and Nutrition Research Report No. 13), U.S. Department of Agriculture.

Wolfe, B., & Behrman, J. (1982). Determinants of child mortality, health and nutrition in a developing country. *Journal of Devlopement Economics, 11*, 163–193.

Chapter 4
Bayesian Geoadditive Mixed Latent Variable Models with Applications to Child Health Problems in Egypt and Nigeria

Khaled Khatab

4.1 Introduction

Childhood morbidity and malnutrition are among the most serious health issues facing developing countries. Analyses of these health outcomes are often based on Demographic and Health Surveys (DHS) datasets which provide reliable information on childhood diseases and undernutrition. The analyses rely on statistical inference with various forms of standard regression models. Because of methodological restraints, it is difficult to detect nonlinear covariate effects, for example of, age, adequately, and it is impossible to recover small-scale, district-specific spatial effects with standard linear regression or correlation analysis. Recent research has applied geoadditive regression models (Fahrmeir and Lang 2001; Fahrmeir et al. 2004). These models can account for nonlinear covariate effects and geographical variation while simultaneously controlling for other important risk factors. They have been used in regression studies of risk factors for acute or chronic undernutrition (e.g., Kandala et al. 2006; Adebayo 2003), for morbidity (Kandala et al. 2006, 2007; Khatab and Fahrmeir 2009) and for mortality (Adebayo and Fahrmeir 2005; Kandala and Ghilagaber 2006).

However, except in Khatab and Fahrmeir (2009), regression analyses are carried out separately for each disease, such as cough or fever, or each undernutrition status such as stunting, wasting or underweight, neglecting possible association or common latent risk factors among these response variables. In this chapter, we take a somewhat different point of view; we apply recently developed geoadditive latent variable models for mixed continuous and discrete responses (Fahrmeir and Raach 2007) considering binary indicators for cough, fever and diarrhea as well

K. Khatab (✉)
Faculty of Health and Wellbeing, Centre for Health and Social Care Research,
Sheffield Hallam University, Sheffield, United Kingdom
e-mail: K.Khatab@shu.ac.uk

N.-B. Kandala and G. Ghilagaber (eds.), *Advanced Techniques for Modelling Maternal and Child Health in Africa*, The Springer Series on Demographic Methods and Population Analysis 34, DOI 10.1007/978-94-007-6778-2_4,

as Z-scores for stunting and underweight as observable outcomes of latent health and nutrition status. This allows to simultaneously account for association between these indicators and to assess the common influence of certain risk factors, nonlinear effects of covariates such as age of child, and geographical variation on the latent variables morbidity and malnutrition. The issues addressed are illustrated with data from the 2003 Demographic and Health Surveys of Egypt and Nigeria but the models and methods used are equally applicable to similar data from other countries.

A background of the present study is reported in previous works (Khatab and Fahrmeir 2009; Khatab 2010). Effects of the different covariates on response variables diarrhea, fever, and cough (indicating child's health status) and stunting and underweight (indicating malnutrition status) were analysed using separate geoadditive latent variable models (Raach 2005; Fahrmeir and Raach 2007).

Further, we apply recently developed geoadditive latent variable models for mixed continuous and discrete responses, which is the main focus of this chapter. Models with one and with two latent variables are estimated using mixed indicators (binary indicators for "health status", and continuous indicators for "nutrition status") and the results are compared. The methods are applied to the 2003 DHS data from Egypt (El-Zanaty and Way 2004) and Nigeria (National Population Commission and ORC Macro 2004). Some of these ideas on joint spatial modelling to identify common and specific risk factors and profiles using shared-component models can be found in Chap. 15.

Computations are carried out using the MCMC package in R (Raach 2005).

4.2 Basic Ideas of Latent Variable Models

Latent variable models provide an important tool for the analysis of multivariate data. When the joint distribution of a set of random variables is specified by a statistical model it becomes a latent variable model if some of them are unobservable (Bartholomew 1987).

There are many reasons why latent variables might be introduced into a model in the first place and how their presence contributes to statistical investigation. One reason is to reduce dimensionality. The information contained in the interrelationships of some variables can be useful, to an approximation, in a much smaller set. This improves the ability to see structures in the data. That is the idea behind factor analysis models and more recent applications of parametric structural models (Bartholomew 1987). Secondly, latent variable models play a prominent role in many fields to which statistical methods are applied, such as social science, psychology and politics. There are two sorts of variables to be considered in terms of latent variable models: variables which can be directly observed, known as manifest variables, and latent variables, which cannot be measured directly.

Many constructs that are of interest to social scientists cannot be observed directly. Examples are preferences, attitudes, behavioral intentions, and personality traits. Such constructs can solely be measured indirectly by means of observable indicators, such as questionnaire items which are designed to elicit responses related to an attitude or preference. There are various types of scaling techniques which have been developed for deriving information on unobservable constructs of interest from the indicators. A latent variable model can be a nonlinear, path analysis or graphical. In addition to the manifest variables, the model can include one or more unobserved or latent variables which represent the constructs of interest. There are two assumptions defining the causal mechanisms underlying the responses. The first one assumes that the responses on the indicators are the result of an individual's position on the latent variable. The second is that the manifest variables have nothing in common after controlling for the latent variable. This is usually referred to as the principle of local independence.

The main purpose of factor analysis is to determine the correlations between a set of observed variables that can be interpreted by a few number of latent variables, and how that could be identified. The factor analysis model can be found in two ways

1. a model, which allows for ordinal or binary indicators. Typically researches have used ordinal data in classic factor analysis models, which are assumed to be normally distributed.
2. a latent variable model including covariates which influence the indicators or the latent variables. Most statistical studies assume that the influence of the covariates on the indicators and on the latent variable is strictly linear.

The original form of factor analysis has its roots in Psychology (Spearman 1904). Spearman hypothesized that performance for each set of intellectual tasks is shared with performance for all other intellectual tasks; the general intellectual ability cannot be directly obtained, and therefore there is a need for a latent variable.

The Latent Variable Models (LVM) presented in this chapter includes binary and continuous indicators.

Further, the model is based on a Bayesian framework where all unknown population parameters are considered as random.

In order to understand the idea of LVM, we have to distinguish between two types of variables: the observable variables which are called indicators or manifest variables, and the unobservable variable which is called latent variable.

LVMs are mostly used in the fields of psychology and social science because most of the variables in these areas cannot be directly quantifiable. LVM are also used in the field of medicine, where patients suffer from disease syndromes which are of a variety of effects such as Fetal Alcohol syndrome, and Downs Syndrome, which are taken as indicators in many teratology studies (Holmes et al. 1987).

4.2.1 General Formulation

Let y' be a vector of p manifest variables (or indicators), $y' = (y_1, y_2, \dots, y_p)$. One wants to find a set of latent factors $\upsilon' = (\upsilon_1, \upsilon_2, \dots, \upsilon_q)$ with a smaller number of components $q < p$ than the observed variables that contain essentially the same information. If both the response variables and the latent factors are normally distributed with zero means and unit variances, this leads to classic factor model (see Jöreskog and Goldberger 1975). We will distinguish between two different sets of covariates.

- covariates that affect the indicators directly $w' = (w_1, w_2, \dots, w_k)$
- covariates that affect the indicators indirectly $x' = (x_1, x_2, \dots, x_r)$

Covariates can be of any type, such as metrical, categorical (dummy variables) or ordinal.

4.2.2 Latent Variable Models Using One factor

Here, we briefly discuss the types of models that will be studied in this chapter. There are three observed variables $y' = (y_1, y_2, y_3)$ which are indicators of a single latent variable υ_1. The observed variables can be binary as in the case of health indicators or continuous as in the case of the malnutrion indicators.

The basic idea of latent variable models or the factor analysis is that the multidimensional vector of p manifest variables y can be represented by one or more latent factor υ with a lower dimension of q. Consequently factor analysis reduces the dimensionality of the data in such a way that the interrelationships among the observed variables are preserved as much as possible.

The basic factor analytic model for Gaussian response consists of so-called *measurement model*

$$y_i = \Lambda \upsilon_i + \varepsilon_i,$$

$$\upsilon_i \sim N(0, I), \quad \varepsilon_i \sim N_p(0, \Sigma), \tag{4.1}$$

for each observation i. Λ is a $p \times q$ dimensional matrix of regression coefficients which are called factor loadings and indicate the relationship between the latent variable υ, and the indicators (manifest variable) y_i. The term ε_i represents a p-dimensional error term. This is the *case when the model* does not *include any covariates effects.*

However, we need to extend the basic factor model for the following reasons; On the one hand, it is useful to include explanatory variables w which affect the observed variables directly. On the other hand, it is interesting to know how the explanatory variables modify the latent factor, and hence affect the observed variables indirectly (indirect effects x). This chapter focuses on both types of exploratory variables (direct and indirect effects) as we are interested in how variables, e.g. demographic variables, affect the latent variables.

Most structural models following Jöreskog and Goldberger (1975), distinguish between two conceptually distinct parts of latent models, namely a structural part and a measurement part.

The structural part of a model specifies the relationships among the latent variables and the measurement part specifies the relationship of the latent to the observed variables. The *measurement model* (with direct effects) is given by

$$y_i = \Lambda \upsilon_i + A w_i + \varepsilon_i. \tag{4.2}$$

where w_i are effects which directly affect the observed manifest variables and A is the matrix of regression coefficients.

The part of the model that links a set of observed covariates with the latent variables, the *linear structural model* is given by

$$\upsilon_i = \gamma x_i + \zeta_i. \tag{4.3}$$

where x_i are indirect effects which modify the latent factors, and hence affect the observed variables. The matrix γ contains the regression coefficients of the indirect covariates x.

The latent variable υ_1 and the observed variable w_i account for the associations among the y variables. The direct relationship between w_1 and y_1 allows the mean level (thresholds) for variable y_i to be different for different values of the w_1 variable.

Finally, $x' = (x_1, x_2)$ affect the latent variable υ_1. Note that variable x needs to be different from variable w for identification reasons.

4.3 Measurement Model and Structural Model

4.3.1 Measurement Model for the Binary Indicators:

The binary variables y_{ij} are taken to be manifestations of some underlying continuous unobserved variables y_{ij}^*.

The connection between the binary variable y_{ij}, $j = p_1 + 1, \ldots, p$ and the underlying variable y_{ij}^* is

$$y_{ij} = 1 \Leftrightarrow y_{ij}^* > t_j.$$

$$y_{ij} = 0 \Leftrightarrow y_{ij}^* \leq t_j$$

Because of the identification restriction, the t_j thresholds of all indicators j are fixed to zero and $var(\varepsilon_i) = 1$.

The relationship between the y_i^* variables and the latent variables υ in the *measurement model* excluding direct effects is given by

$$y_{ij}^* = \alpha_0 + \Lambda \upsilon_i + \varepsilon_{ij}, \quad \varepsilon_{ij} \sim N_p(0, I).$$

where Λ is a matrix containing the factor loadings, indicating strength of relationship between latent factors and indicators.

The relationship between the y_i^* variables and the latent variables υ_i in the measurement model including direct effects is given by

$$y_{ij}^* = \alpha_0 + \Lambda \upsilon_i + Aw_i + \varepsilon_{ij} \quad \varepsilon_{ij} \sim \mathrm{N}_p(0, \Sigma) \tag{4.4}$$

The direct covariates are summarized in the d-dimensional vector $w_i = (w_{i1}, .., w_{id})'$ and the $p \times q$-dimensional matrix A.

The direct effects provide additional information about data structure and increase the strength of dimensionality through the relationship between y_{ij}^* and w_i, used in the analyses later. Here ε_i is distributed normally $\varepsilon_i \sim N_p(0, \Sigma)$ and $\Sigma = diag(\sigma_1^2, \ldots, \sigma_p^2)$, υ is a $(1 \times p)$ vector of latent variables that explain the relationships among the indicators. The $p \times q$ matrix Λ is the matrix of factor loadings which indicate the relationship between the latent variables and the indicators, and λ_0 is the intercept.

We assume that responses are conditionally independent and Bernoulli-distributed. Thus, the model of the binary indicators can be written as

$$y_{ij}|\upsilon_i \sim Bin(1, \pi_{ij}), \quad j = p_1 + 1, \ldots, p, \tag{4.5}$$

and follow a probit model

$$\Phi_{ij} = P(y_{ij} = 1|\upsilon_i) = \Phi(\lambda'_j \upsilon_i + a'_j w_i), \tag{4.6}$$

where Φ denotes the standard normal distribution function, with the same latent variables υ_i, as in (4.4) but using the effect of the covariates instead the matrix. We also assume that all responses y_{ij}, $j = 1, \ldots, p$, are conditionally independent given the latent variables υ_i, so that association between responses is introduced through the common latent variables.

In such models, the correlations between the y_i variables are explained by both latent variables and covariates, instead of the latent variable alone.

4.3.2 Measurement Model for the Continuous Indicators

For continuous (Gaussian) indicators there is no need for underlying variable, so that

$$y_{ij}^* = y_{ij} + \varepsilon_{ij}; \quad \varepsilon_{ij} \sim N(0, \sigma_j^2),$$

The logistic distribution function could also be used instead of the standard normal distribution function; however we use the standard normal distribution function because the parameter estimates for both function lead to similar results in prediction (Moustaki et al. 2004).

4.3.3 Structural Model

Structural models relate latent variables to further covariates which have only indirect effects on the observable responses. Traditional linear structural models (e.g. Moustaki et al. 2004; Skrondal and Rabe-Hesketh 2004) assume (latent) Gaussian linear models

$$\upsilon_{ir} = x_i' \beta_r + \delta_{ir}, \quad r = 1, \ldots, q \tag{4.7}$$

with i.i.d Gaussian errors $\delta_{ir} \sim N(0, 1)$. Here x_i is the vector of covariates with direct effects on the latent variables. For identifiability reasons β_r must not contain an intercept term (it is included already in the measurement model), and the error variance var (δ_{ir}) has to be fixed to 1.

The linear structural model (4.7) implies that the means of the latent variables are linearly dependent on the covariates x_i. This can be a severe restriction in real-life research settings as in our application. For instance, continuous covariates such as age of child, body mass index of mothers, and age of mothers at birth, a strictly linear effect on the mean may not be appropriate. Also, the latent variables "malnutrition" and "morbidity" may be influenced by geographically varying effects. To incorporate these we employ more versatile geoadditive structural models

$$\upsilon_{ir} = x_i' \beta_r + f_{r1}(z_{i1}) + \ldots + f_{rk}(z_{ik}) + f_{r,geo}(s_i) + \delta_{ir}, \quad r = 1, .., q \tag{4.8}$$

where $f_{r1}(z_{i1}), \ldots, f_{rk}(z_{ik})$ are smooth, nonparametric functions (effects) of continuous covariates $z_1, \ldots, z_k$ like age of child, and $f_{r,geo(s_i)}$ is the geographical (spatial) effect of location or geographical region $s_i \in \{1, \ldots, S\}$, where individual i lives.

Such geoadditive models have been previously suggested for observable univariate responses y of different types, (Fahrmeir et al. 2004), and have been applied for analyzing malnutrition or disease indicators separately (Kandala et al. 2007). Further application appear in Kandala (2002), Kandala et al. (2001), Khatab and

Fahrmeir (2009), and Khatab (2010). Geoadditive latent variable models, combining separate regression models to a joint multivariate model, have been suggested recently in a Bayesian framework (Fahrmeir and Raach 2007). The appendix section shortly reviews methods for modelling of the unknown function $f_1, \dots, f_k$ and f_{geo} and points out some identifiability issues.

4.4 Latent Variable Models for Mixed Response Variables

We first introduce the scalar latent variable υ, "health and undernutrition status". We consider a one-dimensional latent variable with different types of covariates. Extension to two-dimensional latent variables with two types of responses and different types of covariates are presented in the next section. The response variables consist of five indicators: *fever, diarrhea, cough, stunting and underweight*.

The *measurement model* using one latent variable is given by

$$y_{ij}^* = \lambda_0 + a_j{}'w_i + \lambda_j \upsilon_i + \varepsilon_{ij}, \quad i = 1, \dots, n, \quad \varepsilon_{ij} \sim N(0, \sigma_j^2) \tag{4.9}$$

for two metrical indicators and

$$y_{ij}^* = \lambda_0 + a_j{}'w_i + \lambda_j \upsilon_i + \varepsilon_{ij}, \quad \varepsilon_{ij} \sim N(0, 1)$$

for the underlying variables y_{ij}^* corresponding to the three binary indicators y_{ij}, $j = 1, 2, 3$.

The form of the *structural model* is

$$\upsilon_i = u_i'\alpha + f_1(x_{i1}) + \dots + f_3(x_{i3}) + f_{geo}(reg_i) + \delta_i \tag{4.10}$$

The models include the direct vector of covariates w_i for each individual response variable. The direct vector w_i includes the categorical covariates *water, educ, toilet, urban, trep and elect* in the LVM for Egypt (Table 4.3). In the case of Nigeria, it includes the covariates *male, educ, radio,* and *water* (Table 4.4). The indirect vector u includes *male, anvis, work, and radio* in the latent variable mixed models for Egypt, and *urban, work, terp, avis, toilet,* and *elect* for Nigeria.

The *measurement model* using two latent variables is given by

$$\begin{pmatrix} y_{i1}^* \\ y_{i2}^* \\ y_{i3}^* \\ y_{i4}^* \\ y_{i5}^* \end{pmatrix} = \begin{pmatrix} \lambda_{i1} \\ \lambda_{i2} \\ \lambda_{i3} \\ \lambda_{i4} \\ \lambda_{i5} \end{pmatrix} + \begin{pmatrix} a_1' \\ a_2' \\ a_3' \\ a_4' \\ a_5' \end{pmatrix} \cdot \begin{pmatrix} w_1 \; w_2 \; w_3 \; w_4 \; w_5 \end{pmatrix} + \begin{pmatrix} \lambda_{11} \; \lambda_{12} \\ \lambda_{21} \; \lambda_{22} \\ \lambda_{31} \; \lambda_{32} \\ \lambda_{41} \; \lambda_{42} \\ \lambda_{51} \; \lambda_{52} \end{pmatrix} \cdot \begin{pmatrix} \upsilon_1 \\ \upsilon_2 \end{pmatrix} + \begin{pmatrix} \varepsilon_{i1} \\ \varepsilon_{i2} \\ \varepsilon_{i3} \\ \varepsilon_{i4} \\ \varepsilon_{i5} \end{pmatrix} \tag{4.11}$$

The *structural model* for the analysis uses two latent factors:

$$\begin{pmatrix} \upsilon_1 \\ \upsilon_2 \end{pmatrix} = \begin{pmatrix} u'_{i1}\alpha_1 \\ u'_{i2}\alpha_2 \end{pmatrix} + \begin{pmatrix} f_{11}(Chage_i) \\ f_{21}(Chage_i) \end{pmatrix} + \begin{pmatrix} f_{12}(BMI_i) \\ f_{22}(BMI_i) \end{pmatrix} + \begin{pmatrix} f_{13}(Mageb_i) \\ f_{23}(Mageb_i) \end{pmatrix} + \begin{pmatrix} f_{14}(reg_i) \\ f_{24}(reg_i) \end{pmatrix} + \begin{pmatrix} \delta_{i1} \\ \delta_{i2} \end{pmatrix} \tag{4.12}$$

where *Chage is* Child's age in months, *BMI is* Mother's body mass index, and *Mageb is* Mother's age at birth. Further, *reg* is the spatial covariate, which refers to governorate or regions where respondent resides.

4.4.1 Selection Cariteria

To decide which covariates should be included in the measurement models and which should be in the structural models, we follow the strategy below:

As a first step, we apply separate geoadditive probit models for health indicators and separate geoadditive Gaussian models for the malnutrition indicators. The results are reported in Khatab and Fahrmeir (2009) and Khatab (2010).

In the second step, we apply geoadditive probit LVMs to analyze the data. Although the Deviance Information Criterion (DIC) is now commonly accepted as a standard tool for selecting probit or logit models, its performance for LVM model choice is not yet well understood.

4.4.2 Models Section

If the effects of covariates turned out to be significantly different (in terms of confidence intervals) for the three diseases, we decided to keep them in the measurement model, otherwise covariates were included in the geoadditive predictor of the structural equation for the latent variable. All nonlinear effects and the spatial effect are included in the structural model.

4.5 Applications

4.5.1 Childhood Diseases

Diarrhea

Diarrheal disease, caused by poor condition of water and sanitation, is a common public health problem in developing countries. It is a variety of micro-organisms

Table 4.1 Overview of the morbidities in Egypt

Health Indicators	Observation	Mean	Std.Dev	No diseases	Had diseases
Diearhea	6,348	0.210	0.407	5,013(78.97)	1,335(21.03)
Fever	6,348	0.323	0.467	4,297(67.69)	2,051(32.31)
Cough	6,348	0.255	0.436	4,725(74.43)	1,623(25.57)

Table 4.2 Overview of the morbidities in Nigeria

Health Indicators	Observations	Mean	Std.Dev	No diseases	Had diseases
Diearhea	5,186	0.179	0.383	4,257(82.09)	929(17.91)
Fever	5,186	0.309	0.462	3,583(69.09)	1,603(30.91)
Cough	5,186	0.235	0.407	3,967(76.49)	1,219(23.51)

including viruses, bacteria, and protozoan's that cause diarrhea, affecting people's health through loss of water and electrolytes. This leads to dehydration and, in disastrous preconditions, to death.

In Egypt, the widespread use of oral rehydration therapy has successfully reduced the severity of diarrheal episodes and sharply reduced the number of subsequent deaths. However, overall diarrheal disease has not declined. In the 2003 DHS, mothers were asked whether any of their children less than 5 years of age had had diarrhea at any time during the 2-week period before the survey.

Fever

Infection is the most common cause of fever in children. Most fevers in babies and children are caused by a viral (germ) infection. Common viral and bacterial illnesses like colds, gastroenteritis, ear infections, croup, and bronchitis are the most likely illnesses to cause fever.

Cough

Cough and breathing difficulties are common problems in young children. Recent literature indicates that breastfed children who had a cough or cold may have difficulties in feeding. Breastfeeding however, could help fight diseases. Along with diarrhea, acute respiratory infection (ARI), particularly pneumonia, is a common cause of death in infants and young children.

Tables 4.1 and 4.2 provide overview of the morbidities in both countries.

4.5.2 Childhood Malnutrition

Childhood undernutrition is amongst the most serious health issues facing developing countries. It is an intrinsic indicator of well-being, but it is also associated with morbidity, mortality, impaired childhood development, and reduced labor productivity (Sen 1999; UNICEF 1998; Pelletier 1998; Svedberg 1996). Three anthropometric variables are measured through z-scores for wasting, stunting and underweight, defined by

$$Z_i = \frac{AI_i - MAI}{\sigma}, \tag{4.13}$$

where AI refers to the individual anthropometric indicator (e.g. height at a certain age), MAI refers to the median of a reference population, and σ refers to the standard deviation of the reference population. Each of the indicators measure somewhat different aspects of nutritional status. Note that higher values of a z-score indicate better nutrition and vice versa. Therefore, a decrease of z-scores indicates an increase in malnutrition. This has to be taken into account when interpreting the results. The reference standard typically used for the calculation is the National Center for Health Statistics-Center for Disease Prevention (NCHS-CDC) Growth Standard that has been recommended for international use by WHO. The reference population are children from the USA. More exactly, up to an age of 24 months these are children from white parents with high socio-economic status, while older children are from a representive sample of all US children.

Stunting

Stunting is an indicator of linear growth retardation relatively uncommon in the first few months of life. However it becomes more common as children get older. Children with *height-for-age* z-scores below minus two standard deviations from the median of the reference population are considered short for their age or stunted.

Underweight

Underweight is a composite index of stunting and wasting. This means children may be underweight if they are either stunted or wasted, or both. In a similar manner to the two previous anthropometric incidences, children may be underweight when their z-score is below minus two standard deviations.

Categorical Covariates

Tables 4.3 and 4.4 provide information on categorical socioeconomic and bio-demographic covariates, their categories, frequencies, and the coding used in the regression models for Egypt and Nigeria, respectively. Although wealth index was

Table 4.3 Overview of the factors analysed in the case study for Egypt

Factor	N(%)	Coding effect
Place of residence		
Urban	2,237(33.58 %)	1
Rural	4,424(66.42 %)	−1.ref
Child's sex		
Male	3,487(52.35 %)	1
Female	3,174(47.65 %)	−1.ref
Working		
Yes	1,209(18.15 %)	1
No	5,452(81.85 %)	−1.ref
Mother's Education		
No,		
Incomp.prim,		
Comp.prim,		
Incomp.sec	4,194(62.97 %)	1
Compl.sec,		
Higher	2,467(37.04 %)	−1.ref
Pregnancy's treatment		
Yes	697(10.46 %)	1
No	5,964(89.54 %)	−1.ref
Drinking water		
Controlled	5,374(80.68 %)	1
Not controlled	1,287(19.32 %)	−1.ref
Missing	1 %	
Had radio		
Yes	5,374(80.68 %)	1
No	1,559(19.32 %)	−1.ref
Has electricity		
Yes	6,203(93.12 %)	1
No	458(6.88 %)	−1.ref
Toilet facility		
Own flush toile facility	1,768(28 %)	1
Other and no toilet facility	4,511(71.8 %)	−1.ref
Missing	1 %	
Antenatal visit		
Yes	4,181(63 %)	1
No	2,342(35 %)	−1.ref
Missing	2 %	

included in previous works of the author, in the present chapter we include only radio, electricity, type of toilet, and drinking water in order to facilitate comparison of results in the two countries.

Table 4.4 Overview of the factors analysed in the case study for Nigeria

Factor	N(%)	Coding effect
Place of residence		
Urban	2,118(35.13 %)	1
Rural	3,911(64.87 %)	−1.ref
Child's sex		
Male	3,062(50.79 %)	1
Female	2,967(49.21 %)	−1.ref
Working		
Yes	3,835(63.61 %)	1
No	2,172(36.39 %)	−1.ref
Mother's Education		
No,		
Incomp.prim,		
Comp.prim,		
Incomp.sec	5,294(87.81 %)	1
Compl.sec,		
Higher	735(12.19 %)	−1.ref
Pregnancy's treatment		
Yes	1,001(16.6 %)	1
No	5,028(83.40 %)	−1.ref
Drinking water		
Controlled	1,899(32 %)	1
Not controlled	4,096(67 %)	−1.ref
Missing	1 %	
Had radio		
Yes	4,466(74.08 %)	1
No	563(25.97 %)	−1.ref
Has electricity		
Yes	2,715(45.03 %)	1
No	3,314(54.97 %)	−1.ref
Toilet facility		
Own flush toile facility	590(10 %)	1
Other and no toilet facility	5,335(88.5 %)	−1.ref
Missing	1.5 %	
Antenatal visit		
Yes	2,412(40 %)	1
No	1,264(21 %)	−1.ref
Missing	29 %	

Child's Age (Chage)

The age of a child has a significant effect on its morbidity as reported in many previous studies. According to the World Health Organization (WHO) children should receive all recommended vaccines by 12 months of age.

Mother's Body Mass Index (BMI)

Body mass index (BMI) varies with the woman's age, and it is somewhat higher among urban women than among rural women. Studies show that this coexistence of under- and overnutrition exists not only at the societal but also the household level. The range of overweight mothers is remarkably large, even within a region. For instance, 55 % of mothers are overweight in Egypt.

Mother's Age at Birth (magb)

This is an important variable to fertility because it marks the onset of the childbearing process. Delay in magb may indicate late establishment of marriage and hence implies shortening of the reproductive period and consequential reduced fertility.

Spatial Covariates

The information of the geographic location (governorate or regions) where the child lives at the time of interview is a significant contribution of the DHS data set to understanding child disease and malnutrition in both countries. In the case of Egypt, there are 20 governorates included. For Nigeria, 37 regions have been considered.

4.6 Case Study of Egypt

In this section, the latent variable models has been applied using data from the 2003 Egypt Demographic and Health Survey (El-Zanaty and Way 2004). The aim of the analysis is investigate the relationship between the indicators of diseases and the indicators of undernutrition in Egypt based on the analyses which have been presented in Khatab and Fahrmeir (2009) that focused on the childhood morbidity in Egypt, and Khatab (2010) that investigate childhood malnutrition in Egypt.

4.6.1 Model Estimation with One Factor Analysis

The modeling focused at this stage on the estimation using the binary indicators (fever, diarrhea, and cough) and the continuous indicators (stunting and underweight), with one latent variable.

In order to decide which of the covariates should be included in the measurement model as direct parametric effects, or in the structural equation as indirect effects via their impact on the latent variables, mentioned criteria are taken into account.

The covariates *male, antenatal visit, radio* and *work* were associated with childhood diseases and childhood undernutrition, so we kept them in the structural equation in the case study of Egypt.

Our analysis started using only one latent variable. The results for the estimation of factor loadings, parametric indirect and direct effects for Egypt are presented in Table 4.5.

The factor loadings in Table 4.5 show that the latent variable has a stronger influence on the first three indicators that belong to the health status than on the nutritional status (*stunting* and *underweight*).

The parametric indirect effects for male, antenatal visit and work have a significant effect on the child health indicators in Egypt. Regarding the parametric direct effects, covariate *urban* is associated with indicators *cough, diarrhea, stunting* and underweight, whilst treatment during pregnancy is associated with the second indicator; and the education level of mother has a positive effect on the indicators of *stunting* and *underweight.*

In addition, none of the covariates which have parametric effects were associated with the indicators of *fever*.

With regards to the nonparametric effects, Fig. 4.1 shows the nonlinear and spatial effects. These results are expected, as the indicators of diseases are clearly represented through the latent variable, so the results are consistent with the results of the prevoius sudy, which has focused on the childhood modrbidity in Egypt (Khatab and Fahrmeir 2009).

The nonlinear effect of child's age indicates that the prevalence of diseases was found to be highest among children 0–12 months of age. As for the effect of a mother's BMI, it has a slight effect on the latent variable; however, there is a higher effect through the interval between 27 and 30. The pattern of mother's age shows that younger mothers (12–20) have a higher effect on the health staus of child comapare to their counterparts (20–35 years of age).

The spatial effect for Egypt indicates that higher risks are associated with some rural areas in the Nile Delta and in Sinai as well.

Again, looking at the estimated mean factor loadings in Table 4.5 we can draw the following conclusions: First, the latent variable has significant effect on all five indicators. Second, as we expected, disease and malnutrition indicators are positively associated. Strictly speaking, disease indicators and z-scores for stunting and underweight are negatively correlated, because by definition z-scores for stunting and underweight decrease with increasing undernutrition.

Third, the latent variable loads much higher onto the disease indicators than onto the malnutrition indicators. Therefore, we reanalyse the data with a LVM with two latent variables in the next subsection. Because the latent variable loads mainly on the disease indicators, these results are comparably close to the ones obtained with the results for the LVM with two latent variables, so we defer interpretation to the following subsection.

Table 4.5 Estimates of factor loadings, parametric indirect and direct effects of the LVMM with one latent variable for Egypt

Parameter	Mean	Std	2.5 %	97.5 %
Factor loadings				
1. Fever λ_{11}	1.247*	0.089	1.094	1.420
2. Cough λ_{21}	0.811*	0.047	0.724	0.901
3. Diarrhea λ_{31}	0.816*	0.043	0.734	0.897
4. Stunting λ_{41}	−0.132*	−0.134	−0.182	−0.084
5. Underweight λ_{51}	−0.133*	0.021	−0.015	−0.074
Parametric indirect effects				
Male	0.168*	0.038	0.036	0.247
Anvis	0.221*	0.064	0.098	0.339
Work	0.123*	0.053	0.0168	0.238
Radio	−0.164	0.108	−0.275	0.072
Parametric direct effects				
Water(a_{11})	0.122	0.088	−0.037	0.295
Educ(a_{12})	−0.065	0.049	−0.157	0.028
Toilet(a_{13})	−0.107	0.128	−0.452	0.116
Urban(a_{14})	0.047	0.068	−0.082	0.183
Trepr(a_{15})	0.076	0.097	−0.108	0.272
Elect(a_{16})	−0.313	0.279	−0.838	0.211
Water(a_{21})	0.061	0.067	−0.065	0.195
Educ(a_{22})	−0.055	0.041	−0.140	0.015
Toilet(a_{23})	−0.089	0.120	−0.348	0.108
Urban(a_{24})	−0.22*	0.063	−0.348	−0.098
Trepr(a_{25})	0.193*	0.073	0.039	0.340
Elect(a_{26})	0.191	0.071	−0.467	0.532
Water(a_{31})	−0.02	0.067	−0.178	0.112
Educ (a_{32})	−0.033	0.038	−0.128	0.037
Toilet(a_{33})	−0.029	0.116	−0.277	0.184
Urban(a_{34})	0.151*	0.056	0.044	0.265
Terpr(a_{35})	0.015	0.079	−0.139	0.165
Elect(a_{36})	−0.096	0.231	−0.516	0.357
Water(a_{41})	0.006	0.050	−0.090	0.108
Educ(a_{42})	0.066[a]	0.026	0.015	0.118
Toilet(a_{43})	0.029	0.084	−0.121	0.208
Urban(a_{44})	0.123[a]	0.037	0.054	0.203
Terpr(a_{45})	−0.009	0.057	−0.108	0.098
Elect(a_{46})	−0.171	0.168	−0.519	0.153
Water(a_{51})	0.013	0.039	−0.065	0.099
Educ (a_{52})	0.052[a]	0.022	0.013	0.095
Toilet(a_{53})	−0.035	0.070	−0.197	0.119
Urban(a_{54})	0.13[a]	0.036	0.069	0.199
Trepr(a_{55})	−0.023	0.0335	−0.126	0.079
Elect(a_{56})	−0.088	0.1455	−0.351	0.200

*Estimate significant at 5 % level

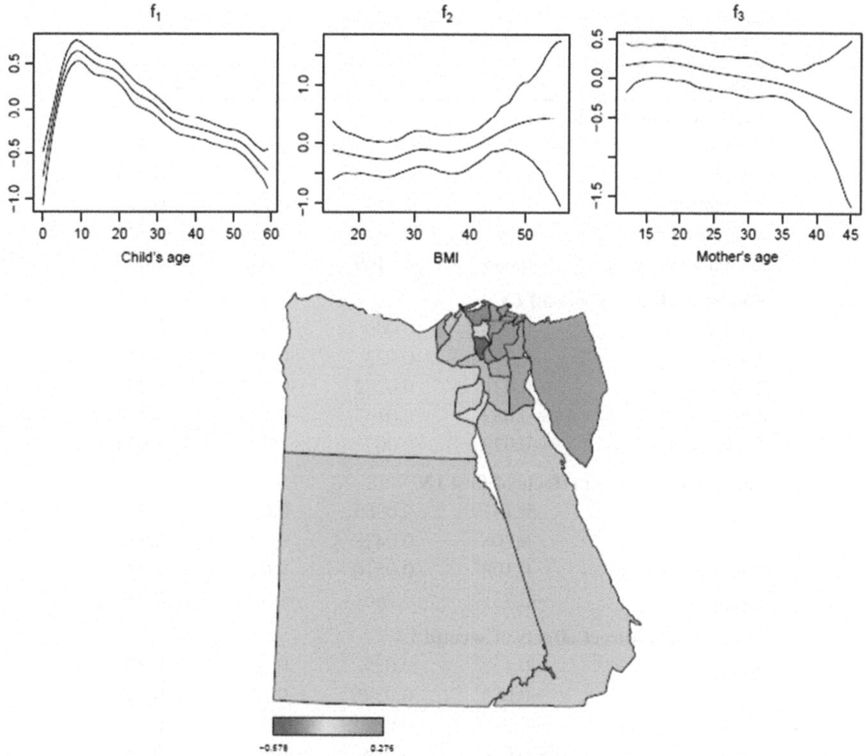

Fig. 4.1 Non-linear effects from top to bottom: child's age, mother's BMI, mother's age at birth and spatial effects (for model LVMM using five indicators), on the indicators of a latent variable "health status" and "undernutrition status" of children for Egypt using only one latent variable

4.6.2 Model Estimation with Two Latent Variables

In this section, we analyze determinants of childhood diseases and childhood undernutrition using two latent variables.

The factor loadings estimates as shown in Table 4.6 observed that the first latent variable loads onto the first three indicators (health indicators), whilst indicators 4 and 5 (nutritional status) are explained by the second latent variable. This was to be expected, because the two different sets of indicators are supposed to measure two different latent constructs. Further, it is indicated that the interpretation for the LVMs with two factors are more reasonable compared to that of one factor model.

Both factor loadings and coefficients of the parametric indirect covariates of the first latent factor are very similar to the estimates of the single latent factor model given in Table 4.6. Regarding the factor loadings of the second latent variable, the indicator *underweight* has high factor loading of 0.975.

The results in Table 4.6 also show that the influences of the covariates *anvis*, *male*, *radio* and *work* are noticeable for the first latent variable, whilst the second

Table 4.6 Estimates of factor loadings of the LVMM with two latent variable and only five indicators for Egypt

Parameter	Mean	Std	2.5 %	97.5 %
Factor Loadings of First LV				
1. Fever λ_{11}	1.221*	0.092	1.07	1.496
2. Cough λ_{21}	0.810*	0.0438	0.721	0.903
3. Diarrhea λ_{31}	0.816*	0.0441	0.737	0.914
4. Stunting λ_{41}	−0.066*	0.0179	−0.106	−0.019
5. Underweight λ_{51}	−0.048	0.0109	−0.051	0.039
Factor loadings of second LV				
1. Fever λ_{12}	0.000	0.000	0.000	0.000
2. Cough λ_{22}	0.033	0.023	−0.058	0.046
3. Diarrhea λ_{32}	−0.031	0.0222	−0.054	0.039
4. Stunting λ_{42}	−0.657*	0.0145	−0.325	−0.260
5. Underweight λ_{52}	−0.975*	0.007	1.061	1.099
Parametric indirect effects of first LV				
Male	0.1319*	0.0385	0.056	0.207
Anvis	0.206*	0.0428	0.127	0.288
Work	0.108*	0.0510	0.0133	0.205
Radio	−0.737*	0.366	−1.359	−0.0512
Parametric indirect effects of second LV				
Male	0.152*	0.025	0.101	0.200
Anvis	−0.085*	0.0296	−0.140	−0.025
Work	−0.0159	0.036	−0.0870	0.052
Trepr	−0.020	0.036	−0.089	0.054
Elect	0.040	0.047	−0.0527	0.123
Radio	0.147	0.133	−0.0982	0.398
Parametric direct effects of both LVs				
Water(a_{11})	0.138	0.085	−0.0257	0.291
Educ(a_{12})	−0.051	0.0504	−0.149	0.038
Toilet(a_{13})	−0.110	0.145	−0.398	0.175
Urban(a_{14})	0.031	0.068	−0.1002	0.164
Trepr(a_{15})	0.082	0.0917	−0.095	0.262
Elect(a_{16})	−0.311	0.267	−0.839	0.208
Water(a_{21})	0.079	0.073	−0.064	0.221
Educ(a_{22})	−0.053	0.0413	−0.130	0.024
Toilet(a_{23})	−0.059	0.125	−0.297	0.176
Urban(a_{24})	−0.211*	0.0610	−0.338	−0.090
Trepr(a_{25})	0.192*	0.077	0.044	0.349
Elect(a_{26})	0.018	0.251	−0.512	0.464
Water(a_{31})	−0.023	0.074	−0.162	0.119
Educ(a_{32})	−0.036	0.040	−0.113	0.028
Toilet(a_{33})	−0.023	0.119	−0.282	0.191
Urban(a_{34})	0.152*	0.059	0.0446	0.276
Trepr(a_{35})	0.014	0.08	−0.136	0.170
Elect(a_{36})	−0.112	0.234	−0.595	0.360

(continued)

Table 4.6 (continued)

Parameter	Mean	Std	2.5 %	97.5 %
Water(a_{41})	−0.019	0.049	−0.109	0.084
Educ(a_{42})	0.061*	0.0219	0.023	0.104
Toilet(a_{43})	−0.007	0.083	−0.175	0.155
Urban(a_{44})	0.036	0.0352	−0.033	0.099
Water(a_{51})	−0.025	0.031	−0.0718	0.037
Educ(a_{52})	0.048*	0.009	0.0278	0.064
Toilet(a_{53})	−0.02	0.068	−0.194	0.132
Urban(a_{54})	0.11*	0.034	0.065	0.194
Trepr(a_{55})	−0.068	0.042	−0.151	0.013
Elect(a_{56})	−0.73	0.132	−0.327	0.160

*Estimate significant at 5 % level

latent variable is associated with *anvis* and *male*. The results of the parametric direct covariates are quite similar to the estimates with a single latent variable. The results are also consistent with those from separate analysis of childhood diseases and childhood malnutrition (Khatab and Fahrmeir 2009; Khatab 2010).

The patterns of the covariates child's age, mother's BMI and mother's age resemble the patterns of the model with one latent variable (Fig. 4.1 is reproduced in the left panel of Fig. 4.2), whilst the influence of these covariates on the second latent variable looks different. Apparently, the nonlinear effects on the second latent variable are associated with the indicators of nutritional status.

Sensitivity Analysis

It is known that the Markov Random Field prior for spatial covariates works well if there are many neighbors for the spatial units. However, this is not the case for Egypt, where there are few governorates and neighbors. Therefore, we carried out a sensitivity analysis for the choice of the prior for the spatial effects. It turned out that the results of the spatial effects remained stable for the separate models and also for the latent variable models (Fig. 4.3).

4.7 Case Study of Nigeria

4.7.1 Model Estimation with One Factor Analysis

For Nigeria, the results (Table 4.7) lead to the same conclusion as for Egypt, where the estimates of factor loadings for the diseases affect the latent variable more than the indicators of undernutrition. The results show that the indicators of undernutrition have a slightly stronger effect on the latent variable. The results of the

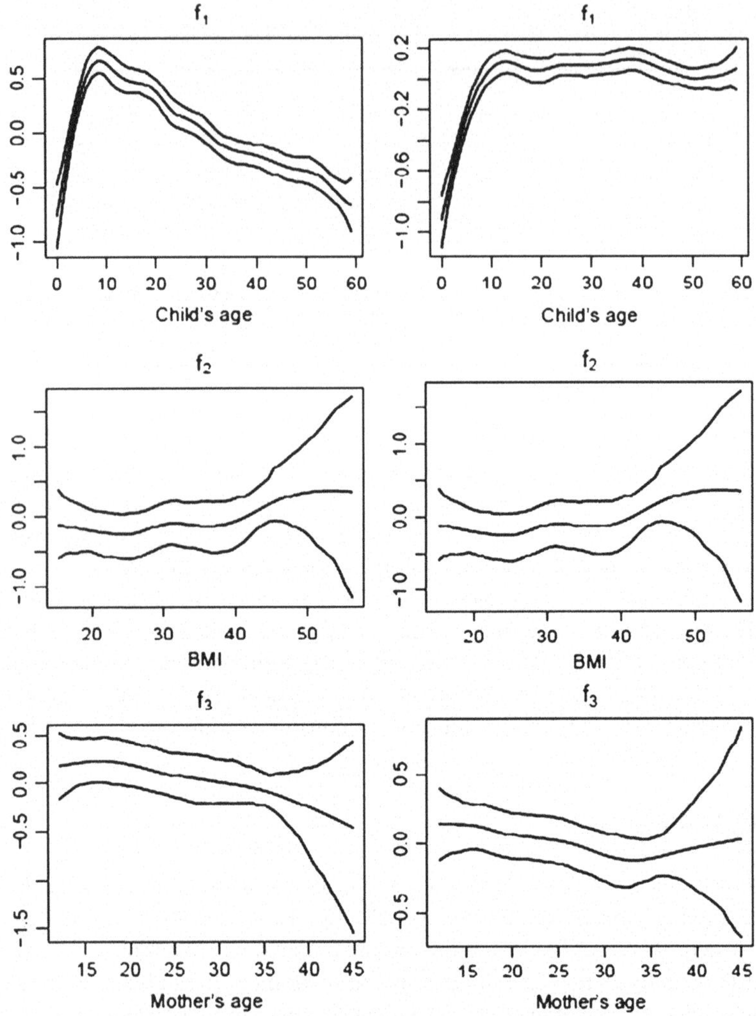

Fig. 4.2 Estimates of nonparametric effect of nonlinear covariates from top to bottom: child's age, mother's BMI, and mother's age at birth for the first (*left*) and second (*right*) latent variables for Egypt

indirect parametric covariates show that only *urban* and *treatment during pregnancy* have significant effect on the latent variable. As for the direct parametric covariates, *male, education level* and *radio* are associated with indicator 4 *(stunting)*, whilst only the level of education is associated with indicator 2 *(cough)*.

The pattern of the nonparametric effects for the nonlinear effects of a child's age shows that the health status of children worsens until about 12 months of age (Fig. 4.4). The effect of BMI seems to be a little higher for mothers with a BMI

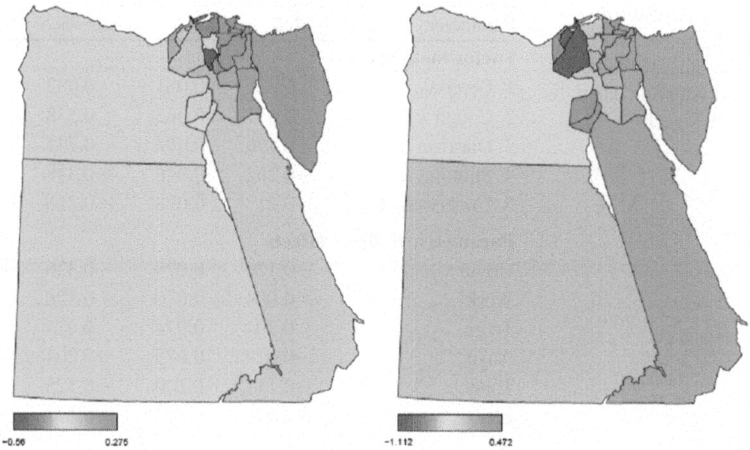

Fig. 4.3 Estimates of the nonparametric effect of spatial covariate for the first (*left*) and second (*right*) for Egypt

under 20. Children from younger mothers, as in Egypt, are more likely to have problems in their health status. We found that the high risk of the latent variable health and nutritional status is pronounced in the northeastern part of Nigeria.

4.7.2 Model Estimation with Two Latent Variables

As shown in Table 4.8, In Nigeria, the second latent variable has the highest influence on the indicator *stunting*, with factor loading of 1.165. The influence of *urban* and *trepr (treatment during pregnancy)* is associated with the first latent variable, however, the second latent variable is more influenced by the covariates *avis* and *elect*. Most of the coefficients of parametric direct covariates are insignificant with the exception of the *child's sex* which affects the indicator *stunting* and the covariate *education level* which affects the indicators of *diarrhea* and *stunting*. Else, the results in Table 4.8 are very similar to those of the single latent variable model in Table 4.7.

4.8 Summary and Discussion

In this chapter we have formulated a latent model for joint analysis of childhood diseases and malnutrition in two African countries to highlight shared specific risk factors which affect the diseases and malnutrition status in those countries.

The main goal was to assess the extent of spatial variation among risk of diseases and nutritional status.

Table 4.7 Estimates of factor loadings, parametric indirect and direct effects of the LVMM with one latent variable for Nigeria

Parameter	Mean	Std	2.5 %	97.5 %
Factor loadings				
1. Fever λ_{11}	0.821*	0.081	0.682	0.989
2. Cough λ_{21}	0.651*	0.063	0.538	0.781
3. Diarrhea λ_{31}	0.896*	0.084	0.741	1.087
4. Stunting λ_{41}	−0.262*	0.046	−0.348	−0.171
5. Underweight λ_{51}	−0.21*	0.028	−0.246	−0.136
Parametric indirect effects				
Urban	−0.179*	0.079	−0.326	−0.017
Work	0.004	0.070	−0.126	0.147
Trepr	0.204*	0.074	0.053	0.331
Anvis	−0.039	0.085	−0.204	0.126
Toilet	−0.111	0.100	−0.325	0.078
Elect	−0.018	0.077	−0.171	0.127
Parametric direct effects				
Male(a_{11})	−0.006	0.068	−0.141	0.128
Educ(a_{12})	0.024	0.077	−0.125	0.181
Radio(a_{13})	−0.030	0.040	−0.105	0.047
Water(a_{14})	0.044	0.095	−0.130	0.243
Male(a_{21})	0.016	0.061	−0.102	0.134
Educ(a_{22})	0.151*	0.070	0.020	0.282
Radio(a_{23})	0.007	0.039	−0.069	0.086
Water(a_{24})	−0.059	0.093	−0.240	0.113
Male(a_{31})	0.128	0.078	−0.030	0.274
Educ(a_{32})	−0.118	0.094	−0.318	0.051
Radio(a_{33})	−0.044	0.044	−0.136	0.041
Water(a_{34})	−0.050	0.111	−0.249	0.183
Male(a_{41})	−0.218*	0.067	−0.347	−0.100
Educ(a_{42})	0.449*	0.0718	0.308	0.584
Radio(a_{43})	0.090*	0.040	0.012	0.166
Water(a_{44})	0.093	0.095	−0.090	0.274
Male(a_{51})	0.063	0.052	−0.032	0.165
Educ(a_{52})	−0.016	0.056	−0.122	0.085
Radio(a_{53})	0.018	0.030	−0.037	0.076
Water(a_{54})	−0.048	0.069	−0.193	0.087

*Estimate significant at 5 % level

The current study was a follow up of previous studies (Khatab and Fahrmeir 2009; Khatab 2010) where child morbidity and malnutrition in Egypt were modelled separately.

The joint analysis (latent variable models) used in this chapter confirmed most of the previous findings. Additionally, it measured the degree of spatial correlation between the indicators of diseases and those of malnutrition. This is, indeed, one of the appealing features of the model as it permits to assess the association between the diseases and the malnutrition indicators and also distinguishes between the

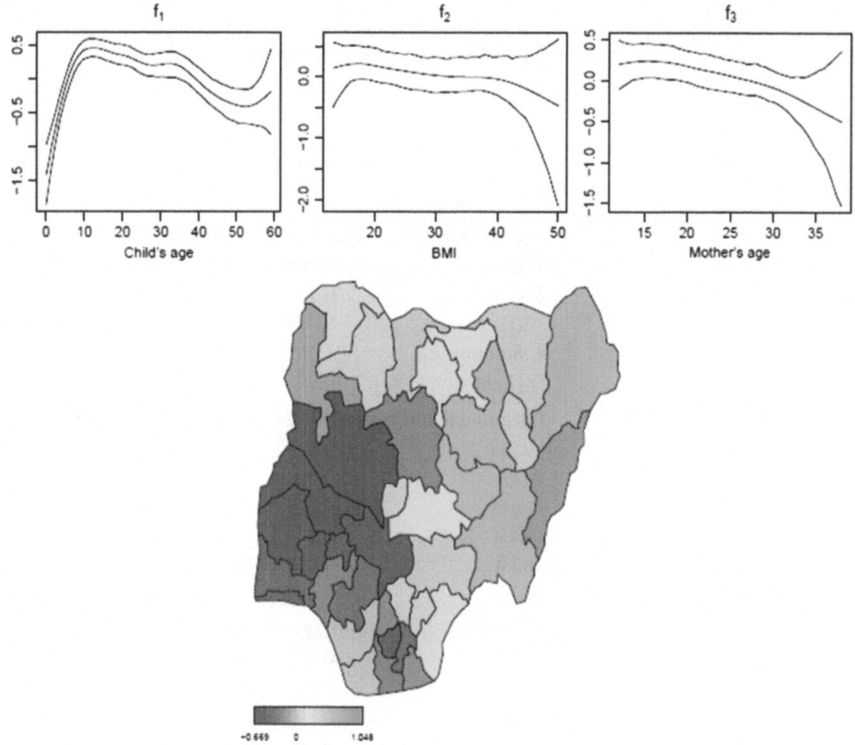

Fig. 4.4 Non-linear effects from top to bottom: child's age, mother's BMI, mother's age at birth and spatial effects (for model LVMM using five indicators), on the indicators of a latent variable "health status" and "undernutrition status" of children for Nigeria using only one latent variable

risk factors associated with each status indicator. In addition, the model allows exploration of how spatial heterogeneity in these factors influences disease and malnutrition patterns.

The epidemiological significance of the findings is that the estimated patterns can be related to known possible explanatory factors or putative sources, thereby guiding policy with regard to targeting interventions.

With regard to the statiscal methodology, geoadditive latent variable models offer new opportunities and insights to analyze child morbidity and malnutrition in developing countries within a joint modelling framework. In our case study for Egypt and Nigeria we found strong support for flexibly modelling the effect of some covariates that have nonlinear influences and for including a spatial effect. The maps could be used for targeting regional development efforts and they may highlight unexpected relationships that would be overlooked in analyses with standard regression or latent variable models (Fig. 4.5).

Compared to separate modelling, the joint model in this chapter offers several advantages. First, it offers a flexible regression modelling of highly correlated response variables within a unified framework, thus improving efficiency and

Table 4.8 Results of LVMM using two latent variable for Nigeria

Parameter	Mean	Std	2.5 %	97.5 %
Factor loadings of first latent variable				
1. Fever λ_{11}	0.957*	0.083	0.821	1.146
2. Cough λ_{21}	1.032*	0.091	0.868	1.208
3. Diarrhea λ_{31}	0.77*	0.065	0.665	0.901
4. Stunting λ_{41}	−0.025	0.048	−0.118	0.073
5. Underweight λ_{51}	−0.155*	0.037	−0.226	−0.090
Factor loadings of second latent variable				
1. Fever λ_{12}	0.000	0.000	0.000	0.000
2. Cough λ_{22}	0.253*	0.045	0.164	0.336
3. Diarrhea λ_{32}	−0.088*	0.0355	−0.1588	−0.014
4. Stunting λ_{42}	1.165*	0.028	1.109	1.224
5. Underweight λ_{52}	0.958*	0.0238	0.910	1.006
Parametric indirect effects of first LV				
Urban	−0.144*	0.067	−0.277	−0.020
Work	0.010	0.068	−0.108	0.160
Trepr	0.243*	0.074	0.091	0.380
Anvis	−0.037	0.076	−0.171	0.111
Toilet	−0.075	0.099	−0.287	0.109
Elect	−0.023	0.074	−0.170	0.121
Parametric indirect effects of second LV				
Urban	0.021	0.060	−0.103	0.141
Work	0.105	0.060	−0.014	0.219
Trepr	0.093	0.0613	−0.030	0.218
Anvis	0.359*	0.063	0.234	0.474
Toilet	0.143	0.080	−0.012	0.304
Elect	0.159*	0.064	0.029	0.287
Parametric direct effects of both LV				
Male(a_{11})	−0.0073	0.066	−0.135	0.1230
Educ(a_{12})	−0.039	0.078	−0.186	0.130
Radio(a_{13})	−0.052	0.042	−0.137	0.034
Water(a_{14})	0.041	0.103	−0.168	0.245
Male(a_{21})	0.032	0.074	−0.104	0.168
Educ(a_{22})	0.068	0.087	−0.100	0.242
Radio(a_{23})	−0.024	0.048	−0.115	0.068
Water(a_{24})	−0.056	0.110	−0.261	0.185
Male(a_{31})	0.115	0.0707	−0.023	0.256
Educ(a_{32})	−0.154*	0.081	−0.312	−0.006
Radio(a_{33})	−0.066	0.038	−0.142	0.011
Water(a_{34})	−0.06	0.102	−0.266	0.137
Male(a_{41})	−0.242*	0.063	−0.374	−0.119
Educ(a_{42})	0.185*	0.066	0.0565	0.326
Radio(a_{43})	0.028	0.039	−0.052	0.105
Water(a_{44})	0.072	0.0897	−0.102	0.230
Male(a_{51})	−0.061	0.047	−0.1472	0.042
Educ(a_{52})	0.048	0.054	−0.052	0.153
Radio(a_{53})	0.027	0.029	−0.030	0.082
Water(a_{54})	−0.005	0.072	−0.144	0.139

*Estimate significant at 5 % level

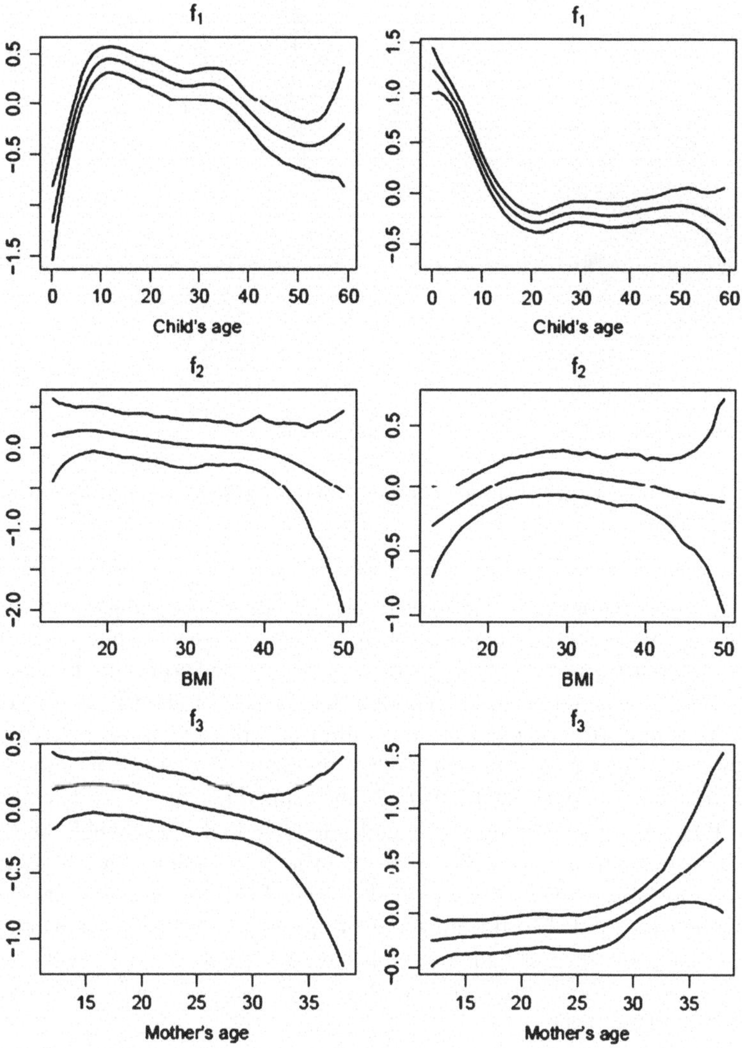

Fig. 4.5 Estimates of nonparametric effect of nonlinear covariates from top to bottom: child's age, mother's BMI, and mother's age at birth for the first (*left*) and second (*right*) latent variable for Nigeria

precision of parameter estimates. This, in turn, allows to include more indicators in the model as response variables. Further, the model is able to deal with the different type of indicators such as binary, continuous, ordinal, etc. In addition, not only the probit model can be applied in terms of the latent variable model, but also the Poisson and some other families of the distributions can be implemented.

In Egypt, rural areas in the Nile Delta and some other provinces there or in Lower Egypt are associated with malnutrition in children. One reason, as some

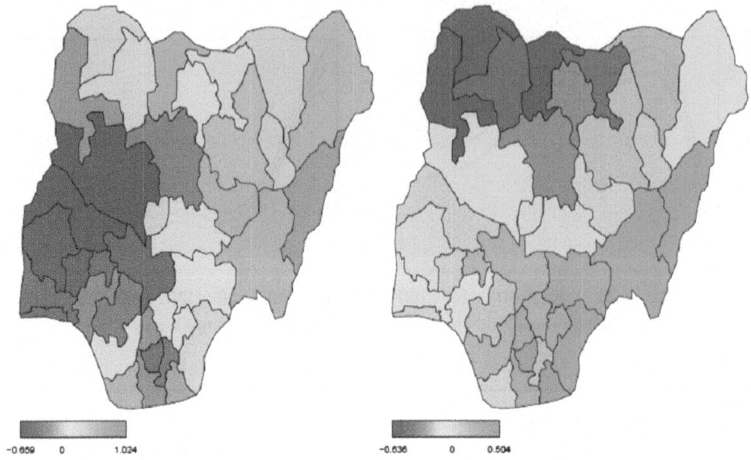

Fig. 4.6 Estimates of the nonparametric effect of spatial covariate for the first (*left*) and second (*right*) for Nigeria

previous studies reported, is that obesity among adults, particularly women, has reached very high proportions in Egypt in the last few years, while malnutrition rates in children (in the first 2 years of life) remain stubbornly high. The 1998 national food consumption survey reported that 16.7 % of children 2–6-years-old were underweight. Overweight and obesity affected 1.6 % of 2–6-year old children. The prevalence of stunting in preschool children ranged from 13 % in Lower Egypt to 24 % in Upper Egypt (Khatab 2010). At the same time, rates of early childhood malnutrition remain stubbornly stable and relatively high. The double burden of obesity and malnutrition is clearly evident. In addition, public awareness of the increasing prevalence of obesity and of diet-related chronic disease is increasing, and attention has turned to documenting the problem. On the other hand, most studies relating diarrhea and malnutrition have been conducted in economically marginal regions, where young children have high rates of diarrhea diseases and severely faltering growth.

In Nigeria (Fig. 4.6), there is a sizeable difference between pronounced disease in the eastern parts of the country and significantly better health status in the northern, and central parts. We can see from the results that southeastern regions and some regions in the north part are associated with a high rate of childhood disease. That is because, as suggested by previous studies, a high level of pollution is present due to petroleum production in those regions. For this reason, the pollution in this area affected the health of children through water pollution that influences access to drinkable water sanitation (see Adebayo 2002; Adebayo and Fahrmeir 2005).

The results indicate that, mostly districts in the northeast and southeast positively associated with *height-for-age* and *weight-for-age*. The results also reveal striking regional variations, with the northeast, south and southeast in much worse situations in terms of stunting and underweight than the northwest and southwest. On the other hand, the children who live in the northwest part of the country are more likely to be wasted than their counterparts in other parts of country.

There are both conceptual and technical problems associated with information on prevalence of fever, diarrhea and cough obtained retrospectively from cross-sectional studies. First, seasonal differences of occurrence in diarrhea are difficult to be taken into account in such studies. Longitudinal studies may be more appropriate to in different seasons. Second, during the survey, neither the children were examined nor mothers were given a precise definition of what constitutes an episode of various diseases. On the other hand, we have no sufficient information about the children who have died before the survey, and whether the cause of death was the diseases reported here or not.

The questions in the DHS measure the mother's perception of her child's health rather, than morbidity according to clinical examination. This may create variations among different socio-economic groups because perception of illness is not the same across different social groups. Third, loss of memory of events as well as misinterpretation of the reference period can also contribute to the problems associated with the prevalence of diarrhea (Bateman and Smith 1991).

To sum up, Latent Variable Models offer a new methodology for considering special types of diseases and malnutrition as indicators for latent morbidity and to flexibly model covariate and spatial effects on this latent variable. Compared with separate geoadditive models for the indicator variables, latent variable models can be advantageous from a statistical and a substantive perspective. Common latent variables automatically induce association between indicator variables not covered by covariates.

Acknowledgments The research underlying this paper is part of a research project obtained during my work period at the Munich University with Prof. Ludwig Fahrmeir. Part of this paper has been presented and discussed in the Statistics and Life Sciences Conference, Munich, Germany (March 2008) and other part has been prepared and discussed for the 57th International Statistical Institute Conference in Durban, South Africa, 2009.

My thanks go to Prof. Ludwig Fahrmeir, for his insightful comments, helpful advice and his discussions which helped me very much in editing this work. Comments from an anonymous referee are also gratefully acknowledged. Finally, I want to thank Prof. Thomas Kraus, Institute of Occupational and Social Medicine, Medical Faculty, RWTH Aachen University for his support in the final phase of this work.

Appendix

Priors and Identifiability

Priors for regression coefficients α_j and β_j are flat, i.e. $p(\alpha_j) \propto 1$, $p(\beta_j \propto 1)$, or weakly informative Gaussian, which is the standard prior in linear regression models. Similarly, inverse Gamma priors are usually chosen for error variances σ_j^2 in Gaussian measurement models.

Concerning factor loadings λ_j, we first have to deal with the well known identifiability problem in factor analysis and latent variables models. Any transformation from λ'_j to $\tilde{\lambda}'_j = \lambda_j{}'V$ and from υ_i to $\upsilon^2{}_i = V'\upsilon_i$ with an orthogonal matrix V leads to the same predictor because $\tilde{\lambda}'_j \tilde{\upsilon}_i = \lambda'_j \upsilon_i$. To avoid this identifiability problem we choose the matrix $\Lambda = (\lambda'_1, .., \lambda'_p)'$ of factor loadings to be a lower block triangular matrix of full rank and positive diagonal elements as recommended by Geweke and Zhou (1996) and Aguilar and West (2000). To avoid so-called Heywood cases, we assume a standard normal prior for these factor loadings, which is a standard choice in applications.

The nonparametric effects $f_{r1}, \ldots, f_{rk}$ for continuous covariates $z_1, \ldots, z_k$ in the structural equations (4.8) are modelled as (Bayesian) P-splines. Dropping indices to simply the notation, a function f is approximated through a polynomial spline

$$f(z) = \Sigma_{c=1}^{d} \gamma_c B_c(z), \tag{4.14}$$

where $B_1(z), \ldots, B_d(z)$ are B-spline basis functions. Smoothness of the function f is achieved by assuming a (second order) random walk model.

$$\gamma_{c=1} - 2\gamma_{c-1} + \gamma_{c-2} = u_c \sim N(0, \tau^2) \tag{4.15}$$

for the sequence of B-spline coefficients. The variance τ^2 controls the amount of smoothness and is estimated (together with all other parameters) by assuming an inverse Gamma prior.

More information about Bayesian P-spline regression is given in Lang and Brezger (2004) and Fahrmeir et al. (2004).

The geographical effects $f_{geo}(s)$ for regions $1, \ldots, S$ are modelled through Markov random field priors, a popular model in disease mapping (Besag et al. 1991) and in spatial statistics (Rue and Held 2005). The basic idea is that adjacent regions should have a similar impact on the latent variables, whereas two regions far apart from each other need not exhibit such a similarity. We assume the standard Markov random field prior

$$f_{geo}(s) | f_{geo}, s' \neq s \; N \left(\Sigma_{s' \in N_s} \frac{f_{geo(s')}}{n_s}, \frac{\tau^2_{geo}}{n_s} \right), \tag{4.16}$$

where $N(s)$ is the set of neighboring regions s' of s, i.e. share a common boundary with region s, and n_s is the number of neighboring regions. Hence, the conditional mean of $f_{geo(s)}$ is an average of the spatial effects $f_{geo(s')}$ of all adjacent regions. As for P-splines, the variance τ^2_{geo} controls smoothness of geographical effects and, again, obeys an inverse Gamma prior.

Identification Problems

There are two sources of identification problems.

The first is associated with modelling of ordinal variables, but our focus is in this chapter was on binary indicators. The second is related to the uniqueness of factor loadings matrix Λ and factor scores.

For the binary indicators the t_j of all indicators j are fixed to zero and $var(\varepsilon_i)$ =1 in order to solve the identification problem. For more details see Raach (2005).

Uniqueness of Factor Analysis and Scores

Consider a transformation of the model

$$y_i^* = \lambda_0 + \Lambda T^{-1} T \upsilon_i + A w_i + \varepsilon_i \tag{4.17}$$

with a $q \times q$ non-singular matrix T (e.g. Bartholomew 1987), i.e. where ΛT^{-1} is a loading matrix, new latent scores $T\ \upsilon_i$ and $V(\upsilon_i) = T\Psi T'$.

Without any restrictions for Λ or Ψ, a different number of models may be created. Since the matrix T consists of q^2 elements, we have to set q^2 restrictions in the model. For this reason the latent scores have a standard normal distribution, and no correlations among the latent variables exist.

In the traditional exploratory factor analysis, the variance matrix of the latent scores can be chosen to be q-dimensional identity matrix I_q, leading to $\upsilon_i \sim N_q(0, I_q)$.

For this reason, the latent scores have a standard normal distribution, and no correlations among the latent variables could exist. The model is invariant under transformations with orthogonal $q \times q$ matrix V of form $\tilde{\Lambda} = \Lambda V'$, and $\tilde{\upsilon}_i = V \upsilon_i$ since this transformations can keep the variance of latent scores without any changing ($V(\upsilon_i) = V I_k V' = \Psi$). The factor loadings matrix Λ is chosen to be a lower block triagonal matrix of full rank and positive diagonal elements (Geweke and Zhou 1996) using free parameters $f = pq - \frac{q(q-1)}{2}$.

Prior Distributions

This section discuses briefly a complete specification of the prior distributions for all parameters included in illustration of the present chapter. Since the prior distributions of the underlying variables y^* and the latent variables υ are implicitly determined by the prior distributions of all other parameters and the distributional assumptions about ε_i and ξ_i, we have to specify prior distributions for the parameter vector $\theta = vec\{\lambda_0, \Lambda, A, \Sigma, \beta, \gamma, \tau\}$. If we assume that the individual parts of the model are stochastically independent, then the prior distribution yields

$$p(\theta) = p(\lambda_0, \Lambda, A).p(\Sigma).p(\tau).p(\beta, \gamma).$$

The following subsections present briefly the prior distributions of the measurement model $p(\lambda_0, \Lambda, A)$, $p(\Sigma)$ and $p(\tau)$ and of the structural model $p(\beta, \gamma)$.

Prior Distribution of Intercept, Factor Loading and Direct Effects

Regarding the intercepts factor loadings and direct effects we define a $p.(1+q+d)$ dimensional vector $\overline{\Lambda}$ which contains all parameters of λ_0, Λ and A arranged $\overline{\Lambda} := (\Lambda_{10}, \Lambda_{11}, a_{11}, ..a_{1d}, ..., \lambda_{p0}, \lambda_{p1}, ..., \lambda_{pq}, a_{p1}, .., a_{pd})$. The prior distribution selected for λ is a $p.(1+q+d)$ dimensional multivariate normal density with the mean $\overline{\lambda}^*$ and the precision matrix $\overline{\Lambda}$ which are chosen according to prior information, i.e.

$$\overline{\lambda}\, N \sim (\overline{\lambda}^*, \overline{\Lambda}^{*-1})$$

$$p(\overline{\lambda}) \propto constant.$$

We chose noninformative priors for the intercepts λ_0 and the regression coefficients A of direct effects (see Fahrmeir and Raach 2006). The conjugate prior distribution of the vector of regression coefficients γ_r is a m-dimensional multivariate normal density with mean γ_r^* and precision matrix Γ_r^*, $\gamma_r \sim N(\gamma_r^*, \Gamma_r^{*-1})$. In our analysis, we always choose noninformative priors for all regression parameter γ_r, hence all values of Γ_r^* are set to zero.

Prior Distribution of Structural Model

Prior Distribution for Smoothing Functions

A prior for smoothing functions $f_{r1}, ..., f_{rg}$ is based on a Bayesian P-spline approach (Eilers and Marx 1996).

Prior Distribution for Spatial Effect

The prior of spatial effect is based on Markov random field (Besag 1974; Besag and Kooperberg 1995).

Fully Posterior Inference

A vector of parameters can be estimated after all parameters are arranged in the parameter vector θ.

$$\theta = vec\{\lambda_0, \Lambda, A, \Sigma, \beta, \gamma, t\}.$$

Hence the posterior distribution is

$$p(\theta|y, w, x, u) \propto p(\theta).p(y|\theta, w, x, u).$$

The complete parameter vector is obtained by adding the underlying variables and latent variables to the parameter vector θ leading to a posterior distribution

$$p(\theta, y^*, z|y, w, x, u) \propto p(\theta)p(y, y^*|\theta, w, x, u)$$

Sampling from the posterior distribution is done through MCMC algorithms. There are three different MCMC algorithms that can be used and that essentially differ in the way of estimating the cutpoints in the case of ordinal indicators (Raach 2005; Fahrmeir and Raach 2007).

References

Adebayo, S. B. (2003). *Semiparametric Bayesian regression for multivariate responses*. Ph.D. Thesis, Hieronymus Verlag, Munich.

Adebayo S. B., & Fahrmeir, L. (2002). Analyzing child mortality in Nigeria with geoadditive survival models. SFB 386, discussion paper 303, University of Munich, Germany.

Adebayo, S. B., & Fahrmeir, L. (2005). Analysing child mortality in Nigeria with geoadditive survival models. *Statistics in Medicine, 24*, 709–728.

Aguilar, O., & West, M. (2000). Bayesian dynamic factor models and variance matrix discounting for portfolio allocation. *Journal of Business and Economic Statistics, 18*, 338–357.

Bateman, O. M., & Smith, S. (1991). A comparison of the health effects of water supply and sanitation in urban and rural Guatemala. In Proceeding of DHS world conference, Washington, DC, 5–7 Aug 1991, v. Columbia: Macro International InC, pp. 745–756.

Besag, J. (1974). Spatial interaction and the statistical analysis of lattice systems. *Journal of the Royal Statistical Society, Series, B36*, 192–236.

Besag, J., & Kooperberg, C. (1995). On conditional and intrinsic autoregressions. *Biometrika, 82*, 733–746.

Besag, J., York, Y., & Mollie, A. (1991). Bayesian image restoration with two applications in spatial statistics (with discussion). *Annals of the Institute of Statistical Mathematics, 43*, 1–59.

Bartholomew, D. J. (1987). *Latent variable models and factor analysis* (2nd ed.). London/New York: Charles Griffin and Company Ltd./Oxford University Press. Bartholomew, D.J., & Knott, M. (1999). Arnold, London.

Eilers, P. H. C., & Marx, B. D. (1996). Flexible smoothing with B-splines and penalties (with comments). *Statistical Science, 11*, 89–121.

El-Zanaty, F., & Way, A. A. (2004). *2003 Egypt interim demographic and health survey*. Cairo: Ministry of Health and Population [Egypt], National Population Council, El-Zanaty and Associates, and ORC Macro.

Fahrmeir, L., Kneib, T., & Lang, S. (2004). Penalized structured additive regression of space-time data: A Bayesian perspective. *Statistica Sinica, 14*, 731–761.

Fahrmeir, L., & Lang, S. (2001). Bayesian inference for generalized additive mixed models based on Markov random field priors. *Applied Statistics (JRSS C), 50*, 201–220.

Fahrmeir, L., & Raach, A. (2006). A Bayesian semiparametric latent variable model for mixed responses. Discussion paper 471, revised for Psychometrika.

Fahrmeir, L., & Raach, A. (2007). A Bayesian semiparametric latent variable model for mixed responses. *Psychometrika, 72*, 327–346.

Geweke, J., & Zhou, G. (1996). Measurnig the pricing error of the arbitrage pricing theory. *Review of Financial Studies, 9*, 557–587.

Holmes, L. B., Harvey, E. A., Kleiner, B. C., Leppig, K. A., Cann, C. I., Munoz, A., & Polk, B. F. (1987). Predictive value of minor anomalies: Use incohort studies to identify teratogens. *Teratology, 36*, 291–297.

Jöreskog, K. G., & Goldberger, A. S. (1975). Estimation of a model with multiple indicators and multiple causes of a single latent variable. *Journal of the American Statistical Association, 70*, 631–639.

Kandala, N. B. (2002). *Spatial modelling of socio-economic and demographic determinants of childhood undernutrition and mortality in Africa*. Ph.D. Thesis, Shaker Verlag, Munich.

Kandala, N. B., Ji, C., Stallard, N., Stranges, S., & Cappuccio, F. P. (2007). Spatail analysis of risk factors for childhood morbidity in Nigeria. *Journal of Tropical Medicine, 77*(4), 770–778.

Kandala, N. B., Lang, S., Klasen, S., & Fahrmeir, L. (2001). Semiparametric analysis of the socio-demographic determinants of undernutrition in two African countries. *Research in Official Statistics, 4*(1), 81–100. 217.

Kandala, N. B., Magadi, M. A., & Madise, N. J. (2006). An investigation of district spatial variations of childhood diarrhoea and fever morbidity in Malawi. *Social Science & Medicine, 62*, 1138–1152.

Kandala, N. B., & Ghilagaber, G. (2006). A geo-additive Bayesian discrete time survival model and its application to spatial analysis of childhood mortality in Malawi. *Quality and Quantity, 40*, 935–957.

Khatab, K. (2010). Childhood malnutrition in Egypt using geoadditive probit and latent variable model. *American Journal of Tropical Medicine and Hygiene, 82*(4), 653–663.

Khatab, K., & Fahrmeir, L. (2009). Analysis of childhood morbidity with geoadditive probit and latent variable model: A case study for Egypt. *American Journal of Tropical Medicine and Hygiene, 81*, 114–128.

Lang, S., & Brezger, A. (2004). Bayesian P-splines. *Journal of Computational and Graphical Statistics, 13*, 183–212.

Moustaki, I., Jöreskog, K. G., & Mavridis, D. (2004). Factor models for ordinal variables with covariate effects on the manifest and latent variables: A comparison of LISREL and IRT approaches. *Structural Equation Modeling, 11*, 487–513.

National Population Commission (NPC) [Nigeria] and ORC Macro. (2004). *Nigeria demographic and health survey 2003*. Calverton: National Population Commission and ORC Macro.

Pelletier, D. (1998). Malnutrition, morbidity, and child mortality in developing countries. In United Nations (Ed.), *Too young too die: Genes or gender?* New York: United Nations.

Raach, A. W. (2005). *A Bayesian semiparametric latent variable model for binary, ordinal and continuous response*. Dissertation, edoc.ub.uni-muenchen.de

Rue, H., & Held, L. (2005). *Markov random fields: Theory and applications*. Boca Raton: Chapman & Hall/CRC.

Sen, A. (1999). *Development as freedom*. Oxford: Oxford University Press.

Skrondal, A., & Rabe-Hesketh, S. (2004). *Generalized latent variable modeling*. Boca Raton: Chapman and Hall.

Spearman, C. (1904). General intelligence objectively determined and measured. *The American Journal of Psychology, 15*, 201–293.

Svedberg, P. (1996). Gender bias in Sub-Saharan Africa: Reply and further evidence. *Journal of Development Studies, 32*, 933–943.

UNICEF. (1998). *The state of the world's children*. New York: UNICEF.

Chapter 5
Mapping Socio-economic Inequalities in Health Status Among Malawian Children: A Mixed Model Approach

Lawrence N. Kazembe

5.1 Introduction

There has been a long interest in public health on the linkage between health and socio-economic determinants, with many studies published from developed countries, for example in Europe and USA (Braveman and Tarimo 2002; Wagstaff 2000; Black et al. 2003). The studies commissioned by World Health Organization (WHO) on socio-economic determinants of health also spells out the importance of socio-disparities in health, and its impact on socio-economic development (Wagstaff 2000; Zere and McIntyre 2003). In these studies, the following have been identified as key determinants of health: deprivation or SES, education, race or ethnicity, and rurality. For years, routine public health statistics have been reported, in Europe and United states, by social factors (mainly income and education), race or ethnicity. These have facilitated monitoring of socio-economic disparities in health, and allowed comparison among social classes. In contrast, in developing countries, studies that examine differences in risk, stratified by education or income are relatively few, and where these have been considered there is no explicit investigation of socio-economic patterning (Fotso and Kuate-Defo 2005; Hong 2007).

Furthermore, comparatively few studies have mapped socio-economic inequalities in childhood health (Congdon 2003). Differences in risk that suggest a socio-economic patterning at a particular area would support targeted interventions in areas highlighted to be hotspots of ill health. Although it is well-known that socioeconomic factors such as income and education are significant determinants of individual health, the clear differences in risk across different socio-economic

L.N. Kazembe (✉)
Department of Statistics and Population Studies, University of Namibia, P/Bag 13301, 340 Mandume Ndemufayo Avenue, Pionerspark, Windhoek, Namibia
e-mail: lkazembe@unam.na

N.-B. Kandala and G. Ghilagaber (eds.), *Advanced Techniques for Modelling Maternal and Child Health in Africa*, The Springer Series on Demographic Methods and Population Analysis 34, DOI 10.1007/978-94-007-6778-2_5,

strata have not been studied in African scenario. In particular, there is interest to understand the complex relationship between deprivation and childhood health in Africa.

Health outcomes are highly dependent on geographical location. Proper account of spatial clustering of the response is needed. The sources of spatial heterogeneity are many. The inclusion of spatial effects permits modelling unobserved or unmeasured covariate information on the community level. Analysing their geographical interrationship can help policy makers understand spatial patterns and identify differences in disease burden across areas. Although this has a rich applications in cases arising in developing countries, few such studies focused on problems from developing countries exist. Investigations in the past have revealed geographical variation in the distribution of risk in childhood morbidity (Kandala 2006; Kandala et al. 2006). In some instances, spatial profiles of risk happen to be similar. For example, rural areas are associated with poorer health, impoverished neighbourhoods are at relatively increased risk. Indeed, epidemiological overlap and co-morbidity seem to be the norm than not. The impact of control efforts can be substantial if interventions are spatially targeted (Carter et al. 2000). Recognizing the areas where the risk overlap would assist in scaling-up of resources. Identifying geographical differences in the risk may assist in planning integrated interventions, thus reducing the cost of providing interventions and avoid duplications of systems aimed at delivering resources.

The aims of this study are: (i) to jointly model the geographical distribution of the four leading causes (diarrhoea, fever, stunting and underweight) of child morbidity, (ii) to investigate the association of SES with the four ill-health conditions stated above. SES is fitted as a spatially varying covariate, controlling for other risk factors on the four causes, and (iii) to explore patterns of spatial correlation. We conducted a multilevel spatial study with district (a third-level of administration) and sub-districts (a fourth-level of administration) in Malawi as units of analysis. This study takes advantage of the existing national surveys like the demographic and health survey, which reports data on a number of variables including those on childhood health, and socio-economic variable which can be construed as possible socio-determinants of health. In addition, these surveys collected geo-referenced data, which makes applications of spatial epidemiological techniques a possibility.

We applied a multinomial model to analyse spatial patterns of childhood co-morbidity in Malawi, in what is called a multi-categorical response models (Kneib and Fahrmeir 2006). We considered the joint occurrences of (i) diarrhoea and fever, (ii) diarrhoea and stunting, (iii) fever and stunting and (iv) stunting and underweight as outcomes. Each of the joint outcome is considered as a response category of a multinomial random variable. Note that such responses may be modelled in different ways. Multivatiate models are such an alternative, see for example Fahrmeir and Raach (2007) who introduced a latent class model to model multiple indicators. However, multicategorical models, such as the multinomial logistic model, are widely used in the social sciences, as either choice or classification models, for instance in demographic analysis of life-course events, fertility preferences and contraceptive use (Steele et al. 2004). In several of these models, spatial patterns have not been considered.

In our modelling strategy, we included both individual covariates and a structured latent variable at two geographical levels (district and subdistrict). Our approach here recognises the fact that several health outcomes occur simultaneously, largely because of common risk factors, and probably due to overlap between multiple risk factors, or that one disorder creates an increased risk for the other (Kazembe and Namangale 2007; Fenn et al. 2005). In many sub-Saharan African countries, diarrhoea, malaria, and malnutrition cause and inflict the largest burden National Statistical Office and ORC Macro (2004), and they are often common forms of co-morbidities (Källander et al. 2004; Mulholland 2005). Indeed, their co-existence is largely blamed to expedited early and high childhood mortality (Fenn et al. 2005; Mulholland 2005; Källander et al. 2004; Black et al. 2003). Our model, further, extends a novel application of spatially-varying coefficients models to capture the changing pattern of SES in space (Fotheringham et al. 2002; Gamerman et al. 2003; Gelfand et al. 2006).

Modelling and inference is done through use of the empirical Bayes (EB) approach via penalised likelihood techniques (Kneib and Fahrmeir 2006; Fahrmeir et al. 2004; Tutz 2004). However, fully Bayesian (FB) approach is possible (Fahrmeir and Lang 2001). For example, Tutz (2004) developed a class of generalised semiparametric mixed models and proposed penalized marginal likelihood approach for the estimation of parameters. Fahrmeir et al. (2004) considered a penalised geoadditive model for space-time data with inference performed using an empirical Bayes (EB) approach.

Now the rest of this chapter is structured as follows. Section 5.2 describes model development, while Sect. 5.3 gives details of model fitting. In Sect. 5.4, we apply the techniques to real data from 2006 Malawi Multiple Indicator Cluster Surveys data. Section 5.5 gives the results. The final section is the conclusion.

5.2 Model Development

5.2.1 The Multinomial Model

A multinomial random variable applies where an event, Y, ends up with three or more outcomes $1, \ldots, J$ ($J > 2$). Specifically suppose. Y has unordered categories, we assume

$$Y \sim \text{multinomial } (1, p(v_{i,}\alpha)) \quad \text{for } i = 1, \ldots, n,$$

such that $p(v_i, \alpha) = (p_1(v_i, \alpha), \cdots, p_J(v_i, \alpha))'$, and $P(y_i = j|\alpha) = p_j(v_i, \alpha)$, given some covariates $v = (v_1, \ldots, v_p)'$ and corresponding parameter set α.

The most common approach to estimate multinomial probabilities is through the logistic model

$$p(v_i,\alpha) = P(y_i = j|\alpha) = \begin{cases} \dfrac{\exp(\eta_{ij})}{1+\sum_{h=1}^{J-1}\exp(\eta_{ih})} & j = 1,\cdots,J-1 \\ \dfrac{1}{1+\sum_{h=1}^{J-1}\exp(\eta_{ih})} & j = J \end{cases} \tag{5.1}$$

where $\eta_{ij} = v'\alpha_j$ is the linear predictor. The last category J is considered as a reference classification outcome. The likelihood L would take the form

$$L = \prod_{i=1}^{n}\prod_{j=1}^{J}[p(v_i,\alpha)]^{y_{ij}}$$

with log-likelihood

$$\log L = \sum_{i=1}^{n}\sum_{j=1}^{J} y_{ij}\log[p(v_i,\alpha)].$$

In this classical multinomial logit model all covariates are assumed to be independent of the category while effects are category-specific. Extensions of the classic model allows for the inclusion of category-specific covariates w_{J-1} leading to the predictor $\eta_{ij} = v'\alpha_j + w_j\theta$.

Since the observations are associated with location of residence, it is desirable to account for spatial correlation and heterogeneity. Modelling of heterogeneity and spatially structured variation may be obtained by introducing random effects. Similarly, nonlinear effects are introduced in the model through smoothing functions. The predictor (5.1) is expanded to include all possible explanatory variables like fixed, nonlinear and spatial covariates, giving a semi-parametric predictor (Tutz 2004),

$$\eta_{ij} = v'\alpha_j + w_j\phi + \sum_{k=1}^{q} f_{jk}(x_{ij}) + f_{spat}(s_j) \tag{5.2}$$

where α are fixed effects corresponding to $w_j = (w_{j1},\cdots,w_{jp})'$, $f_{jk}, k = 1,\ldots,q$ are unknown smooth functions, for each response category j, of continuous covariates $x_{ij} = (x_{k11},\cdots,x_{kql})'$ that enter nonlinearly, and $f_{spat}(s_j)$ is the spatial component of the model that captures random effects of area $s_j, s \in \{1,\ldots,S\}$.

The component $f_{spat}(s_j)$ is split further into spatially structured and unstructured random effects, $f_{str}(s_j)$ and $f_{unstr}(s_k)$ respectively, to capture any residual variation, within or between area, in health status that is not explained by components of the model. Further, define $\gamma = (\phi,\ \alpha')'$ as the overall vector of fixed regression coefficients, and let

$$U = \begin{pmatrix} u'_1 \\ \vdots \\ u'_{J-1} \end{pmatrix} = \begin{pmatrix} v' & 0\, w'_1 - w'_J \\ \ddots & \vdots \\ 0 & v' w'_{J-1} - w'_J \end{pmatrix}$$

be the corresponding design matrix constructed from the covariates w_k and category-specific covariates v'. Then, after reindexing, we can rewrite the predictor (5.2) in generic matrix notation as

$$\boldsymbol{\eta}_j = \boldsymbol{U}\boldsymbol{\gamma}_j + \boldsymbol{X}_1\boldsymbol{\beta}_{j1} + \boldsymbol{X}_2\boldsymbol{\beta}_{j2} + \cdots + \boldsymbol{X}_l\boldsymbol{\beta}_{jl} + \cdots + \boldsymbol{X}_{str}\boldsymbol{\beta}_{j,str} \tag{5.3}$$

which reduces to $\boldsymbol{\eta}_j = \boldsymbol{P}\boldsymbol{\theta}_j$, where $\boldsymbol{P} = (\boldsymbol{U}, \boldsymbol{X}_1, \boldsymbol{X}_2, \ldots, \boldsymbol{X}_{unstr}, \boldsymbol{X}_{str})$ are appropriate design matrices for each fixed, metrical and spatial effect respectively, and $\boldsymbol{\theta}_j = (\boldsymbol{\gamma}_j, \boldsymbol{\beta}_{j1}, \boldsymbol{\beta}_{j2}, \ldots, \boldsymbol{\beta}_{j,str})$ is a high dimensional parameter vector. The elements $\boldsymbol{X}_1, \boldsymbol{X}_2, \ldots, \boldsymbol{X}_l, \ldots, \boldsymbol{X}_{str}$ and $\boldsymbol{\beta}_{j1}, \boldsymbol{\beta}_{j2}, \cdots, \boldsymbol{\beta}_{jl}, \cdots, \boldsymbol{\beta}_{j,unstr}, \boldsymbol{\beta}_{j,str}$ are such that $\boldsymbol{f}_l = \boldsymbol{X}_l\boldsymbol{\beta}_{jl}$. The most compact form of the predictor $\boldsymbol{\eta}$ is obtained by

$$\boldsymbol{\eta} = \begin{pmatrix} \eta_1 \\ \vdots \\ \eta_{J-1} \end{pmatrix} = \boldsymbol{U}\boldsymbol{\gamma} + \boldsymbol{X}_1\boldsymbol{\beta}_1 + \boldsymbol{X}_2\boldsymbol{\beta}_2 + \ldots + \boldsymbol{X}_l\boldsymbol{\beta}_l + \ldots + \boldsymbol{X}_{str}\boldsymbol{\beta}_{str}$$

5.2.2 *Modelling Spatial Structure*

We fitted the following three models. The first model fitted was where SES is considered as a fixed variable while adjusting for bio-demographic factors, and using districts and sub-districts as the spatial units in a simple conditional autoregressive (CAR) model. Second, within the CAR framework, we explored the idea of modelling SES as a spatially varying coefficient covariable. Third, we introduced latent class models to automatically control for correlation at two scales within a framework of a multilevel model or random intercepts.

Random Effects Model

Spatial correlation between areas is achieved by incorporating suitable random effects into $\boldsymbol{\beta}_{str}$. This is specified using Markov Random Field (MRF) priors. The MRF is defined as

$$\boldsymbol{\beta}_{str} | \{\boldsymbol{\beta}_{str}, \tau^2_{str}\} \sim N\left(0, \tau^2_{str} Q^{-1}\right) \tag{5.4}$$

where τ^2_{str} is the unknown precision parameter which controls the degree of similarity, and Q is the spatial precision matrix. The (i, j)-th element of the spatial precision matrix Q is given by

$$Q = \begin{cases} m_s, & s = r \\ -1, & s \sim r \\ 0, & \text{elsewhere} \end{cases}$$

where $s \sim r$ denotes that area s is adjacent to r which is assigned -1, m_s is the number of adjacent areas to s. We define areas as neighbours if they share a common border. Thus area s, given neighbouring area r, has the following conditional distribution (Besag et al. 1991)

$$\boldsymbol{\beta}^2_{str} | \{\boldsymbol{\beta}^r_{str}, s \neq r\} \sim N\left(\frac{1}{m_s} \sum_{r \in \delta s} \boldsymbol{\beta}^r_{str}, \frac{\tau^2_{str}}{m_s}\right) \tag{5.5}$$

where s and r are adjacent areas in the set of all adjacent areas (δ_s) of area s, and m_s are the number of adjacent areas.

For completeness, we specify other prior assumptions required in order to model the relationship depicted in (5.3). Essentially, this is the second stage of the hierarchy. For the fixed regression parameters, γ, a suitable choice is the diffuse prior, $p(\gamma) \propto constant$. The smooth functions of continuous covariates are modelled using a second-order random walk prior given by $\beta_l | \beta_{l-1}, \beta_{l-2}, \tau^2_l \sim N\left(2\beta_{l-1} - \beta_{l-2}, \tau^2_l\right)$ for $l = 3, \ldots, j$ with noninformative priors for the initials. Again τ^2_l controls the amount of smoothing, with larger values leading to less smoothing. In order to capture unstructured spatial random effects (β_{unstr}), we assumed exchangeable normal priors, $\beta_{unstr} \sim N\left(0, \tau^2_{unstr}\right)$, where τ^2_{unstr} is a variance component that allows for over-dispersion and heterogeneity.

Spatially-Varying Coefficient Model

The second model fitted is spatially varying coefficients (SVC) model. The SVC model allows the regression parameters for the lth covariate and jth joint health condition, $\beta_{jl} = \left[\beta_{jl}(s_1), \ldots, \beta_{jl}(s_S)\right]'$, to be different in different locations. Thus SVC is an extension of model (5.2),

$$\boldsymbol{\eta}_j = \cdots + f_{spat}(s_j) x_l + \cdots$$

and can be seen as interaction terms, where the effect of x_l varies smoothly over the domain of s_j. In other words, geographical location acts as an effect modifier of x_l. Models of this kind are also known as geographically weighted regression, see Fotheringham et al. (2002); Gamerman et al. (2003); Gelfand et al. (2006). Again the evaluation function $f_{spat}(s_j)x_l$ can be written as matrix $\boldsymbol{g} = \boldsymbol{Z\beta}$, such that $\boldsymbol{g} = \left(x_1 f_{spat}(s_1), \ldots, x_n f_{spat}(s_n)\right)' = \text{diag}(x_1, \ldots, x_n)\boldsymbol{X} = \boldsymbol{Z}\boldsymbol{\beta}$, where $\boldsymbol{Z} = \text{diag}(x_1, \ldots, x_n)\boldsymbol{X}$. Again, a random walk prior can be assigned to the vector of regression coefficients β. Note that the varying coefficients can also be interpreted as a two-dimensional surface $f_{spat}(s_j x_l) = f_{spat}(s_j)x_l$. Therefore the predictor can be written as

$$\boldsymbol{\eta}_j = \cdots + f_{spat}(s_j, x_l) + \cdots$$

and therefore can be approximated by the tensor product of the one-dimensional penalised splines (P-splines). If we assume that the unknown surface $\boldsymbol{\beta}_{str} = f(s_j, x_l)$, then

$$f(s_j, x_l) = \sum_{p=1}^{m_1} \sum_{v=1}^{m_2} \beta_{pv} B_{1,p}(s_j) B_{2,v}(x_l) \tag{5.6}$$

where $B_{11}, \ldots, B_{1m_1}$ are the basis functions in s_j direction and $B_{21}, \ldots, B_{2m_2}$ in x_l direction. The design matrix $\mathbf{X}_k$ is now $n \times m_1 \cdot m_2$ dimensional and consists of products of basic functions. Priors for β_{pv} are based on spatial smoothness priors as specified in Besag and Kooperberg (1995). A two-dimensional first order random walk has been shown to work well (Lang and Brezger 2004). This is based on the four nearest neighbours and is specified as

$$\beta_{pv}|\cdot \sim N\left(\frac{1}{4}(\beta_{p-1,v} + \beta_{p+1,v} + \beta_{p,v-1} + \beta_{p,v+1}), \frac{\tau_{pv}^2}{4}\right) \tag{5.7}$$

for $p,v = 2, \ldots, m-1$ and appropriate changes for corners and edges. This prior is a direct generalization of a first order random walk in one dimension. Its conditional mean can be interpreted as a least squares locally linear fit at knot position ς_p, ς_v given the neighbouring parameters. In many applications it is desirable to additionally incorporate one dimensional main effects. Again, similar to the one dimensional case additional identifiability constraints have to be imposed on the functions.

Multilevel Models: Exploring Spatial Correlation and Heterogeneity at District and Sub-district Levels

Assuming that the outcome is clustered at a sub-district and district administrative levels, two area-specific random effects can be introduced in (5.2) to model their effects. The predictor then becomes

$$\eta hijk = x'_{hij}\beta_k + \theta_{hik} + \phi_{hk} \tag{5.8}$$

for sickness status k, of child j in subdistrict i within district h. The components θ_{hik} and ϕ_{hk} are area-specific random effects for the subdistrict and district respectively, which can further be split into spatially structured variation and unstructured heterogeneity.

5.3 Penalised Likelihood Inference

Inference for the semiparametric model is based on the empirical Bayesian approach, also called the mixed model methodology (Brezger et al. 2005; Fahrmeir et al. 2004). The EB approach is achieved by recasting the predictor model (5.3) as generalized linear mixed model (GLMM) after appropriate reparametrization. This provides the key for simultaneous estimation of the functions f_l and the variance parameters τ_l^2 in the empirical Bayes approach. To rewrite model (5.3) as mixed model, we assume that β_l has dimension d_l and the corresponding penalty matrix has rank $h_l < d_l$. Each parameter vector β_l is partitioned into a penalized $\left(\beta_l^{pen}\right)$ and unpenalized $\left(\beta_l^{unp}\right)$ part yielding a variance component model (Brezger et al. 2005; Fahrmeir et al. 2004),

$$\beta_l = \Psi_l^{unp}\beta_l^{unp} + \Psi_l^{pen}\beta_l^{pen} \tag{5.9}$$

for some well defined $d_l \times (d_l - h_l)$ matrix Ψ_l^{unp} and a $d_l \times h_l$ matrix Ψ_l^{pen}. The following priors are assumed. For the penalized part, an i.i.d Gaussian prior is suitable, while for the unpenalized part we assume a flat prior:

$$p\left(\beta_l^{pen}\right) \sim N\left(0, \tau_l^2 I_{hl}\right) \quad \text{and} \quad p\left(\beta_l^{unp}\right) \propto const. \tag{5.10}$$

Applying decomposition (5.9) to all the components of predictor (5.3) yields

$$\eta = X^{unp}\beta^{unp} + X^{pen}\beta^{pen}. \tag{5.11}$$

We have obtained in (5.11) a GLMM with fixed effects β^{unp} and random effects β^{pen}. The posterior, in terms of the GLMM representation, is given by

$$p(\beta^{unp}, \beta^{pen}|data) \propto L(data, \beta^{unp}, \beta^{pen}) \prod_{l=1}^{g} \left(p\left(\beta_l^{pen}|\tau_l^2\right)\right) \tag{5.12}$$

where $L(\cdot)$, again, denotes the likelihood which is the product of individual likelihood contributions and $p\left(\beta_l^{pen}|\tau_l^2\right)$ as defined above. Estimation of regression coefficients and variance parameters is carried out using iteratively weighted least squares and approximate restricted maximum likelihood. Such details are given in Lin and Zhang (1999). Fahrmeir et al. (2004) further derived numerically efficient formulae that allow for handling large data sets.

5.4 Application: Modelling Health Status Among Malawian Children

5.4.1 Case Data

We used as a case study data collected as part of the 2006 Malawi Multiple Cluster Indicators Survey (MICS). MICS was designed to provide estimates of health and demographic indicators at the national and regional levels, and allow for regional and urban-rural comparisons. A two-stage stratified sampling design was implemented to collect the data. A total of 1,040 enumeration areas (EAs) as defined in the Malawi Population and Housing Census of 1998 were selected, stratified by urban/rural status with sampling probability proportional to the population of the EA. Each EA was geo-referenced. A fixed number of households were randomly selected in each EA. All women aged 15–49 were eligible for interview. A total of 32,220 women were interviewed with a response rate of 98 %. The data was realized through an interviewer – administered questionnaire.

The outcome variables were derived from self-reported sickness status of each child for the four ill-health conditions (fever, diarrhoea, stunting and underweight), as reported by the care-givers (often mothers), experienced within 2 weeks prior to the survey date. The first two outcomes were based on a mother's self-report on the child, based on the following questions: "Does the child have fever now/Did the child have fever during the last 2 weeks" and "Did the child have diarrhoea in the last 2 weeks". Stunting and underweight were based on the transformed Z-scores on the height-for-age and weight-for-age measurements respectively done on the child. A child was considered stunted or underweight if $Z < -2$. Table 5.1 shows a cross-classification of diarrhoea, fever

Table 5.1 Fixed effects estimates and 95 % credible intervals (CI) from the multivariate spatial model of childhood fever, diarrhoea and stunting morbidity in Malawi, 2006

				Child stunted		
Child ill with fever				No	Yes	Total
Yes	Child had diarrhoea	Yes	Count	1,562	1,408	2,970
			% of Total	19.4	17.5	36.9
		No	Count	2,713	2,373	5,086
			% of Total	33.7	29.5	63.1
	Total		Count	4275	3,781	8,056
			% of Total	53.1	46.9	100
No	Child had diarrhoea	Yes	Count	1,285	1,141	2,426
			% of Total	8.6	7.6	16.3
		No	Count	6,934	5,563	12,497
			% of Total	46.5	37.3	83.7
	Total		Count	8,219	6,704	14,923
			% of Total	55.1	44.9	100

and stunting. Evidently, the proportion experiencing multi-comorbidity is relatively large ($p = 17.5$ %, $n = 14{,}923$). The proportions of co-morbidities of fever and diarrhoea, and fever and stunting are 19.4 % and 29.5 % respectively, higher than co-morbidity of diarrhoea and stunting (7.6 %). A multi-categorical response was constructed as follows: (1) if the child was sick of both diarrhoea and fever (DF), (2) if the child had diarrhoea and was stunted (DS), (3) if the child had fever and was stunted (FS), (4) if the child was stunted and underweight (SUN), and (5) if the child experienced no disease and not malnourished within the observation period. Note that detailed single disease analyses have been dealt with elsewhere, see Kandala et al. (2006), and our reporting shall deal with the five diseases combinations.

The following individual covariates were included in the analysis: (1) age of the child categorized as (a) 1–5 months, (b) 6–11 months, (c) 12–23 months, (d) 24–35 months and (e) 36–59 months (reference group); (2) received vitamin A within 6 months prior to the survey date (yes = 1, no = 0); (3) type of place of residence (rural = 1, urban = 0); (4) crowding indicator based on the whether household size exceeded 5, which is the median household size in Malawi (yes = 1, no = 0), (5) region of residence (1 = north, 2 = centre, 3 = south), (6) mother's education level (1 = none, 2 = primary, 3 = secondary or higher), and (7) wealth ranking (1 = lowest, 2 = lower, 3 = medium, 4 = higher, and 5 = highest). The "no" category was the reference group for all binary variables above. Individual data were nested within two areas: 364 subdistricts and 31 districts.

5.4.2 Implementation

Let Y_{ijk} and π_{ijk} be the sickness status and probability of co-morbidity of diarrhoea and fever ($k = 1$), co-morbidity of diarrhoea and stunting ($k = 2$), co-morbidity of fever and stunting ($k = 3$), co-morbidity of stunting and underweight ($k = 4$), no disease ($k = 5$) of child j, $j = 1, \ldots, n_i$ in area i, $i = 1, \ldots, S$. We fit the following four sets of multinomial logistic models. The first model ($M1$) is purely spatial,

$$\text{M1a: } \eta_{ijk} = f_{str}(TA_j) + f_{unstr}(TA_j).$$

$$\text{M1b: } \eta_{ijk} = f_{str}(TA_j) + f_{unstr}(TA_j) + f_{str}(district_j) + f_{unstr}(district_j).$$

In this model we introduce spatial smoothness priors to capture spatial correlations at district and sub-district level. This is achieved by assuming CAR priors (5.5). Further, the model permits unstructured heterogeneity. This model investigates whether there is substantial spatial variation in the joint health conditions, and if the answer is yes whether this variation can be explained by socio-economic status and bio-demographic factors.

The second model, $M2$, is a spatial parametric model, which adjusts for covariates,

$$\text{M2a: } \eta_{ijk} = x_{ij}{}'\beta_j + f_{str}(TA_j) + f_{unstr}(TA_j) + f_{str}(district_j) + f_{unstr}(district_j).$$

With this model, we assess how much of the spatial variation is attenuated by the inclusion of fixed effects of all considerable covariates. Here the effects of SES are estimated as fixed effects. In model *M2b* we estimate the spatial effects at both district and sub-district levels.

In the third model *M3*, we fit a spatial semi-parametric model with age of child assumed nonlinear and the rest of the variables assumed fixed,

$$\text{M3: } \eta_{ijk} = x_{ij}'\beta_j + f(age) + f_{str}(TA_j) + f_{unstr}(TA_j)$$

For the nonlinear effects we use a second-order random walk prior. Model *M3* investigates the bias of fitting restrictive linear model, *M2*.

In the last model *M4*, we fit a spatially varying coefficient model with SES assumed space varying, through components $SES^* f_{str}(TA_j)$ and $SES^* f_{str}(district_j)$. The rest of the variables are estimated as in model *M3*,

$$\begin{aligned}\text{M4: } \eta_{ijk} = x_{ij}'\beta_j + f(age) + f_{str}(TA_j) + f_{unstr}(TA_j) + SES^* f_{str}(TA_j) \\ + SES^* f_{str}(district_j).\end{aligned}$$

Implementation of these models was carried out in `BayesX` (Brezger et al. 2005). In `BayesX`, regression coefficients are estimated iteratively. For each model fitted, convergence is achieved when the change in regression parameters is 0.0001 and terminated at 400 iterations if convergence is not achieved. However, all models converged at less than 25 iterations. We compare the fitted models using Akaike Information criterion (AIC). This is defined as sum of the log-likelihood and the degrees of freedom (*df*). The log-likelihood measures the goodness of fit whereas the *df* measures model complexity. The smaller the AIC, the better the fit of the model.

5.5 Results

5.5.1 Random Effects Model

Figure 5.1 shows the observed geographical variations in childhood fever, diarrhoea and stunting at district level for both highest and lowest levels of SES. There is evidence of similarities in geographical patterning of the three conditions for lowest levels of SES, in contrast to the patterning at highest levels of SES. Table 5.2 shows the relationship between the disease outcomes with SES. The health outcomes significantly associated by SES ($\chi^2 = 293.81$, $p < 0.001$). Figure 5.2 provides evidence of the relationship between the health classification and geographical context, at sub-district level, measured through latent variables. It is revealing to note that the varying risk has some degree of similarities in an area. Such variation may largely be due to differences in population composition and structure, or there

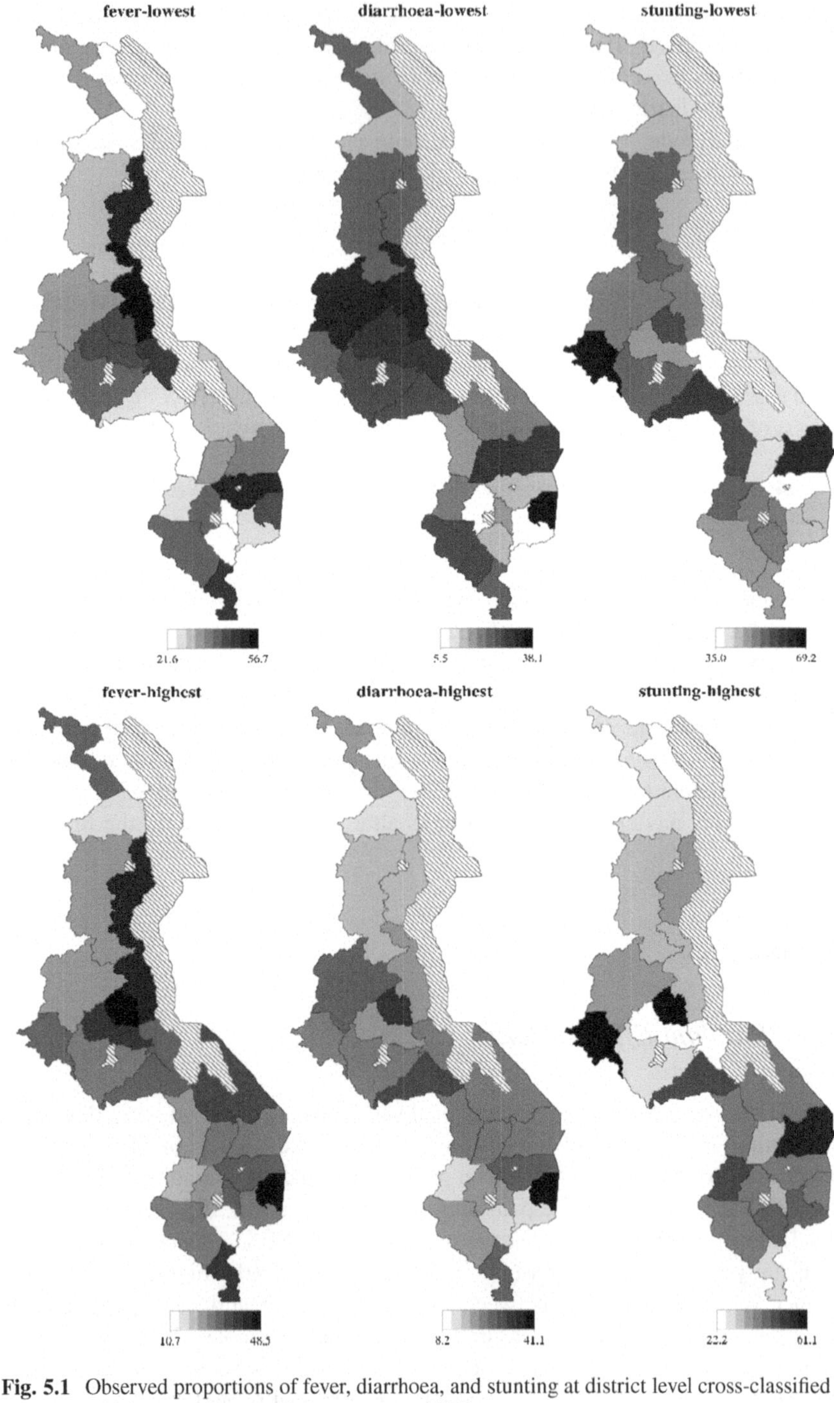

Fig. 5.1 Observed proportions of fever, diarrhoea, and stunting at district level cross-classified by *lowest* and *highest* wealth quintiles, a measure of SES

Table 5.2 Cross-tabulation of co-morbidities with socio-economic status (SES), maternal education and rural-urban differentials

		Co-morbidities[a]						
Wealth quintile		DF	DS	FS	SUN	None	Total	χ^2 (*p*-value)
	Lowest	6.9[b]	3.1	10.9	19.0	59.0	5,202	293.81 (<0.001)
	Lower	7.6	3.2	10.4	17.1	60.8	4,960	
	Medium	7.2	2.8	11.7	15.7	61.6	4,946	
	Higher	6.2	3.1	9.6	13.7	66.0	4,432	
	Highest	5.4	2.9	6.9	10.2	73.4	3,698	
Maternal education	None	6.6	3.2	11.2	18.9	60.1	5,168	209.58 (<0.001)
	Primary	6.9	3.0	10.3	15.8	64.0	15,307	
	Secondary	6.8	3.5	7.5	7.8	74.4	2,449	
Area	Urban	5.8	2.7	6.9	12.1	72.6	2,347	82.28 (<0.001)
	Rural	6.9	3.1	10.6	16.1	63.3	20,647	

[a]*DF* diarrhoca and fever, *DS* diarrhoea and shtunting, *FS* fever and stunting, *SUN* stunting and underweight
[b]Number are percentage

may be substantial area effects, which can be explained by factors considered here. In this model, the highest risk for diarrhoea and fever (outcome I) was in Mulanje (South), Mchinji (Centre) and Karonga (North). For outcome II (diarrhoea and stunted), we observe that risk is highest in the central region and parts of Mangochi district. Similar patterns were observed at district level for outcome III (fever and stunted). The varying risk of joint stunted-underweight condition were highest in Dedza and South-eastern region (Fig. 5.3).

The fit of the model, as assessed through AIC, shows it improved when covariates were included in the model (Table 5.3). This baseline model yielded $AIC = 49615.97$, higher compared to the AIC obtained under model $M2$, which includes covariates ($AIC = 49429.22$). Model $M4$ performs far better than the other two ($AIC = 47469.43$). We therefore dwell our discussions on this model ($M4$).

Table 5.4 gives estimates of fixed effects for the four joint outcomes based on model $M4$. Outcome I, the joint diarrhoea-fever condition, was positively associated with age of the child, socio-economic ranking at lowest to medium levels, but no significant difference was obtained at higher level of SES compared to those at highest level of SES. The central region, relative to the northern region, was positively associated with outcome I. Similarly, crowded households were positively associated with the joint condition of diarrhoea and fever. For the second outcome, diarrhoea combined with stunting was negatively associated with age of less than 6 months and was positive for ages between 6 and 47 months relative to those aged 49–60 months. Nevertheless there was no significant association with SES, maternal education, crowded households, vitamin A or place of residence. The joint fever-stunted condition (outcome III) was observed to be associated with age, negatively for those aged <6 months, and positively for those above age 12–47 months. We also noted a positive association of this category with SES, rural residence and

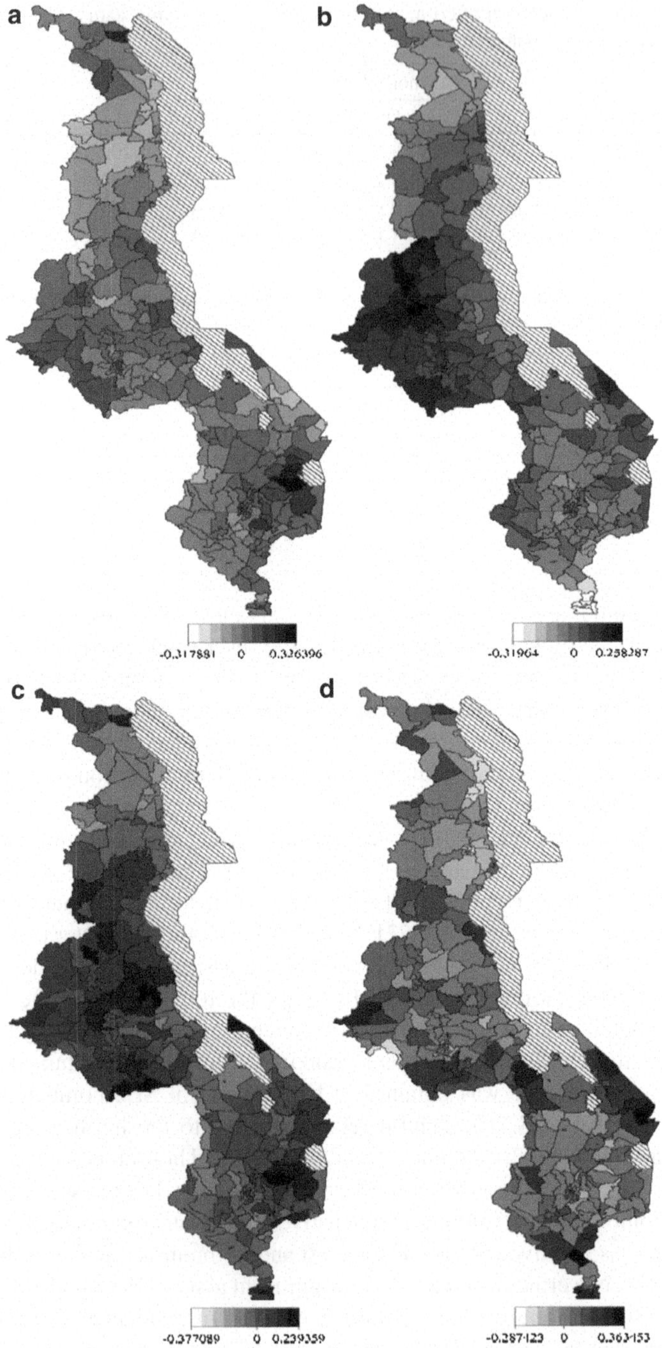

Fig. 5.2 Association between health outcomes and geographical location at sub-district level based on model $M1$. Plot (**a**) outcome I (diarrhoea and fever); (**b**) outcome II (diarrhoea and stunted); (**c**) outcome III (fever and stunted); (**d**) outcome IV (stunted and underweight)

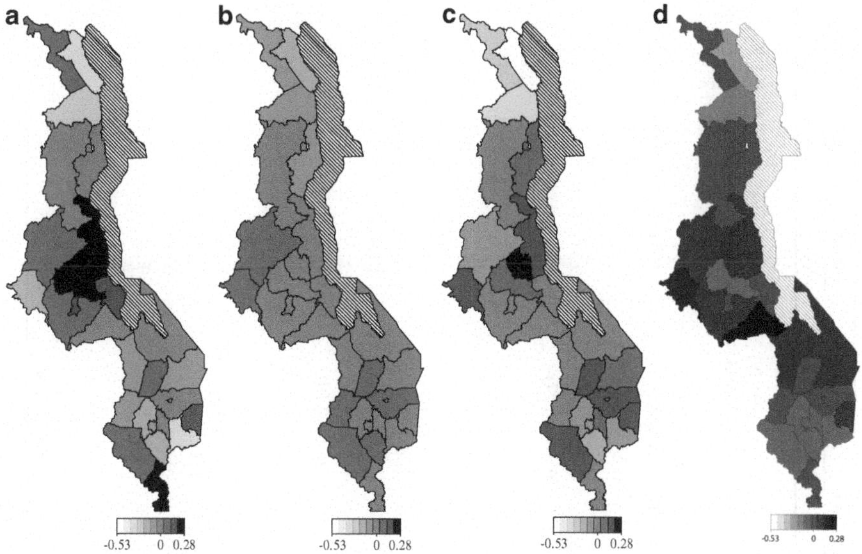

Fig. 5.3 Total residual spatial effects in the latent variable model. Shown are posterior modes at district level for DF (*plot* **a**), DS (*plot* **b**), FS (*plot* **c**) and SUN (*plot* **d**)

Table 5.3 Model comparison values based on Akaike information criterion (AIC) for selected multinomial models[a]

Model	Description	Log likelihood	Degrees of freedom	AIC
*M*1	Random effects at districts and sub-district	49,125.23	245.37	49,615.97
*M*2	Fixed + Random effects	48,944.50	242.36	49,429.22
*M*3	Space-varying SES + Random effects	48,902.30	346.46	49,595.22
*M*4	Fixed + Nonlinear + Space-varying SES	46,872.61	298.41	47,469.43

[a]See Sect. 5.4.2 for details on models fitted

maternal education. For the last outcome, a combination of stunted and underweight, a significant relationship was observed with age of the child, SES, region, maternal education and crowded households. However, for all joint health outcomes, age of child was better estimated as nonlinear effects (Fig. 5.4). Indeed, considering the values of log-likelihood, AIC (Table 5.3), the model with nonlinear effects (*M*4) was better than the other two (*M*1 and *M*2). Note that for all outcomes the risk increased with age up to age 15–20 months and then started decreasing at about age of 20 months. However, for diarrhoea-fever condition this effect seemed to fall much earlier, at about 10 months (Fig. 5.3).

Table 5.4 Regression coefficient summaries for the best model (Model 4) fitted to data on children co-morbidity of diarrhoea, fever, stunting and underweight

	Diarrhoea, Fever		Diarrhoea, Stunted		Fever, Stunted		Stunted, Underweight	
Variable	Mode[a]	95 % CI	Mode	95 % CI	Mode	95 % CI	Mode	95 % CI
Age(months)								
<6	0.33	(0.19, 0.47)	−0.26	(−0.42, −0.11)	−0.55	(−0.43, −0.29)	−1.29	(−1.46, −1.12)
6–11	0.99	(0.88, 1.12)	0.49	(0.37, 0.61)	−0.038	(−0.14, 0.062)	−0.20	(−0.28, −0.11)
12–23	0.66	(0.56, 0.79)	0.61	(0.50, 0.72)	0.33	(0.25, 0.40)	0.31	(0.24, 0.38)
24–35	0.36	(0.24, 0.47)	0.24	(0.11, 0.35)	0.12	(0.041, 0.19)	0.18	(0.11, 0.25)
36–47	0.12	(0.0074, 0.24)	0.16	(0.044, 0.26)	0.11	(0.030, 0.19)	0.061	(−0.017, 0.13)
48–59	0		0		0		0	
SES								
Lowest	0.11	(0.017, 0.21)	0.076	(−0.050, 0.19)	0.24	(0.15, 0.32)	0.34	(0.27, 0.43)
Lower	0.16	(0.067, 0.26)	0.071	(−0.047, 0.18)	0.18	(0.091, 0.27)	0.27	(0.19, 0.34)
Medium	0.12	(0.018, 0.21)	−0.0078	(−0.14, 0.11)	0.21	(0.13, 0.31)	0.21	(0.13, 0.28)
Higher	0.064	(−0.042, 0.16)	0.035	(−0.082, 0.15)	0.12	(0.035, 0.21)	0.13	(0.049, 0.21)
Highest	0		0		0		0	
Region								
South	0.34	(−0.14, 0.62)	0.17	(−0.16, 0.38)	0.043	(−0.32, 0.27)	0.19	(−0.057, 0.44)
Centre	0.38	(0.057, 0.64)	0.14	(−0.073, 0.34)	−0.0023	(−0.33, 0.24)	0.30	(0.093, 0.56)
North	0		1.00		1.00		1.00	
Residence								
Rural	0.03	(−0.088, 0.13)	0.036	(−0.083, 0.15)	0.10	(0.012, 0.19)	−0.028	(−0.12, 0.069)
Urban	0		0		0		0	
Crowded								
No	0		0		0		0	
Yes	0.071	(0.016, 0.13)	0.024	(−0.045, 0.093)	0.028	(−0.020, 0.076)	−0.046	(−0.086, −0.0041)
Education								
None	−0.033	(−0.13, 0.074)	−0.022	(−0.14, 0.098)	0.10	(0.011, 0.19)	0.35	(0.26, 0.44)
Primary	0.0027	(−0.093, 0.090)	−0.068	(−0.17, 0.036)	0.087	(0.010, 0.17)	0.29	(0.21, 0.37)
Secondary	0		0		0		0	
Vitamin A								
No	0		0		0		0	
Yes	0.093	(−0.00029, 0.19)	0.047	(−0.078, 0.16)	−0.00011	(−0.079, 0.081)	−0.040	(−0.12, 0.035)

SES socio-economic status, *CI* credible interval
[a]Posterior mode

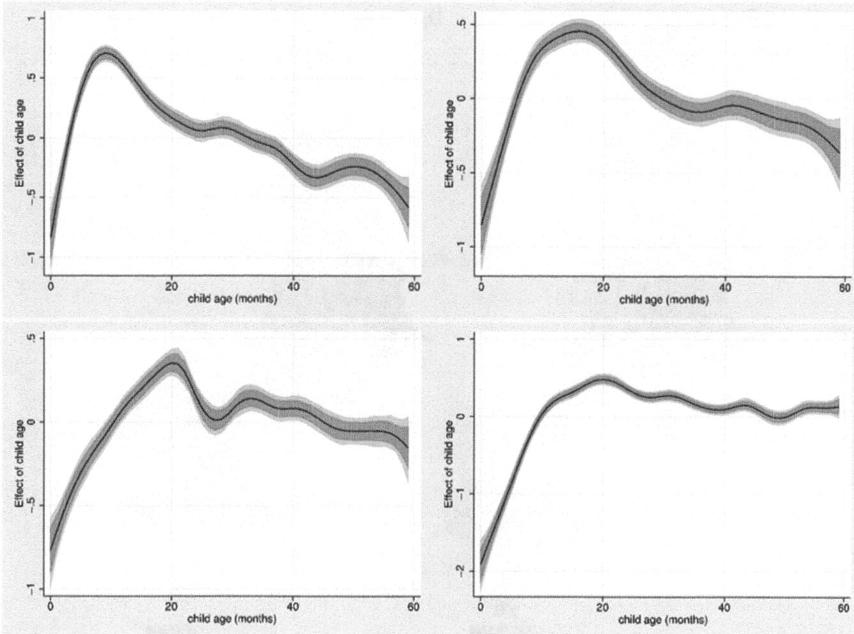

Fig. 5.4 Nonlinear effects of age of the child on co-morbidities of diarrhoea, fever, stunting and underweight

5.5.2 *Space-Varying Coefficient Model*

Figure 5.5 displays spatial effects from a model where a spatially varying coefficient was assumed. The varying effect of SES on the log-odds ranged between −0.095 and +0.13 on the joint diarrhoea-fever condition, with a positive effect in the north near Songwe river, in the central region in one sub-district in Mchinji, and around lake Chilwa in Zomba district (see plot (a)). The combined condition of diarrhoea-stunted is shown in plot (b), and that of fever-stunted (plot c) portrayed a similar risk pattern with regards their association with SES. The risk is highest in the central region and equally lowest in other regions, ranging between −0.66 and +0.39 and from −0.05 to +0.02 for the South or North respectively. Evidently the influence of SES was dominant in the joint diarrhoea-stunted condition as shown by the magnitude of the effects. For outcome IV, the varying risk of SES, range between −0.13 and +0.26, with a few pockets of significantly positive association.

Total residual spatial effects, after accounting for fixed and space-varying effects still remained significant, and are plotted in Fig. 5.6. Plot (a) shows the spatial effects of outcome I (diarrhoea and fever). Here we observe clusters of positive association in the South-eastern region, along Salima and in Chitipa. For outcome II (combined diarrhoea-stunted category), as shown in panel (b), there was evidence of positive clustering in the central region, and isolated areas in Nkhatabay and Mangochi.

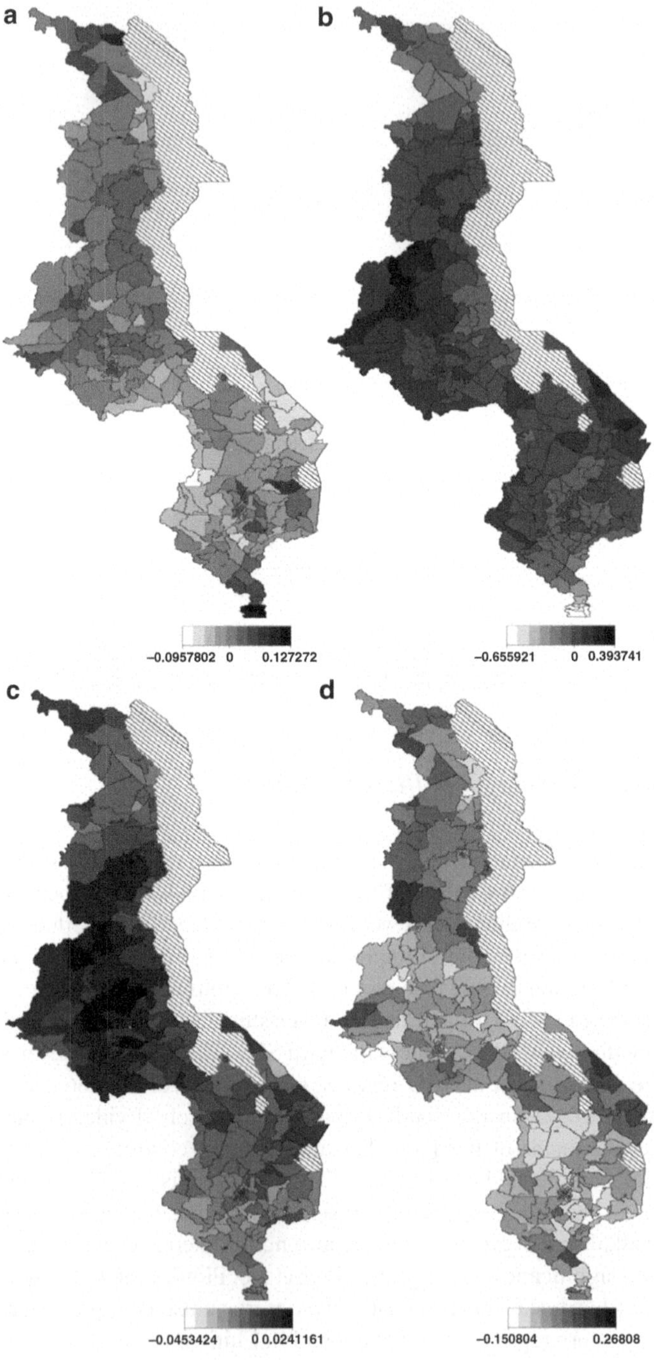

Fig. 5.5 Spatially varying coefficient effects of SES on joint conditions of diarrhea, fever, stunting and underweight, as defined in the text

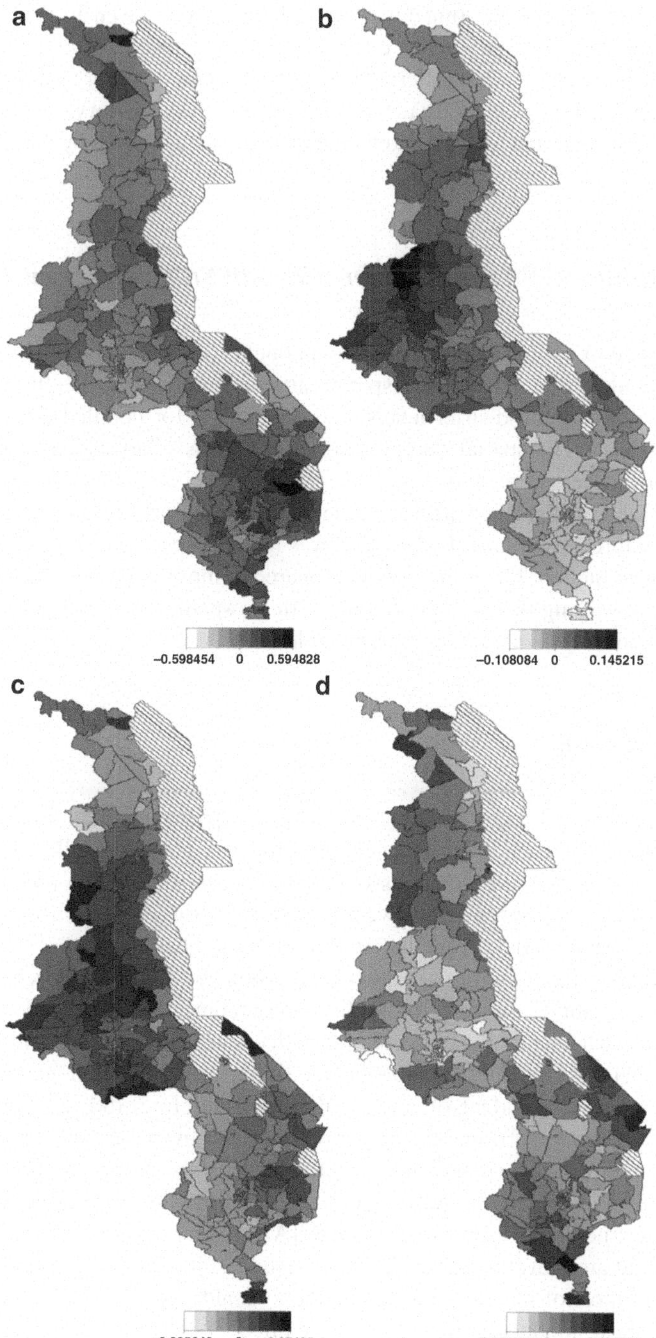

Fig. 5.6 Total residual spatial effects in the latent variable models. Shown are the posterior modes for outcome I-IV as defined in Table 5.4

The residual effects for the joint fever-stunted category is given in panel (c). The effects are again increased in the central region in Dowa, Ntchisi, Salima and Nkhotakota districts. Similar patterns of positive association were obtained in the South in Zomba, Nsanje and Chiradzulu districts. The last category, combination of stunted-underweight had fewer pockets of elevated risk, as shown by dark shades of colour.

5.5.3 Multilevel Structure at District and Subdistrict Level

Table 5.5 presents estimates of variance components for the spatial effects obtained from two models that explore the spatial structure of the four health conditions at both district and sub-district levels (see Sect. 5.4.2 for detailed description of the two models). The spatial components in $M1a$ was relatively large compared to when covariates were added in $M3$. When model $M1a$ is extended to add district spatial structure, the variance components are almost split (see model $M1b$). A similar picture was obtained when SES was fitted as space-varying. The variance components in model $M2b$ were higher compared to those in model $M4$, suggesting again that the varying risks of childhood health are spatially correlated to a number of factors, both at individual and population level.

5.6 Discussion

The concepts of SES and health are pervasive in epidemiological studies, yet an examination of the such a complex relationship has not been fully explored. In this Chapter, we observed a clear association between joint health conditions and social inequality, measured using wealth ranking. Using a version of structured additive regression model, in particular defining joint health status as a categorical outcome, we fitted a multinomial logistic regression model. We explored the socio-economic inequalities existing for each joint outcome, and extended our model to investigate whether the socio-economic effects are spatially varying. Previous studies of neighborhood effects on health status have modeled neighborhoods as if they were independent of one another and therefore, did not consider the interrelations among surrounding neighborhoods. To overcome this shortcoming, this Chapter employed spatial autocorrelation analysis to assess the degree of interrelation among neighborhoods, and incorporated this among-neighborhood effect into a structured additive regression (STAR) model to simultaneously analyze individual and area-level variables. Evidently, the last model that incorporated both does explain most of the variation in childhood health status. This, as assessed by AIC, is the 'best' model among the many we fitted.

The multinomial model presented here is based on the hierarchical framework. At first level of hierarchy we presented a measurement model, followed by prior distributions at second level of hierarchy. This allows to model complex relationships

Table 5.5 Variance of spatial effects at sub-district (TA) and district (D) level for selected models fitted

Variance components	M1a[b]	M1b	M2b	M3	M4
τ^2_{RES}(TA)					
I[c]	0.461(0.153, 0.976)	0.007(0.004, 0.019)	0.072(0.026, 0.130)	0.518(0.105, 0.901)	0.224(0.057, 0.551)
II	0.270(0.082, 0.549)	0.081(0.012, 0.284)	0.044(0.004, 0.098)	0.209(0.095, 0.475)	0.032(0.005, 0.082)
III	0.486(0.276, 0.722)	0.084(0.010, 0.261)	0.041(0.010, 0.083)	0.506(0.342, 0.699)	0.119(0.045, 0.268)
IV	0.276(0.055, 0.517)	0.054(0.001, 0.337)	0.083(0.043, 0.143)	0.098(0.002, 0.378)	0.175(0.010, 0.383)
τ^2_{SVC}(TA)					
I				0.163(0.018, 0.608)	0.044(0.001, 0.265)
II				0.032(0.002, 0.117)	0.152(0.016, 0.344)
III				0.022(0.004, 0.077)	0.006(0.001, 0.018)
IV				0.297(0.043, 0.543)	0.086(0.001, 0.315)
τ^2_{RES}(D)					
I[c]		0.316(0.003, 0.936)	0.122(0.044, 0.253)		
II		0.155(0.007, 0413)	0.014(0.001, 0.053)		
III		0.396(0.013, 0.911)	0.125(0.047, 0.267)		
IV		0.176(0.007, 0.529)	0.042(0.002, 0.118)		
τ^2_{SVC}(D)					
I[c]					0.571(0.263, 1.149)
II					0.075(0.001, 0.288)
III					0.529(0.244, 0.978)
IV					0.175(0.038, 0.583)

[a]See Sect. 5.4.2 for details on models fitted

[b]Posterior modes are given

[c]Response outcome categories: *I* fever and diarrhea, *II* stunted and diarrhea, *III* fever and stunted, *IV* stunted and underweight observed in a child

that may exist, often realized in social science. This paper shows the importance of such advanced tools and statistical techniques to better assess associations that emanate at various levels, both at individual and population levels. In particular, modelling the clustering variation allowed accounting directly for unmeasured risk factors that vary with location. In this work, the geographical unit is the sub-district or district, and because these are not the smallest spatial units, within-area variability is expected, hence the need for both spatially varying coefficient, heterogeneity and clustering random components in a single model. This therefore rules out over-parameterisation of the model and hence the need for multilevel structured models. A possible extension to the model we have considered here is to include area-level risk factors together with individual factors. One limitation of this study is that the data for diarrhoea and fever are self-reported and thus suffer from recall-bias.

Some researchers have argued that the definition of socio-economic status is limited. Therefore a more inclusive definition should include education. The definition of SES as approached here, follows the DHS definition and is systematic approach to determine a household's relative economic status (Rutstein and Kiersten 2004). The importance of wealth is its association with reproductive and maternal health, child mortality and health, and use of public services, and is seen as an enabling factor in health seeking behaviour.

As of the substantive modelling and risk factors obtained in this study, our findings are consistent with what has been obtained before in previous studies (Kazembe and Namangale 2007; Kandala et al. 2006; Kandala 2006). This research has differentiated variability due to both individual and neighborhood effects (that is unmeasured characteristics), see Table 5.5. Our findings, therefore, suggest that the challenge to improve poor child health goes beyond addressing individual factors, but also require to understanding unmeasured covariates for potential effective interventions. Although we employed multinomial model, alternative methods, as presented in the introduction, that employ multivariate responses as opposed to multiple responses exist and much further work remains to be done, including exploring the use of spatial structural equation models (SSEM) as demonstrated in Fahrmeir and Raach (2007).

Acknowledgements We acknowledge permission granted by UNICEF to use the 2006 Malawi MICS data.

References

Besag, J., & Kooperberg, C. (1995). On conditional and intrinsic autoregressions. *Biometrika, 82*, 733–746.

Besag, J., York, J., & Mollie, A. (1991). Bayesian image restoration with two applications in spatial statistics (with discussion). *Annals of the Institute of Statistical Mathematics, 43*, 1–59.

Black, R. E., Morris, S. S., & Bryce, J. (2003). Where and why are 10 million children dying every year? *Lancet, 361*, 2226–2234.

Braveman, P., & Tarimo, E. (2002). Social inequalities in health within countries: Not only an issue for affluent nations. *Social Science & Medicine, 54*, 1621–1635.

Brezger, A., Kneib, T., & Lang, S. (2005). BayesX: Software for Bayesian inference based on Markov Chain Monte Carlo simulation techniques. *Journal of Statistial Software, 14*, 11.

Carter, R., Mendis, K. N., & Roberts, D. (2000). Spatial targeting of interventions against malaria. *Bulletin of the World Health Organization, 78*, 1401–1411.

Congdon, P. (2003). Modelling spatially varying impacts of socioeconomic predictors on mortality outcomes. *Journal of Geographical Systems, 5*, 161–184.

Fahrmeir, L., & Lang, S. (2001). Bayesian inference for generalized additive mixed models based on Markov random field priors. *Journal of the Royal Statistical Society: Series C, 50*, 201–220.

Fahrmeir, L., & Raach, A. (2007). A Bayesian semiparametric latent variable model for mixed responses. *Psychometrika, 72*, 327–346.

Fahrmeir, L., Kneib, T., & Lang, S. (2004). Penalized additive regression for space-time data: A Bayesian perspective. *Statistica Sinica, 14*, 715–745.

Fenn, B., Morris, S., & Black, R. E. (2005). Comorbidity in childhood in Ghana: Magnitude, associated factors and impact on mortality. *International Journal of Epidemiology, 34*, 368–375.

Fotheringham, A., Charlton, M., & Brunsdon, C. (2002). *Geographically weighted regression: The analysis of spatially varying relationships*. Chichester: Wiley.

Fotso, J. C., & Kuate-Defo, B. (2005). Measuring socioeconomic status in health research in developing countries: Should we be focusing on households, communities or both? *Social Indicators Research, 72*, 189–237.

Gamerman, D., Moreira, A., & Rue, H. (2003). Space-varying regression models: Specifications and simulation. *Computational Statistics and Data Analysis, 42*, 513–533.

Gelfand, A. E., Kim, H. K., Sirmans, C. F., & Banerjee, S. (2006). Spatial modelling with spatially varying coefficient processes. *Journal of the American Statistical Association, 98*, 387–396.

Hong, R. (2007). Effect of economic inequality on chronic childhood undernutrition in Ghana. *Public Health Nutrition, 10*, 371–378.

Källander, K., Nsungwa-Sabiiti, J., & Peterson, S. (2004). Symptom overlap for malaria and pneumonia – policy implications for home management strategies. *Acta Tropica, 90*, 211–214.

Kandala, N.-B. (2006). Bayesian geoadditive modelling of childhood morbidity in Malawi. *Applied Stochastic Models in Business and Industry, 22*, 139–154.

Kandala, N.-B., Magadi, M. A., & Madise, N. J. (2006). An investigation of district spatial variations of childhood diarrhoea and fever morbidity in Malawi. *Social Science & Medicine, 62*, 1138–1152.

Kazembe, L. N., & Namangale, J. J. (2007). A Bayesian multinomial model to analyse spatial patterns of childhood co-morbidity in Malawi. *European Journal of Epidemiology, 22*, 545–556.

Kneib, T., & Fahrmeir, L. (2006). Structured additive regression for categorical space-time data: A mixed model approach. *Biometrics, 62*, 109–118.

Lang, S., & Brezger, A. (2004). Bayesian P-splines. *Journal of Computational and Graphical Statistics, 13*, 183–212.

Lin, X., & Zhang, D. (1999). Inference in generalized additive mixed models by using smoothing splines. *Journal of the Royal Statistical Society Series B, 61*, 381–400.

Mulholland, K. (2005). Commentary: Comorbidity as a factor in child health and child survival in developing countries. *International Journal of Epidemiology, 34*, 375–377.

National Statistical Office, ORC Macro. (2005). *Malawi demographic and health survey 2004: Preliminary report*. Zomba: NSO.

Rutstein, S. O., & Kiersten, J. (2004). *The DHS wealth index* (DHS comparative reports, Vol. 6). Calverton: ORC Macro.

Steele, F., Goldstein, H., & Brown, W. (2004). A general multilevel multistate competing risks model for event history data, with an application to a study of contraceptive use dynamics. *Statistical Modelling, 4*, 145–159.

Tutz, G. (2004). Generalized semiparametrically structured mixed models. *Computational Statistics and Data Analysis, 46*, 777–800.

Wagstaff, A. (2000). Socioeconomic inequalities in child mortality: Comparisons across nine developing countries. *Bulletin of the World Health Organization, 78*, 19–29.

Zere, E., & McIntyre, D. (2003). Inequities in under-five child malnutrition in South Africa. *International Journal for Equity in Health, 2*, 7.

Chapter 6
Analysis of Grouped Survival Data: A Synthesis of Various Traditions and Application to Modeling Childhood Mortality in Eritrea

Gebrenegus Ghilagaber

6.1 Introduction

This paper merges together some statistical methods used in the analysis of data involving rates of occurrence of an event. These methods are (1) indirect standardization with the multiplicative model, (2) loglinear regression for count data, and (3) proportional hazards regression for survival data. In many applications these approaches have been portrayed as belonging to distinct fields or as competing methodologies. In this paper it is demonstrated that (1) and (2) actually represent one special case of (3) in two different, but equivalent, parameterizations. One advantage of such synthesis is that computer algorithms developed for one setting can be exploited in another. Accordingly, we demonstrate how the General Loglinear Analysis Procedure in SPSS, and the GENMOD Procedure in SAS may be used to compute estimates of baseline and relative hazards (parameters common in survial analysis) and how these estimates may be interpreted in relation to standardization. The issues addressed are illustrated by empirical analysis of a data set on mortality experiences among 7,055 Eritrean children based on data from the 1995 Eritrean Demographic and Health Survey.

In Sect. 6.2 we describe standard inference procedures for constant and piece-wise constant hazard rates in the case of one populations. This is extended to the case of two populations in Sect. 6.3. Section 6.4 is devoted to a description of the multiplicative hazards model, estimation of its parameters, its relationship to Cox's proportional hazards model, and to Poisson model for count data. Further, we demonstrate how standard programs like SPSS or SAS may be used to estimate its parameters. An empirical illustration is provided in Sect. 6.5 where the data

G. Ghilagaber (✉)
Department of Statistics, Stockholm University, SE-106 91 Stockholm, Sweden
e-mail: Gebre@stat.su.se

N.-B. Kandala and G. Ghilagaber (eds.), *Advanced Techniques for Modelling Maternal and Child Health in Africa*, The Springer Series on Demographic Methods and Population Analysis 34, DOI 10.1007/978-94-007-6778-2_6,

set, dependent and explanatory variables are described and inference procedures – parameter estimation, testing for significance, and goodness-of-fit tests are shown in detail. Section 6.6 summarizes the chapter.

6.2 Maximum Likelihood Estimation of the Hazard Rate

6.2.1 *Estimation of a Constant Hazard Rate*

A simple parametric specification of the hazard function, λ (t), is the exponential model where the hazard rate remains constant over time (is independent of t). Accordingly, the corresponding survivor functions are $f(t) = \lambda \exp(-\lambda t)$, $S(t) = \exp(-\lambda t)$, and $\lambda(t) = \lambda$ for $t > 0$, $\lambda > 0$. In constructing the likelihood function, uncensored observations contribute f(t) while censored observations contribute S(t) to the likelihood. These may be combined as

$$g(t) = [\lambda \exp(-\lambda t)]^{\delta(t)}[\exp(-\lambda t)]^{1-\delta(t)} = \lambda^{\delta(t)} \exp[-\lambda(t)],$$

where $\delta(t)$ is a censoring indicator with value $\delta(t) = 1$ if an individual has experienced the event at time t and $\delta(t) = 0$ if the individual is censored at time t.

Let $T_1, T_2, \ldots, T_n$ be n independent observations of T from an exponential distribution with parameter λ. The contribution to the likelihood of an individual with value t_h (h =1, ..., n), is then given by

$$\Lambda_h = g(t_h) = \lambda^{\delta(t_h)} \exp[-\lambda(t_h)]$$

and, hence, the likelihood function for the entire sample is then given by

$$\Lambda = \prod_{h=1}^{n} \Lambda_h = \prod_{h=1}^{n} \lambda^{\delta(t_h)} \exp[-\lambda\,(t_h)] = \lambda^{D_+} \exp[-\lambda T_+]$$

where $D_+ = \sum_{h=1}^{n} \delta(t_h)$ is the total number of events (say, deaths), among the n observations and $D_+ = \sum_{h=1}^{n} t_h$ is the total exposure time (expressed in days, months, years, or any other suitable unit) contributed by both uncensored and censored observations.

The corresponding log-likelihood is then given by

$$\ln \Lambda = D_+ \ln \lambda - \lambda T_+$$

Differentiating lnΛ with respect to λ we get

$$\frac{\partial}{\partial \lambda} \ln \Lambda = \frac{D_+}{\lambda} - T_+$$

while the second derivative is given by

$$\frac{\partial^2}{\partial \lambda^2} \ln \Lambda = -\frac{D_+}{\lambda^2}$$

The first derivative implies that the maximum likelihood estimator of the hazard (intensity) rate, λ, is given by

$$\hat{\lambda} = \frac{D_+}{T_+}$$

which is a straight forward occurrence/exposure rate.

Further, the 2nd derivative implies that the estimated asymptotic variance of $\hat{\lambda}$ is given by

$$Var\left(\hat{\lambda}\right) = -\frac{1}{\frac{\partial^2}{\partial \lambda^2} \ln \Lambda}\Bigg|_{\lambda=\hat{\lambda}} = \frac{\hat{\lambda}^2}{D_+} = \left(\frac{D_+}{T_+}\right)^2 \frac{1}{D_+} = \frac{D_+}{T_+^2} = \frac{D_+}{T_+}\frac{1}{T_+} = \frac{\hat{\lambda}}{T_+}.$$

Consequently, using standard results for maximum likelihood estimates, we have

$$\frac{\hat{\lambda} - \lambda}{\sqrt{\frac{\hat{\lambda}}{T_+}}} \sim N(0, 1)$$

6.2.2 *Estimation of a Piece-Wise Constant Hazard Rate*

A straightforward extension of the exponential model is the so-called piece-wise exponential model (piecewise-constant hazard model). A piecewise exponential distribution arises from a distribution whose hazard rate is a step function. In other words, for given time points $t_0, t_1, \ldots, t_k$, (where often $t_0 = 0$) the density function is

$$f(t) = \begin{cases} \lambda_1 \exp\left(-\lambda_1 t\right), \ t_0 \le t < t_1 \\ \lambda_2 \exp\left[-\lambda_1 t_1 - \lambda_2\left(t - t_1\right)\right], \ t_1 \le t < t_2 \\ . \\ . \\ . \\ \lambda_k \exp\left[-\lambda_1 t_1 - \lambda_2\left(t_2 - t_1\right) - \ldots - \lambda_k\left(t - t_{k-1}\right)\right], \ t \ge t_{k-1} \end{cases}$$

The corresponding survivor function is given by

$$S(t) = \begin{cases} \exp(-\lambda_1 t), \; t_0 \le t < t_1 \\ \exp[-\lambda_1 t_1 - \lambda_2 (t - t_1)], \; t_1 \le t < t_2 \\ . \\ . \\ . \\ \exp[-\lambda_1 t_1 - \lambda_2 (t_2 - t_1) - \ldots - \lambda_k (t - t_{k-1})], \; t \ge t_{k-1} \end{cases}$$

so that the hazard function is

$$\lambda(t) = \begin{cases} \lambda_1, \; t_0 \le t < t_1 \\ \lambda_2, \; t_1 \le t < t_2 \\ . \\ . \\ . \\ \lambda_k, \; t \ge t_{k-1} \end{cases}$$

When $\lambda_i = \lambda$ for all i we get the exponential model. The likelihood function of the entire sample is then given by (by adjusting the likelihood in the previous subsection):

$$\Lambda = \prod_{i=1}^{k} \lambda_i^{D_i} \exp[-\lambda_i T_i]$$

where D_i and T_i now refer to the total number of events (say, deaths) and exposure units in the ith interval. The (natural) log-likelihood is given by

$$\ln \Lambda = \sum_{i=1}^{k} D_i \ln \lambda_i - \sum_{i=1}^{k} \lambda_i T_i$$

and maximization in the usual manner leads to

$$\hat{\lambda}_i = \frac{D_i}{T_i}, \; Var\left(\hat{\lambda}_i\right) = \frac{\hat{\lambda}_i}{T_i}, \text{ and } \frac{\hat{\lambda}_i - \lambda_i}{\sqrt{\frac{\hat{\lambda}_i}{T_i}}} \sim N(0, 1)$$

6.2.3 Extension to Two Populations

Consider J populations and let D_{ij} be the number of occurrences, say deaths, at age group (duration group) i (i = 1, ...,I) in the jth population for T_{ij} months of observed time (exposure).

Define

$$D_{i+} = \sum_{j=1}^{J} D_{ij},\ D_{+j} = \sum_{i=1}^{I} D_{ij},\ D_{++} = \sum_{i=1}^{I}\sum_{j=1}^{J} D_{ij}$$

and let T_{i+}, T_{+j}, and T_{++} represent similar quantities for the exposure variable T. Usually, the intensity functions are assumed to be piece-wise constant in each of the two populations but may vary between the two populations. In other words, the time to event (death) is assumed to follow piece-wise exponential distribution in each population.

In the context of our notation, the density function of the time to death in age group i for a person in population j is given by

$$f\left(t_{ij}\right) = \lambda_{ij} \exp\left(\lambda_{ij} t_{ij}\right)$$

The corresponding likelihood function is given by

$$\Lambda = \prod_{i=1}^{I}\prod_{j=1}^{J} \lambda_{ij}{}^{D_{ij}} \exp\left[-\lambda_{ij} t_{ij}\right]$$

so that

$$\ln \Lambda = \sum_{i=1}^{I}\sum_{i=1}^{J} \left(D_{ij} \ln \lambda_{ij} - \lambda_{ij} t_{ij}\right)$$

Further,

$$\frac{\partial}{\partial \lambda_{ij}} \ln \Lambda = \frac{D_{ij}}{\lambda_{ij}} - T_{ij}.$$

Thus, the MLE of λ_{ij} is the corresponding occurrence/exposure rate in the (i, j)th cell:

$$\hat{\lambda}_{ij} = \frac{D_{ij}}{T_{ij}}.$$

A standard argument for maximum likelihood estimators proves that the $\hat{\lambda}_{ij}$, are asymptotically stochastically independent, that the estimator $\hat{\lambda}_{ij}$ has the asymptotic mean λ_{ij} (is asymptotically unbiased), and that its asymptotic variance can be estimated by $\frac{\hat{\lambda}_{ij}}{T_{ij}}$.

6.3 The Multiplicative Hazard Model with Two Factors: Imposing a Structure on the Hazard Rate

6.3.1 *The Two-Factor Multiplicative Model*

Assume, in general, that we are interested in some collection of hazard rates λ_{ij} where the factor indexed by i has I levels and factor indexed by j has J levels.

Suppose that the following multiplicative two factor model holds:

$$\lambda_{ij} = \theta_i \alpha_j$$

whereby the age-specific hazard rates are obtained from multiplicative contributions of the ith age (duration) group θ_i, and jth level of the covariate (say, period or birth cohort) α_j. A model of this form has been suggested for many situations. A brief discussion of its merits has been given by Breslow and Day (1975) while Hoem (1987) reviews the statistical theory behind the model.

This model has I + J parameters though a restriction of some kind will be needed to attain identifiability. Here it suffices to mention that α_j measures the relative super-/sub-hazard of death in period j (relative to a baseline level) θ_i is the hazard at duration i in the standard (baseline) level of the covariate.

6.3.2 *Maximum Likelihood Estimation*

To find estimates of the parameters θ_i and α_j when the multiplicative model holds, we first define ω_{ijr} as an indicator of whether the rth sample member having the jth level of the covariate dies ($\omega_{ijr} = 1$) or is alive ($\omega_{ijr} = 0$) in the ith age group (duration). The contribution, to the likelihood, of the sub-sample of individuals in the ith age group and having the jth level of the covariate can then be obtained as

$$\Lambda_{ij} = \prod_r \left(\theta_i \alpha_j\right)^{\omega_{ijr}} \exp\left(-t_{ijr}\theta_i \alpha_j\right) = \left(\theta_i \alpha_j\right)^{D_{ij}} \exp\left(-T_{ij}\theta_i \alpha_j\right)$$

The likelihood for the entire sample will then be the product of the Λ_{ij} over all levels of i and j:

$$\Lambda = \prod_i \prod_j \Lambda_{ij} = \prod_i \prod_j \left\{ \left(\theta_i \alpha_j\right)^{D_{ij}} \exp\left(-T_{ij}\theta_i \alpha_j\right) \right\}$$

so that

$$\ln \Lambda = \sum_i D_{i+} \ln \theta_i + \sum_i D_{+j} \ln \alpha_j - \sum_i \sum_j T_{ij}\theta_i \alpha_j$$

where D_{i+} and D_{+j} are as defined before.

If we differentiate $\ln \Lambda$ with respect to θ_i and separately with respect to α_j and proceed in the normal manner to maximize $\ln \Lambda$, we get the normal equations

$$\boldsymbol{\theta}_i^{(k)} = \frac{D_{i+}}{\sum_j \boldsymbol{\alpha}_j^{(k-1)} T_{ij}}$$

and

$$\boldsymbol{\alpha}_j^{(k)} = \frac{D_{+j}}{\sum_i \boldsymbol{\theta}_i^{(k)} T_{ij}}$$

This is a system of I + J equations that does not have an explicit solution in general. It defines the maximum likelihood estimators θ_i and α_j implicitly, but one cannot write a simple formula for them. When the occurrences D_{ij} and exposures T_{ij} are given, numerical values of the estimators can easily be found from an iteration process, however. One such iteration process is as follows:

Define initial values $\boldsymbol{\alpha}_j^{(0)} = 1$ for all j = 1, ..., J and enter them into the right hand side of the equation for $\boldsymbol{\theta}_i^{(k)}$ to get corresponding first values for the $\boldsymbol{\theta}_i^{(k)}$, as follows:

$$\boldsymbol{\theta}_i^{(1)} = \frac{D_{i+}}{\sum_j \boldsymbol{\alpha}_j^{(0)} T_{ij}} = \frac{D_{i+}}{\sum_j T_{ij}} = \frac{D_{i+}}{T_{i+}}$$

Then, $\boldsymbol{\theta}_i^{(1)}$ is a straightforward occurrence/exposure rate at age group (duration) i when we take no account of the other covariate indexed by j. In other words, it is the crude death rate in age group i (crude because we have not yet standardized for, say, period differences).

Now compute a next approximation to α_j by plugging $\boldsymbol{\theta}_i^{(1)}$ into the equation of $\alpha_j^{(k)}$, i.e. let

$$\boldsymbol{\alpha}_j^{(1)} = \frac{D_{+j}}{\sum_i \boldsymbol{\theta}_i^{(1)} T_{ij}}$$

The denominator gives the expected number of deaths in the jth period had the individuals in this period been subjected to the mortality rates for the entire population at each age ($\boldsymbol{\theta}_i^{(1)}$). In other words, $\alpha_j^{(1)}$ is the effect of the jth period, indirectly standardized with respect to age (duration), using the whole observed subpopulation (T_{ij}) as a standard.

Next, plug $\alpha_j^{(1)}$ back into the equation for $\boldsymbol{\theta}_i^{(k)}$ to get a second approximation $\boldsymbol{\theta}_i$:

$$\boldsymbol{\theta}_i^{(2)} = \frac{D_{i+}}{\sum_j \boldsymbol{\alpha}_j^{(1)} T_{ij}} \qquad i = 1, 2, \ldots, I$$

We note, again, that the denominator in $\boldsymbol{\theta}_i^{(2)}$ gives the expected number of deaths in the ith age group had the individuals in this age group been subjected to the mortality rates for the entire population at each period ($\boldsymbol{\alpha}_j^{(1)}$). In other words, $\boldsymbol{\theta}_i^{(2)}$ is the hazard rate at age group i, indirectly standardized with respect to the period (birth cohort), using the whole observed subpopulation (T_{ij}) as a standard.

The next step would be to continue the iterations until convergence is attained. Upon convergence, we may use the final estimates (say $\boldsymbol{\theta}_i^*$ and $\boldsymbol{\alpha}_j^*$) to get a set of standardized hazard rates

$$\lambda_{ij} = \theta_i^* \alpha_j^*$$

gives the final maximum likelihood estimate of λ_{ij} under the multiplicative structure.

6.3.3 Extension to More Than Two Factors and Goodness-of-Fit Tests

The above model can be extended to include even further factors. With a third factor, for instance, the hazard function becomes

$$\lambda_{ijk} = \theta_i \alpha_j \gamma_k$$

while with four factors we may decompose the model as

$$\lambda_{ijkl} = \theta_i \alpha_j \gamma_k \delta_m$$

and so on.

Further, interaction between two covariates or between a covariate and the duration variable may be included in the model. With four factors where the last two factors interact, the hazard function may be written as

$$\lambda_{ijkl} = \theta_i \alpha_j \phi_{km}$$

while if the interaction is between the time variable and the second factor the model may be written as

$$\lambda_{ijkl} = \theta_{ij} \gamma_k \delta_m$$

At each step, the overall fit of the model and the improvement in fit resulting from adding a set of covariates to the model can be tested by a likelihood ratio test.

6.3.4 Similarities Between the Multiplicative Model and the Cox Model

In the Cox proportional hazards model (Cox, 1972), we deal with expressions like

$$\lambda\left(t|z_1,\ldots,z_k\right) = \lambda_0(t)\exp\left(\sum_j \beta_j z_j(t)\right)$$

where $\lambda\left(t|z_1,\ldots,z_k\right)$ is the hazard rate at time t for an individual with covariate vector $(z_1,\ldots,z_k)$, these covariates being regressors which may depend on time t, $\lambda_0(t)$ is the base-line hazard rate that applies when all covariates have the value of zero, and the β_j's are corresponding regression coefficients to be estimated.

In the multiplicative model, on the other hand, we have expressions like

$$\lambda_{ij} = \theta_i\alpha_j$$

where, without loss of generality, i indexes the (grouped) time variable, while j indexes a categorical covariate.

It is possible to transform the later (multiplicative) model so that it fits into the form of former (Cox) model. Consider a child who is still alive. Let t be his exact age, counted as a continuous variable (here months), and let i(t) be the corresponding level of the grouped time variable. In other words, i(t) represents a categorical value corresponding to t.

Suppose that s/he attains the level j(t) of the categorical covariate indexed by j at time t. Then, the multiplicative model means that we consider the hazard-rate of death at age t to be a discrete hazard model:

$$\lambda(t) = \theta_{i(t)}\alpha_{j(t)}$$

Now define $\lambda_0(t) = \theta_{i(t)}$ and let $z_j(t) = 1$ if the child attains level j(t) at age group i(t) and $z_j(t) = 0$, otherwise. Finally, let $\beta_j = \ln\alpha_j$ for all j. Then $\lambda\left(t|z_1,\ldots,z_k\right)$ in the Cox model is nearly equal to λ_{ij} in multiplicative model (or, equivalently to $\lambda(t)$ in the above discrete model). The only difference is that while the original Cox model is based on the exact failure times, the discrete model is based on grouping the failure times.

Nevertheless, we note here that by defining $z_j(t)$ to be a binary representation of j(t) for all levels but one, of the variable indexed by j (and letting $z_j(t) = 0$ when j(t) equals to the base-line level), it can be shown (see, for instance, Hoem 1993) that the multiplicative model is just a grouped-data version of the Cox proportional hazards model.

6.3.5 *Similarities Between the Multiplicative Model and Poisson Model for Count Data*

In practical applications of the multiplicative model, it is assumed that the populations are sufficiently large, and the events sufficiently rare, so that the data are well represented by the Poisson model. In such a setting, the T_{ij} are regarded as fixed numbers whereas the D_{ij} are subject to random variation according to the Poisson distribution with expectation

$$E\left(\boldsymbol{D}_{ij}|\boldsymbol{T}_{ij}\right) = \lambda_{ij}\boldsymbol{T}_{ij} = \theta_i\alpha_j\boldsymbol{T}_{ij}$$

If, in the multiplicative model above, we assume instead that the number of deaths D_{ij} are independent realizations from a Poisson distribution with parameter (mean)

$$E\left(\boldsymbol{D}_{ij}|\boldsymbol{T}_{ij}\right) = \lambda_{ij}\boldsymbol{T}_{ij} = \theta_i\alpha_j\boldsymbol{T}_{ij}$$

for nonrandom T_{ij}, the likelihood of the total sample, Λ_P say, will be

$$\boldsymbol{\Lambda}_P = \prod_{i=1}^{I}\prod_{j=1}^{J}\frac{\left(\boldsymbol{\lambda}_{ij}\right)^{D_{ij}}\exp\left[\lambda_{ij}\boldsymbol{T}_{ij}\right]}{\left(\boldsymbol{D}_{ij}\right)!}$$

$$= \prod_{i=1}^{I}\prod_{j=1}^{J}\frac{\left(\boldsymbol{\lambda}_{ij}\right)^{D_{ij}}\exp\left[\theta_i\alpha_j\boldsymbol{T}_{ij}\right]}{\left(\boldsymbol{D}_{ij}\right)!}$$

which is proportional to the likelihood (Λ) arising from the multiplicative model. The maximum likelihood estimates of θ_i and α_j under the Poisson setting will, therefore, satisfy the previous estimation equations for the genuine occurrence/exposure rates. In such a case, it becomes unimportant for much of the practical analysis which stochastic mechanism applies for a particular data set. As a result, computer algorithms developed for one setting can often be exploited in another.

6.4 Practical Estimation Using SPSS/SAS: A Log-Linear Parameterization of the Multiplicative Model

Consider the two-factor multiplicative model discussed previously:

$$\lambda_{ij} = \theta_i\alpha_j$$

for i = 1, ..., I and j = 1, ..., J, and with one of the α_j's (often α_J) fixed to be equal to 1 (baseline level of the covariate). Now let

$$A_i = \ln \theta_i$$

and

$$B_j = \ln \alpha_j$$

so that, under the multiplicative model,

$$\ln \lambda_{ij} = \ln \theta_i + \ln \alpha_j = A_i + B_j.$$

Further, let

$$\overline{A} = \frac{\sum_{i=1}^{I} A_i}{I} \text{ and } \overline{B} = \frac{\sum_{j=1}^{J} B_j}{J}$$

be the means of the A_i's, and the B_j's, respectively.

Computer procedures such as the General Log-Linear Procedure in SPSS, and the GENMOD Procedure in SAS, yield estimates of the grand mean effect,

$$\Delta = \overline{A} + \overline{B},$$

the interval-specific effects

$$\boldsymbol{a}_i = A_i - \overline{A},$$

and the effect of the jth level of the covariate,

$$\boldsymbol{b}_j = B_j - \overline{B},$$

such that the highest levels are baseline ($a_I = b_J = 0$). The gm (generalized models) procedure in R yields estimates of the same parameters with the lowest levels as baseline ($a_1 = b_1 = 0$) but it can be recoded to have the last highest levels as baseline and hence make the results directly comparable with those from SPSS and SAS.

Further, the procedures provide estimates of standard errors of the estimates, the corresponding test statistic, and asymptotic 95 % confidence intervals for the estimates a_i and b_j.

Using these estimates, we have

$$\begin{aligned}\ln \lambda_{ij} &= \ln \theta_i + \ln \alpha_j = A_i + B_j \\ &= \left(a_i + \bar{A}\right) + \left(b_j + \bar{B}\right) = \left(\bar{A} + \bar{B}\right) + a_i + b_j \\ &= \Delta + a_i + b_j\end{aligned}$$

The corresponding hazard rates and the relative risks (multiplicative factors) may be estimated as follows:

From the last equation above, we have

$$\boldsymbol{\lambda}_{ij} = \exp\left(\Delta + a_i + b_j\right).$$

By design

$$\boldsymbol{\lambda}_{iJ} = \theta_i \alpha_J = \theta_i(1) = \theta_i.$$

Thus, we have

$$\theta_i = \theta_i(1) = \theta_i \alpha_J = \exp(\Delta + a_i + b_J) = \exp(\Delta + a_i + 0) = \exp(\Delta + a_i).$$

Lastly,

$$\alpha_j = \frac{\lambda_{ij}}{\theta_i} = \frac{\exp\left(\Delta + a_i + b_j\right)}{\exp\left(\Delta + a_i\right)} = \exp\left(b_j\right).$$

The last two equations give the final estimates of baseline- and relative hazards, respectively.

Estimates of the 95 % confidence intervals for these relative risks may be obtained by taking the exponential of the corresponding estimates of the 95 % confidence intervals for the estimates of log-hazards.

Again, the procedure outlined above can be easily extended to the case of more than two factors and to models with interactions.

6.5 Demographic Illustration: Modelling Childhood Mortality in Eritrea

We shall now apply the models of the preceding sections to a numerical data set. For illustration we shall take the data in Table 6.1 which contains deaths (D_{ij}) and exposure months (T_{ij}) at age group i for birth cohort j (i = 1, 2, 3, 4; j = 1, 2). The age groups are subdivisions of the first 5 years after birth for some new born children in two independent birth periods. More details about the source of the data may be found in National Statistics Office [Eritrea], & Macro International Inc. (1995).

6.5.1 Estimation in the Unstructured Case

If we can assume a constant intensity over the entire period (1986–1995), then the maximum likelihood estimate of the hazard rate is given by

$$\hat{\lambda} = \frac{D_{++}}{T_{++}} = \frac{456 + 248}{94188 + 100255} = \frac{704}{194440} = 0.0036206,$$

Table 6.1 Deaths and exposure months in two birth cohorts, Eritrea

	Birth cohort (j)						
	1986–1990 (j = 1)			1991–1995 (j = 2)			
Age (i)	D_{i1}	T_{i1}	$\hat{\lambda}_{i1}$	D_{i2}	T_{i2}	$\hat{\lambda}_{i2}$	$\frac{\hat{\lambda}_{i1}}{\hat{\lambda}_{i2}}$
< 1 year (i = 1)	155	36,913	41.99	143	38,197	37.44	1.12
1–2 year (i = 2)	119	27,164	43.81	66	28,070	23.51	1.86
2–3 year (i = 3)	93	17,939	51.84	25	19,433	12.86	4.03
3–5 year (i = 4)	89	12,172	73.12	14	14,555	9.62	7.60
Total	456	94,188	48.41	248	100,255	24.74	1.96

or 36 deaths per 10,000 person months.

If the death rate is assumed to be constant in each birth cohort but varies between the two cohorts, then we have:

$$\hat{\lambda}_1 = \frac{D_{+1}}{T_{+1}} = \frac{456}{94188} = 0.0048414,$$

or 48 deaths person 10,000 person months,

$$\hat{\lambda}_2 = \frac{D_{+2}}{T_{+2}} = \frac{248}{100255} = 0.0024737,$$

or 25 deaths person 10,000 person months.

Thus, a crude estimate of the overall relative hazard of death in period 1 (1986–1990) relative to that in 1991–1995 is given by

$$RR = \frac{\hat{\lambda}_1}{\hat{\lambda}_2} = \frac{0.0048414}{0.0024737} = 1.96,$$

indicating that the risk of death for those born in 1986–1990 was about twice (1.96 times) that of the younger cohort born 1991–1995. This result should, however, be interpreted with caution because the older cohort was exposed (to the risk of death) for a longer time than the younger cohort.

If, on the other hand, the intensity is allowed to vary over both the age groups and for the two birth cohorts, then we have:

$$\hat{\lambda}_{11} = \frac{D_{11}}{T_{11}} = \frac{155}{36913} = 0.0042 \quad \hat{\lambda}_{12} = \frac{D_{12}}{T_{12}} = \frac{143}{38197} = 0.0037$$

$$\hat{\lambda}_{21} = \frac{D_{21}}{T_{21}} = \frac{119}{27164} = 0.0044 \quad \hat{\lambda}_{22} = \frac{D_{22}}{T_{22}} = \frac{66}{28070} = 0.0024$$

$$\hat{\lambda}_{31} = \frac{D_{31}}{T_{31}} = \frac{93}{17939} = 0.0052 \quad \hat{\lambda}_{32} = \frac{D_{32}}{T_{32}} = \frac{25}{19433} = 0.0013$$

$$\hat{\lambda}_{41} = \frac{D_{41}}{T_{41}} = \frac{89}{12172} = 0.0073 \quad \hat{\lambda}_{42} = \frac{D_{42}}{T_{42}} = \frac{14}{14555} = 0.0010$$

6.5.2 Estimation in the Structured Case (Multiplicative Two-Factor Model)

We now fit the multiplicative model to our data set in Table 6.1. We shall take period 2 (1991–1995) as a reference period. Then, the base-line hazards at age group i, θ_i will reflect this period while the relative risk α_1 is the multiplicative factor (intensity of death in period 1 relative to that in period 2).

The SAS input-code and the corresponding output are shown at the end of present Section. Thus, we have $\Delta = -5.9209$, $a_1 = 0.0053$, $a_2 = -0.1643$, $a_3 = -0.2156$, $a_4 = 0$ (by design), $b_1 = 0.6721$, and $b_2 = 0$ (by design).

Thus, we have

$$\hat{\lambda}_{11} = \exp(\Delta + \boldsymbol{a}_1 + \boldsymbol{b}_1) = \exp(-5.9209 + 0.0053 + 0.6721) = 0.0053$$

$$\hat{\lambda}_{21} = \exp(\Delta + \boldsymbol{a}_2 + \boldsymbol{b}_1) = \exp(-5.9209 - 0.1643 + 0.6721) = 0.0045$$

$$\hat{\lambda}_{31} = \exp(\Delta + \boldsymbol{a}_3 + \boldsymbol{b}_1) = \exp(-5.9209 - 0.2156 + 0.6721) = 0.0042$$

$$\hat{\lambda}_{41} = \exp(\Delta + \boldsymbol{a}_4 + \boldsymbol{b}_1) = \exp(-5.9209 + 0 + 0.6721) = 0.0022$$

$$\hat{\lambda}_{12} = \exp(\Delta + \boldsymbol{a}_1 + \boldsymbol{b}_2) = \exp(-5.9209 + 0.0053 + 0) = 0.0027$$

$$\hat{\lambda}_{22} = \exp(\Delta + \boldsymbol{a}_2 + \boldsymbol{b}_2) = \exp(-5.9209 - 0.1643 + 0) = 0.0023$$

$$\hat{\lambda}_{32} = \exp(\Delta + \boldsymbol{a}_3 + \boldsymbol{b}_2) = \exp(-5.9209 - 0.2156 + 0) = 0.0053$$

$$\hat{\lambda}_{42} = \exp(\Delta + \boldsymbol{a}_4 + \boldsymbol{b}_2) = \exp(-5.9209 + 0 + 0) = 0.0027$$

while, the relative risk of death for birth cohort 1 (relative to that of birth cohort 2) is given by

$$\alpha_1 = \frac{\lambda_{i1}}{\theta_i} = \frac{\exp(\Delta + a_i + b_1)}{\exp(\Delta + a_i)} = \exp(b_1) = \exp(0.6721) = 1.9583.$$

The SAS input code is as follows

```
data Erit86_95;
input Age Period Deaths Exposure;
lexposure = log(Exposure);
cards;
```

1 1 155 36913
1 2 143 38197
2 1 119 27164
2 2 66 28070
3 1 93 17939
3 2 25 19433

```
  4 1 89 12172
  4 2 14 14555
run;
proc genmod data=Erit86_95;
class Age Period;
model Deaths=Age Period/dist=poisson link=log
  offset=lexposure type3;
run;
```

The corresponding SAS output is as follows:

Parameter	DF	Estimate	Standard error	95 % Confidence limits		Wald Chi-Square	Pr > ChiSq
Intercept	1	−5.9209	0.1100	−6.1366	−5.7052	2894.86	<.0001
Age1	1	0.0053	0.1143	−0.2188	0.2294	0.00	0.9628
Age2	1	−0.1643	0.1230	−0.4053	0.0768	1.78	0.1816
Age3	1	−0.2156	0.1349	−0.4799	0.0488	2.56	0.1099
Age4	0	0.0000	0.0000	0.0000	0.0000	–	–
Period1	1	0.6721	0.0789	0.5174	0.8268	72.52	<.0001
Period2	0	0.0000	0.0000	0.0000	0.0000	–	–

6.6 Summary and Concluding Remarks

The choice of an appropriate analytic method is a natural question when one is confronted with a specific data-analysis problem. In problems of standardization, for instance, the choice of a standard population and the interpretation of rates standardized with reference to specific population pose problems.

In the present chapter we have described and illustrated a multiplicative hazard model. Further, we demonstrated that this model is (1) a model-based alternative to the problem of standardization and (2) a discrete-data (grouped-data) version of the common proportional hazards model.

When viewed as a model-based indirect standardization, the multiplicative model enables the investigator to test for the importance (significance) of one or more covariates in explaining the behavior under study. Further, its log-linear parameterization enables investigators to estimate its parameters using commonly available software that are developed for other purposes such as contingency table analysis.

References

Breslow, N. E., & Day, N. E. (1975). Indirect standardization and multiplicative models for rates, with reference to the age adjustment of cancer incidence and relative frequency data. *Journal of Chronic Diseases, 28*, 289–303.

Cox, D. R. (1972). Regression models and life-tables (with discussion). *Journal of the Royal Statistical Society B, 34*, 187–220.

Hoem, J. M. (1987). Statistical analysis of a multiplicative model and its application to the standardization of vital rates: A review. *International Statistical Review, 55*, 119–152.

Hoem, J. M. (1993). Classical demographic methods of analysis and modern event-history techniques. *IUSSP: Proceedings of the 22nd International Population Conference, Montreal, Canada 3,* 281–291.

National Statistics Office [Eritrea], & Macro International Inc. (1995). *Eritrea demographic and health survey, 1995*. Calverton: National Statistics Office & Macro International Inc.

Chapter 7
Modelling Immunization Coverage in Nigeria Using Bayesian Structured Additive Regression

Samson Babatunde Adebayo and Waheed Babatunde Yahya

7.1 Introduction

The introduction and usage of different kinds of vaccines have contributed immensely to the eradication of some of the dreaded diseases in many developed countries. Immunization has remained the most cost-effective mechanism through which the outbreak of common diseases is prevented in many developing countries (Odusanya et al. 2000, 2003). More than two million deaths among children are averted all over the world annually through vaccination against some early childhood diseases such as diphtheria, tetanus, pertussis, measles and hepatitis B (Duclos et al. 2009). This improvement in childcare notwithstanding, vaccine preventable diseases still contribute significantly to the global child mortality cases (Centre for Global Development 2005). Particularly in 2002, the World health Organization (WHO) estimated under five mortality cases that are attributable to vaccine preventable diseases to be 1.4 million worldwide. This was about 14 % of total global child mortality all over the world with considerable number of cases being from third-world countries.

In 1974, the Expanded Program on Immunization (EPI) was initiated by the World Health Assembly to assist in coordinating the efforts of public health programmes especially in developing countries to ensure full immunization of

S.B. Adebayo (✉)
Planning, Research and Statistics, National Agency for Food and Drug Administration and Control (NAFDAC), Plot 2032 Olusegun Obasanjo Way, Wuse Zone 7, PMB 5116, Abuja, Nigeria
e-mail: adebayo_sba@yahoo.com

W.B. Yahya
Department of Statistics, University of Ilorin, Ilorin, Nigeria
e-mail: wbyahya@unilorin.edu.ng

N.-B. Kandala and G. Ghilagaber (eds.), *Advanced Techniques for Modelling Maternal and Child Health in Africa*, The Springer Series on Demographic Methods and Population Analysis 34, DOI 10.1007/978-94-007-6778-2_7,

all children under one year of age against common diseases like poliomyelitis, smallpox, diphtheria, tetanus, measles, tuberculosis, pertussis and so on. The EPI further aimed at ensuring that new vaccines and preventive health interventions are extended to children in parts of the world. One of the objectives of the EPI was that by 2010, global routine immunization coverage of all children under one year of age should reach 90 % (Hadler et al. 2004). To ensure that the objectives of the EPI are achieved and sustained especially in poor countries of the world, the Global Alliance for Vaccines and Immunization (GAVI), a coalition of bodies such as United Nations Children Emergency Fund (UNICEF), WHO and the World Bank was created in 1999 (Brugha et al. 2002). This body was enhanced by the establishment of Global Immunization Vision and Strategy (GIVS) (2006–2015) in 2005 at the 58th World Health Assembly. A common objective for establishing both GAVI and GIVS among others is to strengthen national immunization program and improve child and maternal health especially in the third world countries (Bilous et al. 2006).

The huge amount of resources and efforts committed by WHO, UNICEF and World Bank (WHO and UNICEF 2005, 2009) at ensuring full immunization of children all over the world were justified in 2007 when out of 129 million surviving children, a total of 105 million (about 81 %) children under one year of age were vaccinated worldwide with three doses of diphtheria, pertussis and tetanus (DPT3) vaccine while the number of unvaccinated children decreased to 24 million from 33 million reported in the year 2000 (Duclos et al. 2009).

Stemming out of GAVI/GIVS alliance, the impacts and successes of several routine immunization programmes and the EPI initiated in Nigeria have been presented in previous studies, (Clements et al. 2006; Odusanya et al. 2008; Jenkins et al. 2008; WHO 2008a). For instance, significant reduction in the spread of wild polioviruses in 2003 in six notable countries worldwide, was reported by WHO in 2004 (WHO 2004, 2006). Jenkins et al. (2008) discussed the efficacy of monovalent type 1 oral poliovirus vaccine and its immunization coverage in northern Nigeria. It was reported in Jenkins et al. (2008) that immunization efforts contributed significantly to the reduction of the overall number of cases of poliomyelitis by 75 % in Nigeria in 2007. Odusanya et al. (2008) examined some determinants of vaccination coverage in a selected rural area in Nigeria and observed positive association between completeness of vaccination and knowledge of mothers on immunization. Although, about 80 % coverage of DPT/OPV vaccinations was reported, more efforts are still needed for mothers to be fully aware of the need to fully immunize their children against common diseases. Similar results were reported by Oladokun et al. (2010) in their study. In a different study, Ngowu et al. (2008) reported the benefits of immunization and other systemic factors on child mortality reduction in Nigeria. More discussions on immunization coverage and its benefits in Nigeria can be found in Babaniyi and Spiegel (1993); Okoro and Egwu (1994); Odusanya et al. (2000); Centres for Diseases Control (CDC) (1999); and Ambe et al. (2001) among others.

Despite the tremendous improvement in global vaccination coverage as reported in various studies (Patriarca et al. 1991; Dabbagh et al. 2007; Lim et al. 2008; Djibuti et al. 2009; Koumaré et al. 2009; Sanou et al. 2009), 75 % of the unimmunized children worldwide live in African and Asian countries with Nigeria and other African countries and Indian having the highest low coverage of child immunization respectively (Duclos et al. 2009). Apart from socio-cultural factors, the low vaccination profile in some parts of Nigeria is not unconnected with low literacy levels in the affected areas. A typical example was an erroneous belief in some northern parts of the country that vaccinations are designed by the western world to reduce (control) the population of the world, Ambe et al. (2001). This wrong perception of some people about immunization is hitherto impacting negatively on the extent of immunization coverage in those parts of Nigeria, Clements et al. (2006). This has consequently resulted into the existence of many EPI difficult-to-reach (DTR) areas for vaccinations in Nigeria. In 2003 precisely, there was a temporary suspension of all poliovirus immunization in some northern states of Nigeria. This contributed immensely to the high spate of poliomyelitis endemic in the country during the period before poliovirus immunization was reinstituted thereafter (Pallansch and Sandhu 2006). Till date, routine immunization coverage is still low in northern Nigeria.

In spite of the efforts from government and donor agencies, Nigeria, as at present, still ranked among the least successful sub-Sahara African countries with improved records in child survival, (Global Polio Eradication Initiative (GPEI) 2008; IRIN 2007). This is not unconnected with her low level of vaccinations coverage against some common early childhood diseases since low vaccination coverage increases the risks of a child being exposed to various vaccines preventable diseases. The apparent success achieved at reducing measles mortality in some parts of Africa is still fragile because of low level of routine measles immunization coverage (WHO 2008b; Duclos et al. 2009). Therefore, more efforts are still needed to be concentrated at sustaining the current level of vaccination and developing strategies of gaining access into the identified DTR areas for full vaccinations of all the children in Nigeria to be ensured. Accomplishment of this task would surely guarantee remarkable reduction in child (neonatal, infant & under-five) mortality in Nigeria. This would in turn contribute significantly to the attainment of United Nations Millennium Development Goals (MDG 4) that calls for a two-third reduction in child mortality by 2015 as compared to 1990 levels.

Empirical evidence has revealed substantial geographical variations on immunization coverage in Nigeria (NPC [Nigeria] and Macro ICF 2009). In an attempt to address the challenge of low vaccination coverage in Nigeria, this chapter therefore provides detailed analyses of immunization coverage in Nigeria modelling possible trend and geographical variations of vaccination coverage in the presence of other covariates using 1999, 2003 and 2008 Nigeria Demographic and Health Surveys (NDHS) data. We adopt a flexible Bayesian structured additive regression approach which permits joint estimation of trend, non linear effects of continuous covariates, geographical variations and fixed effects of categorical covariates. In the present study, we investigate the influence of bio-demographic variables such as maternal and partner (spouse) educational attainment, mother's age at the birth of child as well as some other socio-economic variables on vaccination coverage in Nigeria using flexible geoadditive models. The approach here permits a joint estimation of the usual linear effects of categorical covariates, nonlinear effects of continuous covariates and small-area district effects on vaccination coverage within a unified structured additive Bayesian framework. This study is aimed at providing policymakers with tools to design effective interventions which can lead to frugal utilization of the scarce resources. The results from this study would guide policy makers at directing the scarce resources to states where they are crucially needed.

Two methods of data analysis were employed in this Chapter. The first approach compares children who received full vaccination with those without full vaccination. Under this setting, a binary outcome variable is obtained in which a probit or logit model is most appropriate. In the second method, we differentiated children who received no vaccination from those who received some and those who received the complete vaccination within the duration. Thus an ordered outcome vaccinations is conceptualized and cumulative probit models are fitted to the data within the Bayesian framework. Details of the two methods are presented in the next sections.

7.2 Data Description

The datasets used for this study are the NDHS data for the 3 years 1999, 2003 and 2008. The Demographic and Health Surveys (DHS) are national representative surveys of men and women of reproductive age and their children in many developing countries of the world. These surveys are funded by *United States Agency for International Development* (USAID) for the purpose of collecting vital up-to-date information on health related matters such as mortality, morbidity, vaccinations and general health conditions of children and their mothers, as well as on many other socio-economic related variables that directly affect the growth and development of the children ((NPC) [Nigeria], 2000; NPC [Nigeria] and ORC Macro 2004).

Information on vaccination coverage and on types of vaccines administered on the children through different immunization schedules are also included in all the NDHS data. The types of vaccines provided free by donor agencies to Nigerian children are *Bacille Calmette Guerin* (BCG) vaccines and *Oral Polio Vaccine* (OPV) to guide against tuberculosis and poliomyelitis respectively. Others are *Diphtheria, Pertussis, and Tetanus* (DPT) and measles vaccines. According to *Nigerian National Program on Immunization* (NNPI) schedule (which is adapted from the WHO immunization schedule), a child is considered to be fully vaccinated if he or she has received a BCG, three doses of DPT (i.e. DPT1, DPT2, DPT3), at least three doses of OPV (i.e. OPV0, OPV1, OPV2), and one dose of measles vaccines (NPC [Nigeria] and ICF Macro 2009).

7.3 Structured Additive Regression Model and Analysis

7.3.1 Structured Additive Regression Model

All analyses in this Chapter are based on Structured Additive Regression (STAR) model proposed by Fahrmeir et al. (2004), Kneib and Fahrmeir (2005), Kneib and Fahrmeir (2006), and Kneib and Fahrmeir (2007), with a flexible geoadditive (Kammann and Wand 2003) predictor accounting for the effects of different types of covariates. STAR embraces the usual famous regression models such as generalized additive models (GAM), generalized additive mixed models (GAMM), generalized geoadditive mixed models (GGAMM), stepwise regression models among others. We consider two outcome variables for immunization coverage in Nigeria. The first being a dichotomous variable, differentiating children aged 12 months and above who received full immunization from their counterparts who did not receive full immunisation (i.e. either some or none) based on the datasets from the 1999, 2003 and 2008 Nigeria Demographic and Health Surveys. This follows a Binomial distribution whose dependence and effect on a predictor of interest can be modelled either through a probit or logit model. Here we chose a probit link for computational reasons as a convenient approach to screen effect of different covariates on the outcome variable. The second outcome variable was considered as an ordered categorical variable; differentiating children who received partial immunization and those who received full immunization from their counterparts who did not receive any. In other words, this results in a 3 – level ordinal outcome. The dependence of this on a predictor of interest can be modelled through a cumulative probit model.

In both cases, a database for analyses was created for children aged 12 months and above. This is to permit proper evaluation of child immunization coverage with the aim of eliciting children who received full immunization. In total, 23, 913 children involved in the surveys were 12 months or older and included in the database.

Generalized linear models (e.g. Fahrmeir and Tutz 2001) assume that, given covariates vector $\boldsymbol{x}$ and unknown parameters β, the distribution of the response variable y belongs to an exponential family, with mean $\mu = E(y|\boldsymbol{x}, \beta)$ linked to a linear predictor η by

$$\mu = h(\eta) \qquad \eta = \mathrm{x}'\beta. \tag{7.1}$$

Here h is a known response function, and β are unknown regression parameters. However, in most practical regression situations, we are often faced with the problem of rigid assumption of linear effect of continuous covariates in the datasets on the predictor. Sometimes, observations may be spatially or temporally correlated. Furthermore, covariates may not be able to sufficiently describe any inherent heterogeneity among individuals or units. To overcome these difficulties, we replace the strictly linear predictor in (7.1) by a structured additive predictor (7.2).

Consider a set of regression observations (y_i, x_i, s_i, v_i), $i = 1, \ldots, n$, where y_i is either a binary or categorical response variable, a vector $x = (x_1, \ldots, x_p)'$ of continuous covariates (say respondents' age), $s_i = (1, \ldots, S)$ the state (district) where respondent i lived during the survey and a further vector $v = (v_1, \ldots, v_q)'$ of categorical covariates. Usually one intends to jointly model the dependence of y_i on continuous, spatial and categorical covariates within the context of generalized additive model (Hastie and Tibshirani 1990).

The predictor η_i for the *structured additive regression* (STAR) model can be defined as

$$\eta_i = \sum_{j=1}^{p} f_j(x_{ij}) + f_{spat}(s_i) + v_i'\beta \tag{7.2}$$

where $f_1, \ldots, fp$ are nonlinear (unknown) smooth functions of the metrical covariates, f_{spat} is the nonlinear effect of spatial covariates and $\beta_i = (\beta_1, \ldots, \beta_q)'$ is a vector of fixed effect parameters for the categorical covariates including *time* (i.e. year of study with 1999 as the reference category). One may further split up spatial effects f_{spat} into spatially correlated (structured) and uncorrelated (unstructured) effects as

$$f_{spat}(s_i) = f_{str}(s_i) + f_{unstr}(s_i).$$

A rationale behind this is that a spatial effect is a surrogate of many unobserved influential factors, some of which may be a strong spatial structure and others may only be present locally.

7.3.2 Model Specification

Model A: According to the World Health Organisation (WHO), each child is expected to have completed an immunization schedule before celebrating his/her first birthday. Through this, a child is considered fully vaccinated if he or she has received a BCG vaccination against tuberculosis, three doses of DPT, vaccine to prevent diphtheria, pertussis, and tetanus; at least three doses of polio vaccine; and one dose of measles vaccine within the first year (NPC [Nigeria] and ICF Macro 2009). A binary variable that describes level of vaccination coverage as

$$y_i = \begin{cases} 1: \text{if a child aged 12 months and beyond has received all the} \\ \text{recommended vaccines} \\ 0: \text{otherwise} \end{cases}$$

was created.

Model B: Here, the immunisation schedule (according to WHO) that a child should receive was categorised into none, partial and full. This was aimed at eliciting information about those children who received partial vaccination separate from those who did not receive any vaccination. Therefore, a three-level ordinal outcome variable describing level of vaccination coverage was created as

$$y_i = \begin{cases} 1 : \text{if a child aged 12 months and beyond has received all the} \\ \text{recommended vaccines,} \\ 2 : \text{if a child aged 12 months and beyond only received some} \\ \text{recommended vaccinations,} \\ 3 : \text{if a child aged 12 months and beyond did not receive any vaccination.} \end{cases}$$

In an attempt to explore possible determinants, trend and spatial variations on level of vaccination coverage in Nigeria between 1999 and 2008, analyses were based on predictor (7.1). For model A, influence of determinants of level of vaccination coverage was modelled through a binary model assuming a probit link within a Bayesian perspective that jointly accounts for nonlinear, time, fixed and spatial effects. Bayesian geoadditive probit model is preferred for computational reasons as a convenient approach to screen a number of different models (Crook et al. 2003). There are considerable computational advantages using the probit formulation and an implementation based on latent variables. In particular, it allows for fast block updates of the parameters representing the non-parametric smoothing functions of the nonparametric effects (Fahrmeir and Lang 2001a; Rue 2001). Furthermore, results using the probit model are qualitatively very similar to logit estimates (Fahrmeir and Tutz 2001). Using the probit link as an approximation to the logit model is very common in many other areas of statistics, for example, in measurement error models as discussed in Carroll et al. (1995, p. 64).

The predictors in these models include non-parametric effect of a metrical covariate (mothers age at the birth of the child – measured in years, and child's age – measured in months), spatial components and linear part in an additive form. Similarly for model B, a cumulative probit model was assumed with the aim of modelling influence of determinants of level of vaccination coverage within a Bayesian perspective that jointly accounts for nonlinear, time, fixed and spatial effects in a similar manner as in model A. In both cases (i.e. models A and B), predictor (7.1) was used to explore the dependence of vaccination coverage on the specified covariates.

7.3.3 Cumulative Probit Model

Let us consider the regression model based on multicategorical outcomes. Such models can be motivated from latent variables such that the response variable y can be observed in ordered categories 1, ..., k. It is postulated that y is a categorized version of a latent variable

$$U = \eta + \varepsilon \tag{7.3}$$

obtained through the threshold mechanism

$$y = r, \ \theta_{r\text{-}1} < U \leq \theta_r, \qquad \mathrm{r} = 1, \ldots, \mathrm{k}$$

with thresholds $-\infty = \theta_0 < \theta_1 < \ldots < \theta_k = \infty$. We assume that the error variable ε has a distribution function F, hence it follows that y obeys a cumulative model

$$p(y \leq r|\eta) = F(\theta_r - \eta), \tag{7.4}$$

where η is the geoadditive predictor described in (7.1) which can be specified for a particular child i. To enhance identifiability, functions are centred about zero, thus the fixed effect parameters automatically include an intercept term. In the application to model B, level of vaccination coverage y is considered as a three-ordered categorical version of the latent continuous variable U. Here ε is assumed to have a standard normal distribution function, i.e.

$$p(y \leq r|\eta = x, s, v) = \Phi(\theta_r - \eta)$$

yielding a cumulative probit model. Cumulative models based on category boundaries or threshold approaches (Edwards and Thurstone 1952) are commonly used in ordinal regression.

7.4 Bayesian Inference

Within a Bayesian context, all parameters and functions are usually considered as random variables upon which appropriate priors are assumed. Independent diffuse priors are assumed on the parameters of fixed effects. For the non-linear effects, Bayesian P-splines prior based on Lang and Brezger (2004); and Brezger and Lang (2006) was assumed. Omitting indices, each function f is represented or approximated through a linear combination

$$p(z) = \sum_{j=1}^{J} \beta_j B_j(z)$$

of B-spline basis functions. Smoothness of function f is achieved by penalizing differences of coefficients of adjacent B-splines (Eilers and Marx 1996) or, in our Bayesian approach, by assuming first or second order Gaussian random walk smoothness priors

$$\beta_1 = \beta_{j-1} + u_1 \qquad \beta_1 = 2\beta_{j-1} - \beta_{j-2} + u_1,$$

with *i.i.d.* errors $u_1 \sim N(0, \tau^2)$. The variance τ^2 controls the smoothness of *f*. Assigning a weakly informative inverse Gamma prior $\tau^2 \sim IG(\varepsilon, \varepsilon)$, ε small, it is estimated jointly with the basis function coefficients.

For the geographical effects $f_{spat}(s)$, $s = 1, \ldots, S$, we assume a Gaussian Markov random field prior. Basically, this is an extension of first order random walk priors to two-dimensional spatial arrays, see Rue and Held (2005) for general information.

For the structured spatial effects $f_{str}(s)$ we chose a Gaussian Markov random field prior which is common in spatial statistics, see Besag et al. (1991).

$$(f_{str}(s) | f_{str}(t); t \neq s, \tau^2) \sim N\left(\sum_{t \in \partial_s} \frac{f_{str}(t)}{N_s}, \frac{\tau^2}{N_s}\right)$$

Unstructured spatial effects are *i.i.d.* random effects.

In order to be able to estimate the smoothing parameters for non linear and spatial effects simultaneously, highly dispersed but proper hyper-priors are assigned to them. Hence for all variance components, an inverse gamma distribution with hyperparameters *a* and *b* is chosen, e.g. $\tau^2 \sim IG(a, b)$. Standard choices of hyperparameters are $a = 1$ and $b = 0.005$ or $a = b = 0.001$.

Similar to Fahrmeir and Lang (2001a, b), posterior samples are drawn from full conditionals of single parameters or blocks of parameters given the rest and the data is enhanced through MCMC simulations. Let α represent the vector of all function evaluations and spatial effects (i.e. $\alpha = (f, f_{spat}, \beta)$) and τ represent the vector of all variance components. For the binomial probit model, Bayesian inference can then be based on the posterior

$$p(\alpha, \tau, \beta | y) \propto p(y | \alpha, \beta) p(\alpha | \tau) p(\tau) p(\beta), \tag{7.5}$$

where $p(y|\alpha, \beta)$ is the likelihood function of the data given the parameters. An additional parameter *U* of the continuous latent variable must be included in the posterior analysis of the cumulative probit models. Therefore, their posteriors can be based on

$$p(\alpha, \tau, \beta, U | y) \propto p(y | U) p(U | \alpha, \beta) p(\alpha | \tau) p(\tau) p(\beta). \tag{7.6}$$

Details about the sampling schemes for both binomial probit and cumulative probit models are discussed in the manual of the software. For the models considered in the applications, all the full conditionals involved have known distributions, hence a Gibbs sampler can be used for the MCMC simulations. Efficiency is guaranteed by Cholesky decomposition for band matrices (Rue 2001). The approach was implemented in BayesX, a statistical package for Bayesian analysis and all computations were performed with the software.

Sensitivity to the choice of priors was investigated in this case-study through different means. First, we compared results from MCMC with similar models using Restricted Maximum Likelihood (REML) approach. Second, hyperpriors for smoothing parameters were varied systematically. Lastly, we considered different priors such as 'Markov Random Field', 'Two dimensional P-spline with first order random walk penalty' which is known as *geospline*, for spatial effects. For model choice and comparison, the deviance information criterion (DIC) which was developed by Spiegelhalter, et al. (2002) was used. BayesX, software for Bayesian inference using structured additive regression models was used for all analyses (Brezger et al. 2009).

Fully Bayesian inference is based on the posterior distribution of the model parameters, which is not of a known form. Therefore, MCMC sampling from full conditionals for nonlinear effects, spatial effects, fixed effects and smoothing parameters was used for posterior analysis. For nonlinear and spatial effects, Metropolis-Hastings algorithms based on conditional prior proposals (Knorr-Held 1999) and iteratively weighted least squares (IWLS) proposals suggested by Brezger and Lang (2006) as an extension of Gamerman and Lopes (2006) were applied. Similar results are obtained from both sampling schemes but we relies on Iteratively Weighted Least Square (IWLS) proposal which has good mixing properties without requiring tuning.

7.5 Data Analysis and Discussions

7.5.1 Analysis

To explore impact of trend, demographic characteristics, continuous variables and spatial effect on level of vaccination coverage in Nigeria between 1999 and 2008, structured additive regression model was fitted. This method of analysis permits joint estimation of time, spatial, nonlinear and fixed effects simultaneously. In this Chapter, all analyses were based on predictor (7.1) for models with outcome variables described as *models A* and *B*. Through this, one would be able to identify possible effect of the predictor on a child receiving full vaccination coverage compared with others who either received partial (i.e. incomplete according to WHO's immunisation schedule) or did not receive any among children who were 12 months and above as at the time of the survey. Covariates were included in the model based on their significance at bivariate level (see Table 7.1).

Model building was guided by the use of Deviance Information Criterion (DIC) proposed by Spiegelhalter et al. (2002). We started the process from a very simple model; where only year of study (trend) was included in the predictor to a complex model involving, trend, demographic characteristics of the respondents (mothers), partner's (husband) educational attainment, random effect of cluster (where respondents were sampled) and that of unstructured spatial effect, structured

Table 7.1 Bivariate analysis of vaccination coverage according to selected characteristics in 1999, 2003 and 2008 Nigeria demographic and health survey

	Level of vaccination coverage				
Variables	None	Partial	Full	P-value[a]	Total respondents
Year of study					
1999	35.9	55.7	8.4	<0.0001	2,109
2003	22.8	71.6	5.6		3,212
2008	29.0	56.9	14.1		18,592
Geopolitical zones					
North Central	11.4	58.9	29.7	<0.0001	2,560
North East	16.3	59.0	24.7		2,304
North West	43.7	53.5	2.8		6,434
South East	27.1	58.1	14.8		4,325
South West	33.6	61.8	4.7		5,457
South South	13.8	66.0	20.2		2,833
Place of residence					
Rural	33.1	58.3	8.6	<0.0001	16,969
Urban	18.0	60.1	21.8		6,944
Sex					
Male	29.0	58.7	12.3	0.579	12,161
Female	28.5	58.9	12.6		11,752
Respondents' education					
None	44.1	52.5	3.4	<0.0001	11,931
Primary	19.5	66.9	13.6		5,561
Secondary	9.0	65.6	25.4		5,256
Higher	4.5	54.2	41.3		1,165
Partners' education					
None	45.3	51.6	3.2	<0.0001	9,579
Primary	22.1	64.2	13.8		5,198
Secondary	16.2	64.6	19.3		5,953
Higher	12.2	60.1	27.8		2,645
Birth order					
More than 4	30.5	60.5	9.0	<0.0001	4,398
Firstborn	28.2	55.2	16.6		11,232
Second to Fourth	30.5	60.5	9.0		8,283
Antenatal visits					
None	47.4	48.8	3.8	<0.0001	6,274
1–9	15.1	67.1	17.8		5,769
More than 9	7.3	64.4	28.3		1,928
Place of delivery					
At home/others	38.2	56.5	5.4	<0.0001	15,902
Hospital	8.8	64.2	27.1		7,844

[a]All test are based on Pearson X^2 test of differences of proportion

Table 7.2 Summary of the DIC as measure of model selection for the fitted models

	Binomial probit			Cumulative probit		
Model predictors	D(bar)	pD	DIC	D(bar)	pD	DIC
M1: trend alone	19,455.39	3.13	19,461.65	55,921.48	4.00	5,929.48
M2: trend + demographic characteristics	15,835.00	17.84	15,870.69	50,146.16	18.85	50,183.87
M3: trend + random effects (state and household) + demographic characteristics	15,313.30	57.87	15,429.04	49,051.03	75.86	49,202.74
M4: m1 + spatial (no random effect)	15,332.20	47.50	15,427.19	49,104.11	49.20	49,202.50
M5: m3 + nonlinear effect of continuous variables	13,845.28	51.71	13,948.70	37,304.78	60.80	37,426.37
M6: spatial + trend + random (state and House hold) + nonlinear of continuous + extended fixed effects	8,134.73	64.48	8,263.70	20,886.75	82.92	21,052.58
M7: spatial + trend + nonlinear of continuous + extended fixed effects	8,130.33	58.06	8,246.46	20,912.07	65.42	21,042.91

spatial effects, nonlinear effect of continuous variables, etc. Some of the fitted models explored are stated below:

M1: η = Trend alone
M2: η = Trend + Demographic characteristics
M3: η = Trend + Random effects (States and cluster)+Demographic characteristics
M4: η = Trend + Spatial effect (i.e. M1 + spatial)
M5: η = M3 + nonlinear effect of continuous variables
M6: η = Trend + Spatial + Random (States and Clusters) + Nonlinear of continuous + extended fixed effects (including partners' educational attainment)
M7: η = Trend + spatial + nonlinear of continuous + extended fixed effects (including partners' educational attainment)

It turned out that, models with predictor M7 is the best in terms of the DIC (see Table 7.2). Therefore, discussion of results in Sects. 7.5.2 and 7.5.3 shall be based on model M7. All analyses are carried out based on BayesX 2.0.1 – software for modelling structured additive regression modelling through a Bayesian perspective (Brezger et al. 2009). This is available under http://www.stat.uni-muenchen.de/~bayesX

7.5.2 *Results*

For the binomial probit model that assumes model A as the outcome variable, Table 7.3 presents findings of the fixed effect model. A significant positive

Table 7.3 Posterior estimates for binomial and cumulative models with predictor M7. Shown are the posterior means, std errors and 95 % credible intervals

	Binomial model with predictor M7				Cumulative probit model with predictor M7			
			95 % credible interval				95 % credible interval	
Variables	Mean	Std error	Lower	Upper	Mean	Std error	Lower	Upper
Constant	−2.160	0.254	−4.460	−3.441	−0.059	0.110	−0.279	0.149
Trend								
Year 1999 (ref)	Ref				Ref			
Year 2003	−0.141	0.143	−0.520	0.020	0.252	0.043	0.163	0.339
Year 2008	0.412	0.096	0.587	0.981	0.315	0.031	0.254	0.376
Geopolitical zones								
North Central (ref)	Ref				Ref			
North East	−0.350	0.494	−1.777	0.122	0.166	0.234	−0.289	0.619
North West	−0.503	0.452	−1.996	−0.155	−0.012	0.212	−0.412	0.399
South East	0.092	0.432	−0.557	1.081	−0.098	0.238	−0.560	0.379
South West	−0.298	0.353	−1.244	0.137	−0.188	0.156	−0.489	0.100
South South	0.072	0.444	−0.638	1.147	0.090	0.255	−0.382	0.631
Place of residence								
Rural (ref)	Ref				Ref			
Urban	0.211	0.065	0.251	0.506	0.169	0.026	0.120	0.220
Sex								
Male (ref)	Ref				Ref			
Female	0.010	0.056	−0.079	0.138	0.028	0.021	−0.013	0.071
Respondents' educ								
None (ref)	Ref				Ref			
Primary	0.239	0.101	0.265	0.678	0.256	0.032	0.195	0.318
Secondary	0.419	0.107	0.591	0.993	0.520	0.040	0.442	0.604
Higher	0.572	0.138	0.758	1.281	0.694	0.062	0.577	0.812
Partners' educ								
None (ref)	Ref				Ref			
Primary	0.180	0.102	0.176	0.578	0.234	0.032	0.173	0.297
Secondary	0.160	0.106	0.134	0.550	0.190	0.033	0.123	0.256
Higher	0.323	0.119	0.406	0.858	0.315	0.045	0.226	0.405
Birth order								
More than 4	Ref				Ref			
Firstborn	0.193	0.120	0.105	0.573	0.001	0.043	−0.085	0.087
Second to Fourth	0.057	0.078	−0.45	0.252	−0.019	0.029	−0.081	0.145
Antenatal visits								
None (ref)	Ref				Ref			
1–9	0.064	0.038	0.031	0.173	0.113	0.016	0.081	0.145
More than 9	−0.053	0.038	−0.153	−0.008	−0.100	0.016	−0.132	−0.068
Place of delivery								
At home/others	Ref				Ref			
Hospital	0.433	0.069	0.634	0.905	0.477	0.029	0.420	0.532
Threshold 1 (θ_1)	NA	NA	NA	NA	0.059	0.110	−0.149	0.279
Threshold 2 (θ_2)	NA	NA	NA	NA	2.234	0.112	2.018	2.463

NA not applicable

trend was observed between 2008 and 1999 compared with 2003 and 1999. Full immunization coverage varies according to the geopolitical zones with North West having significantly lower full vaccination. Residing in urban areas is significantly associated with full immunization coverage as children in urban areas are more likely to be fully immunized compared with their counterparts in rural areas. A significant positive association of respondents' and partners' educational attainment was evident on full vaccination coverage. Firstborns are more likely to have received full vaccination compared with their counterparts who are later than fourth born. Children who were delivered at the hospital are more likely to receive full vaccination coverage compared with those who were delivered at home or other places. Children from mothers who had at most primary, or at most secondary or at most higher education are more likely to receive full vaccination coverage compared with their counterparts with no formal education. Similarly children whose fathers have secondary education or higher are significantly more likely to receive full vaccination compared with those whose fathers have at most primary education of no formal education. Children whose parents received between 1 to 9 antenatal visits are positively associated with receiving full immunization coverage.

Now consider the cumulative probit *model B*. Estimates of the fixed effect parameters are shown in Table 7.3. Similar conclusions can be drawn from the fixed effects as in *model A*. Furthermore, estimates of the threshold parameters θ_1 and θ_2 for categories 'Full vaccination' and 'partial vaccination' respectively are included in Table 7.3. For interpretation of the results of threshold parameters, higher (lower) values correspond to full vaccination. For instance, a positive sign of θ_1 and θ_2 signifies a shift on the latent scale to the left side, yielding a higher probability for category 'full vaccination' and partial vaccination compared with 'no vaccination'. For fixed effects, the directions of findings are similar for cumulative probit models. However, effect of firstborns is not statistically significant.

Turning attention to the nonlinear effects of child's age and mother's age at the birth of the child, Fig. 7.1 presents findings for both *models A* and *B*. From the binomial probit model, a steady decline in full vaccination coverage was evident from children who are 12 months old and beyond. This shows a possible improvement on full vaccination coverage in the recent time compared with the older children. In other words, the younger children are more likely to be fully immunized compared with older children. For cumulative probit model, effect of child's age is almost an approximately zig-zag pattern. On respondents' (mothers) age at birth of the child, the pattern is similar for both binomial probit and cumulative probit models. There is a steady increase in child's immunization coverage up till mother's age birth of 21 years before it stabilises between age 22 and 42 years. This implies that children whose mothers are below 21 years (perhaps teenage mothers) are less likely to receive full immunization coverage compared with those children whose mothers are in the age range 22 and 42 years.

Figure 7.2 displays spatial effects for binomial probit and cumulative probit *models A* and *B* on map of Nigeria. The posterior means are shown in the left columns (a and c) while the corresponding posterior probabilities of significance of spatial effects are shown in the right columns (b and d). Looking at the maps of posterior probabilities, states with white colour are associated with significantly

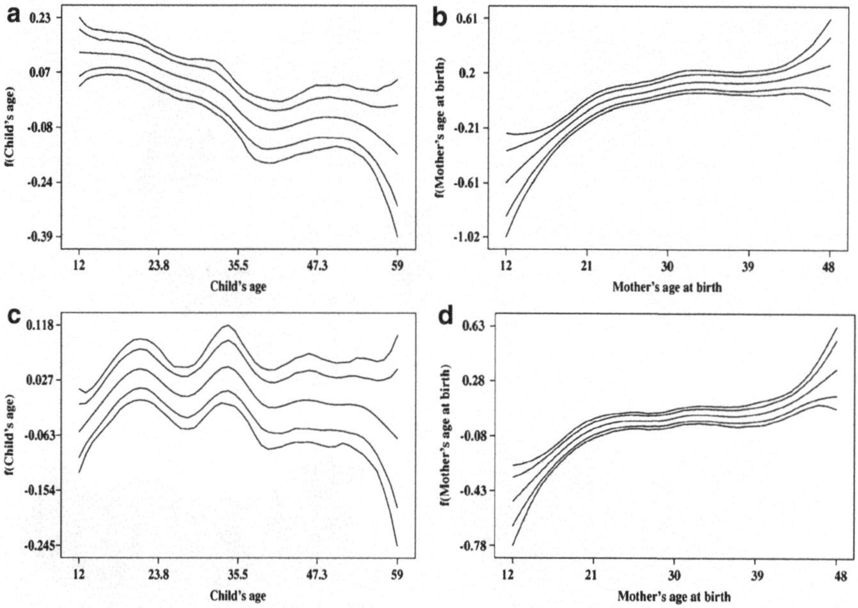

Fig. 7.1 Nonlinear effects of (**a**) Child's age and (**b**) Mother's age at birth [Binomial probit model], (**c**) Chld's age and (**d**) Mother's age at birth with their corresponding 95 % and 80 % credible intervals

high vaccination coverage, states with dark colour are associated with significantly low vaccination coverage while states with grey colour are associated with insignificant spatial effects. In other words, states with white colour have positive credible intervals, states with dark colour have negative credible intervals while states with grey have credible intervals that include zero. For instance, from the cumulative probit model; rather than assuming that all the states in the North East, North West and North Central are significantly associated with low vaccination coverage, this analysis has permitted us to identify that Kano, Sokoto and Zamfara in the North West; Jigawa, Yobe and Borno in North East; and Nassarawa in the North Central are associated with low vaccination coverage. Similarly, Lagos, Oyo, Osun, and Ekiti states in the South West; Ebonyi in the South East and FCT in the North Central are associated with high vaccination coverage. Similar inferences can be drawn from the binomial probit *model A* with Jigawa, Yobe and Benue states significantly associated with no or incomplete vaccination coverage while FCT, Lagos, Osun and Ekiti states are significantly associated with full immunization coverage.

7.5.3 Discussions

Structured additive regression models for binomial and cumulative probit models have been applied to the 1999, 2003 and 2008 Nigeria Demographic and Health Survey data on level of immunization coverage in Nigeria between 1999 and 2008 in

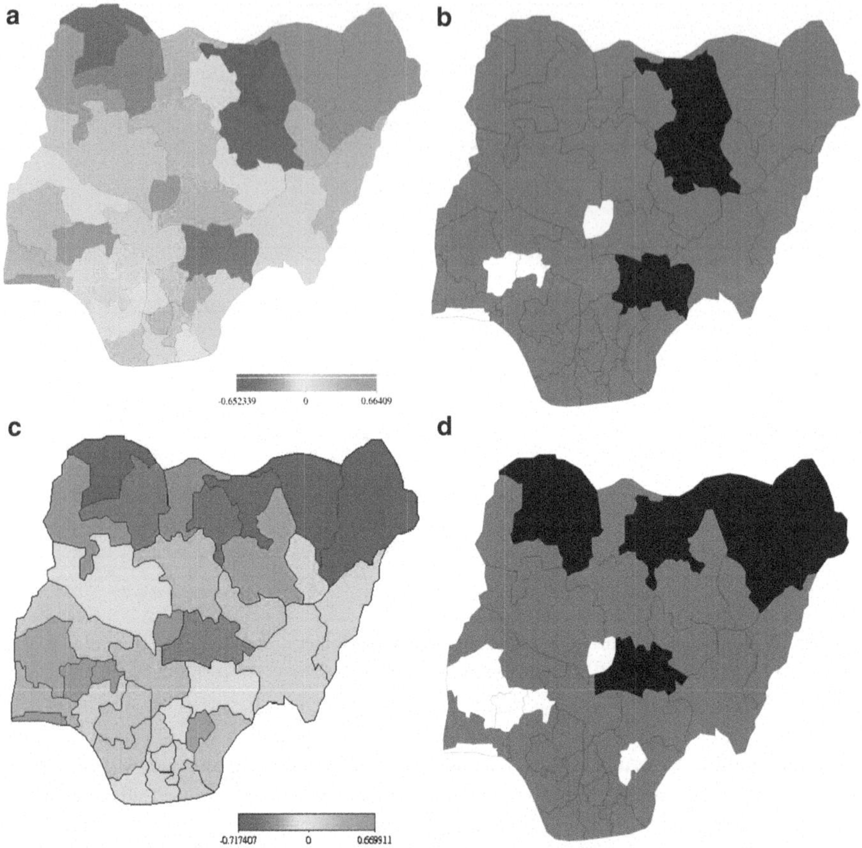

Fig. 7.2 Map of Nigeria showing spatial effect (**a**) and (**c**) for binomial and cumulative probit respectively; and the corresponding map of significance of spatial effects (**b**) and (**d**) for binomial and cumulative probit respectively

this Chapter. In this Section we discuss findings from the analysis and implications for policy formulation on improving immunization coverage in Nigeria. This Chapter has availed us the opportunity to discern states with partial or low immunization coverage with the aim of developing appropriate intervention strategy, which can help in improving immunization coverage.

In this paper, flexible modelling of small area district-specific effects is of great advantage compared to the usual parametric and frequentist approach. For instance, modelling of the effects of the 37 small area districts in Nigeria through a frequentist (parametric approach) would have led to creating 36 dummy variables resulting in superfluous parameters for only one variable. However, Bayesian geoadditive models have distinct advantages for exploring such small area spatial effects by allowing incorporation of spatial effects, nonlinear or time-varying effects of covariates as well as the usual linear effects in a joint model by assigning appropriate smoothness priors to them. Furthermore, this approach of analysis is useful for policy formulation so that governments of the districts (states) where vaccination is done partially or haphazardly can pay more attention to the cause of such. Perhaps it may be necessary to create more awareness on benefits of immunisation in such districts (states) or think of possible improvements. This will further assist government and policy makers on prudent use of the scarce resources, which is prominent in the country.

In this Chapter, the idea behind model B was to identify children who must have dropped out of the exercise. In this case, drop-outs are children who begin the vaccination schedule but do not complete it. Some of the reasons for this may not be unconnected with lack of information, poor services, time constraints; social, cultural or political barriers; misinformation and or distance. Therefore, this paper has revealed that some mothers initiated immunization of their children but dropped out somewhere along the line. So, monitoring drop-outs and devising strategies to prevent them deserve greater attention. With the increased use of expensive vaccines, if a child does not receive all of the doses required for full protection, the resources that have been used to partially vaccinate that child are mostly wasted (USAID 2009).

Reasons for lack of immunization vary from country to country. For instance, studies have shown that most people will use immunization services as long as they know when and where to bring their children to, whether those services are available, accessible, reliable and friendly. Thus the role of communication activities in achieving these conditions is important but not sufficient. Dissemination of information, training, supervision and other ways of improving services need to be employed in a mutually supportive way to promote complete and timely immunization of children and women at large.

Therefore, achievement of immunization goals is affected by the behaviour many groups including politicians, community leaders, health care providers, managers and supervisors, women of reproductive age, parents, children and their families.

7.6 The Impact of Immunization on Child's Health

Another area of maternal and child health issues which has not been sufficiently addressed in the literature is the assessment of all the various immunization vaccines on children's survival. This kind of assessment will serve as a measure to determine whether the core objective of immunizing the children (reduction in children mortality rate through protection of children against the basic early childhood diseases) through the various vaccines has been achieved or not. Thus, It is expected that mortality rate among the groups of children that were fully immunized should be considerably lower than the mortality rate of the unimmunized group of children.

To this end, we obtained from the three waves of the NDHS data discussed here, the number of children that were alive or dead having being vaccinated or unvaccinated against some of the commonly identified early childhood diseases that

Table 7.4 The contingency table showing the cross-classification of children by their full immunization status (fully immunized or non-immunized) and their survival status (dead or alive)

		1999			2003			2008		
		Child's status			Child's status			Child's status		
		Dead	Alive	Total	Dead	Alive	Total	Dead	Alive	Total
Full immunization	No	342	2,918	3,260	772	3,972	4,744	3,201	21,058	24,259
	Yes	0	292	292	0	394	394	0	4,388	4,388
	Total	342	3,210	3,552	772	4,366	5,138	3,201	25,446	28,647

could ordinarily result to child's death if left unchecked. From these statistics, it was possible to compute the conditional probability of survival outcome of a child (alive or dead) given that he or she is fully immunized or non-immunized.

According to NNPI schedule as earlier reported in section 6.2, a child is deemed to have been fully immunized if he or she has received a BCG, the three doses of DPT, one dose of measles and at least the first three doses of OPV vaccines. Based on this recommendation, the survival status (dead or alive) of all the children in each of the NDHS data set was cross-classified against their immunization status (fully immunized or not immunized) the results of which are presented in Table 7.4.

The results from Table 7.4 show that out of 3,552, 5,138 and 28,647 Nigerian children in the 1999, 2003 and 2008 Nigeria demographic and health surveys, only 292 (8.2 %), 394 (7.7 %) and 4,388 (15.3 %) of them were fully immunized against some of the early childhood diseases respectively. These results simply show that less than 20 % of children in Nigerian were fully immunized against the most commonly identified early childhood diseases as at 2008. This has impacted negatively on the survival of the children as revealed in Table 7.4.

It can be observed from Table 7.4 that the conditional probability that a fully immunized child will die is zero. In all the three data sets, all the 292, 394 and 4,388 children that were fully immunized according to 1999, 2003 and 2008 NDHS respectively survived beyond their fifth year of birth. On the other hand, of 3,260, 4,744 and 24,259 children that were not immunized (or not fully immunized) in the 1999, 2003 and 2008 NDHS data, 342, 772 and 3,201 of them died before their fifth year of birth. This translates to significant child mortality rates of 10.5 % in 1999 ($p < 0.0001$; 95 % CI: 0.0947, 0.1161), 16.3 % in 2003 ($p < 0.0001$; 95 % CI: 0.1524, 0.1736) and 13.2 % in 2008 ($p < 0.0001$; 95 % CI: 0.1277, 0.1363) within the group of unimmunized children. Based on these results, it is very clear that more efforts should be directed at ensuring full compliance to the internationally recommended immunization schedule by nursing mothers in Nigeria in order to stem the increasing trend of child mortality.

In addition to the above, we assess the impact of OPV and DPT vaccines on child's survival using the three NDHS data sets. The choice of these two vaccines is informed by their significant impacts on the survival of children during the first 5 years of birth (Taylor et al. 1996).

In Table 7.5, we present the survival status (dead or alive) of all the children in the 1999, 2003 and 2008 NDHS data cross-classified by their OPV immunization

Table 7.5 The contingency table showing the cross-classification of children by their polio immunization status (fully immunized or non-immunized for Polio) and their survival status (dead or alive)

		1999			2003			2008		
		Child's status			Child's status			Child's status		
		Dead	Alive	Total	Dead	Alive	Total	Dead	Alive	Total
Full Polio vaccines	No	342	2,907	3,249	772	4,056	4,828	3,201	21,336	24,537
	Yes	0	303	303	0	310	310	0	4,110	4,110
	Total	342	3,210	3,552	772	4,366	5,138	3,201	25,446	28,647

status (fully immunized or not immunized). Also, tables for the cross-classification of children by their survival status (dead or alive) and their DPT immunization status (fully immunized or not immunized) were obtained, but these were not presented due to space. However, a child is considered to be fully immunized by both OPV and DPT vaccines if he or she has received OPV0, OPV1, OPV2 and DPT1, DPT2, DPT3 vaccines respectively.

In agreement with the results reported in Table 7.4, the results in Table 7.5 generally revealed that all the children that died in 1999, 2003 and 2008 based on the respective data were those children that did not received the full dose of oral polio vaccines as recommended. Interestingly, all the children that received the full OPV survived beyond their fifth year of birth between 1999 and 2008 covered by the data. The results are the same for those children that received full dose of DPT vaccines. In all cases, the proportion of child's deaths due to lack of (full dosage of) OPV and DPT vaccines in the children were all significantly different from zero across the three sets of NDHS data considered ($p < 0.0001$).

7.7 Conclusion

This Chapter has provided readers with opportunity for flexibly modelling of nonlinear effects, spatial effects that incorporate neighbourhood influence, fixed effect and possibly random and interaction effects. In our analysis, we attempted random and interaction effects at an exploratory stage but both were found not to be significant. At another stage of the analysis, effect of continuous covariates i.e. child's age and mother's age at birth was assumed to be linearly related to *models A* and *B* and modelled parametrically. Even though these effects were significant in the parametric models, however, the model with smooth (nonlinear) functions of the covariates was found to be better in terms of the DIC. Evidently effects of child's age and mother's age at birth are non-linear, and an assumption of linear dependence a priori would have been too rigid and resulted in erroneous and spurious conclusions.

Results of the spatial effects for the fitted models showed that there exist substantial geographical variations in level of immunization coverage across Nigeria. While some states were significantly associated with full immunization, some were significantly associated with no or partial immunization coverage. Ensuring full immunization coverage will assist Nigeria in averting deaths in children under five (especially infants) due to preventable causes. Through this, Nigeria can achieve the millennium development goals on reduction of infant and child mortality rates.

Generally, full immunization coverage is still very low in Nigeria. The progressive increase in the percentage of fully immunized children from around 8 % between 1999 and 2003 to about 15 % in 2008 is still not impressive. More serious efforts are still needed from government and non-governmental organizations in the areas of enlightenment campaign to improve significantly on the current achievement if objective number four of the United Nations MDG that calls for a two-third reduction in child mortality by 2015 is to be accomplished in Nigeria.

In conclusion, findings from this Chapter provide insight to policy formulation. Scarce resources have been identified as a major challenge towards implementation of necessary intervention strategies in sub-Saharan African countries, including Nigeria. This Chapter provides policy-makers with tools to enhance appropriate policy formulation on improving access to and coverage of immunization; which can also assist in allocating resources to states or districts where the resources can be effectively utilized. While identifying states that require intensive prevention efforts towards full vaccination, the need for sustenance of the full immunization coverage in states that are associated with full coverage must be ensured by policy-makers in the affected states.

References

Ambe, J. P., Omotara, B. A., & Mandu, B. M. (2001). Perceptions, beliefs and practices of mothers in sub-urban and rural areas towards measles and measles vaccination in Northern Nigeria. *Tropical Doctor, 31*, 89–90.

Agency for International Development USAID. (2009). Immunization essentials: A practical field guide.

Babaniyi, O. A., & Spiegel, R. A. (1993). Status of EPI in Nigeria: Need for sustaining immunization coverage. *Journal of Tropical Pediatrics, 39*(2), 114–116.

Besag, J., York, J., & Mollié, A. (1991). Bayesian image restoration, with two applications in spatial statistics. *Annals of the Institute of Statistical Mathematics, 43*, 1–21.

Bilous, J., Eggers, R., Gasse, F., Jarrett, S., Lydon, P., Magan, A., Okwo-Bele, J. M., Salama, P., Vandelaer, J., Villeneuve, P., & Wolfson, L. J. (2006). A new global immunization vision and strategy. *Lancet, 2006*(367), 1464–1466.

Brezger, A., & Lang, S. (2006). Generalized structured additive regression based on Bayesian P splines. *Computational Statistics and Data Analysis, 50*, 967–991.

Brezger, A., Kneib, T., & Lang, S. (2009). BayesX: Software for Bayesian inference in structured and additive regression models, version 2.0.1. Available under: http://www.stat.uni-muenchen.de/~bayesx

Brugha, R., Starling, M., & Walt, G. (2002). GAVI, the first steps: Lessons for the global fund. *Lancet, 359*, 435–438.

Carroll, R. J., Ruppert, D., & Stefanski, L. A. (1995). *Measurement error in nonlinear models*. London: Chapman and Hall.

Centers for Disease Control and Prevention (CDC). (1999). Progress towards poliomyelitis eradication – Nigeria, 1996–1998. *Morbidity and Mortality Weekly Reports (MMWR), 48*, 312–316.

Centre for Global Development. (2005). *Making markets for vaccines: From ideas to actions*. Washington DC: Centre for Global Development.

Clements, C. J., Greenough, P., & Shull, D. (2006). How vaccine safety can become political – The example of polio in Nigeria. *Current Drug Safety, 1*, 117–119.

Crook, A. M., Knorr-Held, L., & Hemingway, H. (2003). Measuring spatial effects in time to event data: a case study using months from angiography to coronary artery bypass graft (CABG). *Statistics in Medicine, 22*, 2943–2961.

Dabbagh, A., Eggers, R., Cochi, S., Dietz, V., Strebel, P., & Cherian, T. (2007). A new global framework for immunization monitoring and surveillance. *Bulletin of the World Health Organization, 2007*(85), 901–980.

Djibuti, M., Gotsadze, G., Zoidze, A., Mataradze, G., Esmail, L. C., & Kohler, J. C. (2009). The role of supportive supervision on immunization program outcome – A randomized field trial from Georgia. *BMC International Health and Human Rights, 9*(Suppl 1), S11.

Duclos, P., Okwo-Bele, J.-M., Gacic-Dobo, M., & Cherian, T. (2009). Global mmunization: Status, progress, challenges and future. *BMC International Health and Human Rights, 9*(Suppl. 1), S2. doi:10.1186/1472-698X-9-S1-S2.

Edwards, D., & Thurstone, L. (1952). An internal consistency check for scale values determined by the method of successive intervals. *Psychometrika, 17*, 169–180.

Eilers, P. H. C., & Marx, D. B. (1996). Flexible smoothing with B-splines and penalties. *Statistical Science, 11*(2), 89–121.

Fahrmeir, L., & Lang, S. (2001a). Bayesian semiparametric regression analysis of multicategorical time-space data. *Annals of the Institute of Statistical Mathematics, 52*(1), 1–18.

Fahrmeir, L., & Lang, S. (2001b). Bayesian inference for generalized additive mixed models on Markov random field priors. *Applied Statistics, 50*(2), 201–220.

Fahrmeir, L., & Tutz, G. (2001). *Multivariate statistical modelling based on generalized linear models*. New York: Springer Verlag.

Fahrmeir, L., Kneib, T., & Lang, S. (2004). Penalized structured additive regression for space-time data: A Bayesian perspective. *Statistica Sinica, 14*, 731–761.

Gamerman, D., & Lopes, H. F. (2006). *Markov chain Monte Carlo: Stochastic simulation for Bayesian inference* (2nd ed.). New York: Chapman & Hall. ISBN 13: 978-1584885870.

Global Polio Eradication Initiative. (2008). *Wild polio virus 2000–2007*. Retrieved February 16, 2011, from the original report at http://web.archive.org/web/20070927204139/http://www.polioeradication.org/content/general/casecount.pdf

Global polio eradication initiative: Progress 2003. Geneva: World Health Organization. (2004). Accessed September 22, 2008, at [http://www.polioeradication.org/content/publications/2003_progress.pdf]

Hadler, S., Cochi, S., Bilous, J., & Cutts, F. (2004). Chapter 55: Vaccines. *Vaccination programs in developing countries* (4th ed.). Elsevier Inc., United Kingdom

Hastie, T., & Tibshirani, R. (1990). *Generalized additive models*. London: Chapman & Hall.

IRIN (2007). *"Hundreds" dead in measles outbreak*. Retrieved February 16, 2011, at http://irinnews.org/Report.aspx?ReportId=75883

Jenkins, H. E., Aylward, R. B., Gasasira, A., Donnelly, C. A., Abanida, E. A., Koleosho-Adelekan, T., & Grassly, N. C. (2008). Effectiveness of immunization against paralytic poliomyelitis in Nigeria. *The New England Journal of Medicine, 359*, 1666–1674.

Kammann, E. E., & Wand, M. P. (2003). Geoadditive models. *Journal of the Royal Statistical Society C, 52*, 1–18.

Kneib, T., & Fahrmeir, L. (2005). *Supplement to "Structured additive regressionfor categorical space-time data: A mixed model approach."* (Tech. Rep.). Accessed May 23, 2011. Available at http://www.stat.uni-muenchen.de/kneib

Kneib, T., & Fahrmeir, L. (2006). Structured additive regression for categorical space-time data: A mixed model approach. *Biometrics, 62*, 109–118.
Kneib, T., & Fahrmeir, L. (2007). A mixed model approach for geoadditive hazard regression. *Scandinavian Journal of Statistics, 34*, 207–228.
Knorr-Held, L. (1999). Dynamic rating of sports teams. Sonderforschungsbereich 386, paper 98 (1997). http://epub.ub.uni-muenchen.de/
Koumaré, A. K., Traore, D., Haidara, F., Sissoko, F., Traoré, I., Dramé, S., Sangaré, K., Diakité, K., Coulibaly, B., Togola, B., & Maïga, A. (2009). Evaluation of immunization coverage within the Expanded Program on Immunization in Kita Circle, Mali: A cross-sectional survey. *BMC International Health and Human Rights, 9*(Suppl 1), S13.
Lang, S., & Brezger, A. (2004). Bayesian P-splines. *Journal of Computational and Graphical Statistics, 13*, 183–212.
Lim, S. S., Stein, D. B., Charrow, A., & Murray, C. J. L. (2008). Tracking progress towards universal childhood immunisation and the impact of global initiatives: A systematic analysis of three-dose diphtheria, tetanus, and pertussis immunisation coverage. *The Lancet, 372*, 2031–2046.
National Population Commission (NPC) [Nigeria]. (2000). *Nigeria demographic and health survey 1999*. Calverton: National Population Commission and ORC Macro.
National Population Commission (NPC) [Nigeria], & ORC Macro. (2004). *Nigeria demographic and health survey 2003*. Calverton: National Population Commission and ORC Macro.
National Population Commission [Nigeria], & ICF Macro. (2009). *Nigeria demographic and health survey 2008*. Abuja: National Population Commission and ICF Macro.
Ngowu, R., Larson, J. S., & Kim, M. S. (2008). Reducing child mortality in Nigeria: A case study of immunization and systemic factors. *Social Science & Medicine, 67*, 161–164.
Odusanya, O. O., Alufohai, J. E., Meurice, F. P., Clemens, R., & Ahonkhai, V. I. (2000). Low immunization coverage in rural Nigeria. *Nigerian Quarterly Journal of Hospital Medicine, 10*, 118–120.
Odusanya, O. O., Alufohai, J. E., Meurice, F. P., Clemens, R., & Ahonkhai, V. I. (2003). Short term evaluation of a rural immunization program in Nigeria. *Journal of the National Medical Association, 95*, 175–179.
Odusanya, O. O., Alufohai, J. E., Meurice, F. P., & Ahonkhai, V. I. (2008). Determinants of vaccination coverage in rural Nigeria. *BMC Public Health, 8*(381), 1–8. doi:10.1186/1471-2458-8-381.
Okoro, J. I., & Egwu, I. N. (1994). Essential factors in the implementation of an expanded program on immunization in an urban-periurban community in Nigeria. *Asia-Pacific Journal of Public Health, 7*(2), 105–110.
Oladokunm, R. E., Adedokun, B. O., & Lawoyin, T. O. (2010). Children not receiving adequate immunization in Ibadan, Nigeria: What reasons and beliefs do their mothers have? *Nigeria Journal of Clinical Practice, 13*(2), 173–178.
Pallansch, M. A., & Sandhu, H. S. (2006). The eradication of polio – Progress and challenges. *The New England Journal of Medicine, 355*, 2508–2511.
Patriarca, P. A., Wright, P. F., & John, T. J. (1991). Factors affecting the immunogenicity of oral poliovirus vaccine in developing countries: Review. *Reviews of Infectious Diseases, 13*, 926–939.
Rue, H. (2001). Fast sampling of Gaussian Markov random fields with applications. *Journal of the Royal Statistical Society B, 63*, 325–338.
Rue, H., & Held, L. (2005). *Gaussian Markov Random fields: Theory and applications*. London: Chapman and Hall.
Sanou, A., Simboro, S., Kouyaté, B., Gugas, M., Graham, J., & Bibeau, G. (2009). Assessment of factors associated with complete immunization coverage in children aged 12–23 months: A cross-sectional study in Nouna district, Burkina Faso. *BMC International Health and Human Rights, 9*(Suppl 1), S10.

Spiegelhalter, D. J., Best, N. G., Carlin, B. P., & van der Linde, A. (2002). Bayesian measures of model complexity and fit (with discussion). *Journal of the Royal Statistical Society B, 64*, 583–640.

Taylor, M. E, Basu, R. N, Cutts, F., Gasse F, Ndumbe, P., Steinglass, R., & LaForce, J.-M. (1996). *Sustainability of achievements: Lessons learned from universal child immunization*. Report of a Steering Committee. Evaluation and Research Office, UNICEF.

World Health Organisation. (2006). Challenges in global immunization and the Global Immunization Vision and strategy 2006–2015. *Weekly Epidemiological Record, 81*, 190–195. http://www.who.int/wer/2006/wer8119.pdf

World Health Organization. (2008a). Typhoid vaccines: WHO position paper. *Weekly Epidemiological Record, 83*(6), 49–59. http://www.ncbi.nlm.nih.gov/pubmed/18260212

World Health Organization (WHO). (2008b). Progress in global measles control and mortality reduction, 2000–2007. *Weekly Epidemiological Record, 83*, 441–448.

World Health Organisation, & UNICEF. (2009). Immunization coverage in Nigeria. http://www.who.int/immunization_monitoring/data/nga.pdf

World Health Organization (WHO). (2004). Immunization, vaccines and biologicals. http://www.who.int/immunization

World Health Organization, & UNICEF. (2005). GIVS Global Immunization Vision and Strategy 2006–2015. http://www.who.int/vaccines-documents/DocsPDF05/GIVS_Final_EN.pdf website World Health Organization.

Chapter 8
Macro Determinants of Geographical Variation in Childhood Survival in South Africa Using Flexible Spatial Mixture Models

Samuel O.M. Manda

8.1 Introduction

In many societies around the world, social and economic programmes have been put in place aimed at improving the health of the populations. This is premised on evidence that a healthy population is economically more active; thus contributing to efforts meant to lowering levels of poverty (Romani and Anderson 2002). Leading indicators of overall social-economic development and health status of a country are infant (under 1 year) mortality and under-five mortality rates (Romani and Andersen 2002; Bradshaw et al. 2004; Burgard and Treiman 2006). Under-five mortality rate, defined as the number of children younger than 5 years who die out of 1,000 live births, is a Millennium Development Goal 4 (MDG 4) indicator (United Nations 2012). Furthermore, in conditions where HIV/AIDS is pandemic, childhood death rates are important for investigating inequalities regarding HIV policies and services; in particular, differential rates of mother-to-child transmission (MTCT) of HIV (Bradshaw et al. 2004).

Even though childhood mortality rates have generally been declining worldwide, the levels of the decline and the current rates vary considerably across regions. In some regions, for example, the sub-Saharan African (SSA) region, declines in child mortality have either reversed or slowed or stalled in many countries from the early 1990s, making it unlikely that the target of reducing under-five mortality rate by two thirds between 1990 and 2015 will be reached (Fotso et al. 2007). The more wealthier and modernised regions have had faster declines in, and have lower, childhood mortality rates and vice-versa (Heaton and Amoateng 2007; UNICEF 2010). Between 1990 and 2008, the overall world-wide reduction in under-five

S.O.M. Manda (✉)
Biostatistics Unit, South African Medical Research Council, Pretoria, South Africa
e-mail: Samuel.Manda@mrc.ac.za

N.-B. Kandala and G. Ghilagaber (eds.), *Advanced Techniques for Modelling Maternal and Child Health in Africa*, The Springer Series on Demographic Methods and Population Analysis 34, DOI 10.1007/978-94-007-6778-2_8,

mortality rate was 28 %, with a high of 40 % in the industrialised countries and a low average of 22 % in the SSA region. The overall under-five mortality rate is 65 deaths (1,000 live births), with rates of 6 and 144, respectively, in the industrialised and the SSA region (UNICEF 2010).

South Africa (SA) has one of the lowest rates of childhood mortality in the SSA region (SA infant mortality rate is 45; SSA's is 82 (African Population and Health Research Center 2008)). However, the country is one of the few at the start of the 1990s to have experienced a reversal in child mortality decline. The reversal has been attributed to an increase in HIV prevalence in pregnant women within the same period (Hall 2009). The country's low childhood mortality rates mask variation within the country where the rates vary by province, with the Western Cape province having the lowest infant and under-five mortality rates at 30 and 39 per 1,000 live births, while the Eastern Cape province has the highest rates at 61 and 81 per 1,000 live births, respectively (Hall 2009). Ethnicity is an important predictor of differential childhood mortality rates in South Africa as it is indicative of differences in educational, health and social-economic access; a legacy of the then *apartheid* policies (Romani and Anderson 2002; Burgard and Treiman 2006; Heaton and Amoateng 2007).

This chapter uses data from the South African Demographic Health Survey 1998 (SADHS 1998) (Department of Health 2002) and the spatially relevant health district data to investigate geographical variation of childhood mortality in South Africa. In particular, we use socio-economic, demographic and health variables at the district level to explain excess risk in childhood mortality at the district level. Childhood mortality is modelled with time-to-event survival random effects models involving spatially arranged random effects. We do not restrict the conditional distribution of the spatial random effects to be Gaussian but are flexibly modelled using mixtures of Gaussian and double exponential distributions. The resulting residual fitted hazard rates are mapped to help the search for possible persistent spatial correlations, which may suggest links with district-specific covariates. This study therefore provides the benefit of identifying groups of children and places to be targeted with relevant and effective interventions; thus helping stakeholders to prioritise the available resources to places and sub-groups that are in greater need.

8.2 Some Theoretical Considerations

A number of studies in poor and less developed countries have used a number of individual and household factors to model childhood mortality. These include the mother's age, education and occupation, parity, birth interval, breastfeeding duration, sex of child, previous child deaths, and household amenities (Forste 1994; Huang et al. 1997; Manda 1999). In particular, the studies have shown gathered inverse relation between birth intervals and infant and child mortality. There are various mechanisms by which birth intervals might affect childhood mortality.

A short birth interval may erode the reproductive and nutritional resources of the mother leading to a higher incidence of premature and weaker births. Closely spaced children compete for scarce resources such as food and clothing. An increased transmission of infant and child contagious infections among closely spaced siblings may also occur. Early cessation of breastfeeding may expose the child to greater risks of illness from contaminated water and food in conditions where proper substitutes of food are scarce. But the effects of birth intervals and breastfeeding duration on childhood mortality are too complicated to entangle, due to complications arising from different factors (Manda 1999; Kandala and Ghilagaber 2006):

Maternal age at birth of the child and birth order tend to exhibit a U-shaped relationship with childhood mortality (Sastry 1997). Young mothers have reproductive systems that are not completely mature, and this leads to underweight and weaker babies, while older mothers have declining maternal resources due to aging. Young mothers are also less likely to have received adequate prenatal care. High order births have relatively higher childhood mortality because they are born to older women. First-born children are more likely to be born to young mothers. Maternal education and household wealth provide the means with which the mother can ably care for a sick child, and the awareness of preventive modern medicines. In some studies, the survival status of the proceeding child had been used to model family effects where it has been assumed that if mortality risks within a family are correlated, the index child has a higher chance of dying.

On the macro level, countries in the Sub-Saharan Africa region are characterised by some of the highest infant and under-five mortality rates in the world (Balk et al. 2004). The declines, which started in the late 1960s, have stalled in the 1990s, with some countries actually experiencing an increase in childhood mortality. Overall, the region accounts for more than one in three of deaths of children under the age of five (Amouzou and Hill 2004). Within the region, levels and trends in mortality exhibit a considerable heterogeneity. In particular, the western and middle regions experience high childhood mortality rates than the eastern and southern region. A number of contributing factors have been assessed to explain the observed variation in both infant and child mortality across countries. Amouzou and Hill (2004) investigated the effect of three of a country's socioeconomic indicators: per capita income, illiteracy levels among women and the level of urbanisation on child mortality variations across the region's countries. Their results showed a positive association between illiteracy levels among women and negative associations between per capita income, urbanisation and child mortality. On the other hand, Balk et al. (2004) studied environmental and geographical factors such as population density, urban proximity, climate, farming system and disease environment in a spatial analysis of child mortality in West Africa, and found that country-specific variations in child mortality attenuated when these spatially-relevant variables were accounted for in the models.

Sub-nationally, spatial variations in child mortality have also been shown to exist. In a study of childhood mortality in Malawi, Kalipeni (1993) and Kandala and Ghilagaber (2006) found that districts in the Northern region tended to display lower rates of infant mortality than districts in the Central and Southern regions. These spatial variations persisted even after controls for important district level factors, such as female education and agricultural occupation, health facilities and demography (age at first marriage and fertility levels). In Zimbabwe, Root (1997) concluded that population density was an independent predictor of provincial variations of child mortality, with children in the lower-density Ndebele provinces having lower child mortality than their counterparts in the higher-density Shona provinces. Gemperli et al. (2004) found high level of infant mortality in the Central and Eastern parts of Mali, which were partially reduced by the inclusion of socioeconomic and bio-demographic variables at the individual level. In other parts of the world, geographical differentials in child mortality have also been observed, for instance in the Guizghou region, China (Huang et al. 1997) and Bolivia (Forste 1994), which were attributed to poverty differentials.

The few studies that have modelled community heterogeneity effects on child mortality have not controlled for community-specific spatial relevant factors (Sastry 1998; Bolstad and Manda 2001). Gemperli et al. (2004), Balk et al. (2004) and Kandala and Ghilagaber (2006) in their analyses of small-area spatial variation of infant and child mortality in the sub-Saharan region, appended area-specific spatially-relevant factors to individual and household data in the Demographic and Health Survey (DHS) data sets. The spatial analysis studies in Kalipeni (1993), Root (1997) and Balk et al. (2004) did not account for spatial dependence in the data. Moreover, they did not even account for heterogeneity effects in the data across the studied geographical areas to account for extra-variation. The results may have been biased because failure to account for both unstructured and structured heterogeneity could underestimate the standard errors of the parameters, which might inflate their significance. Only a few studies have modelled childhood mortality using correlated spatial effects (Banerjee et al. (2003) and Gemperli et al. (2004)). We follow this up in this study; childhood mortality in the period 0–59 months is modelled using a counting process formulation of a proportional hazards model, which is modified to include spatially correlated frailty effects adjusted for area-specific spatially-relevant factors.

8.3 Flexible Modelling of Area Spatial Effects

8.3.1 Basic Frailty Model

The application of Clayton-type counting process formulations for clustered survival data and gamma frailty are now routinely applied in analyses of clustered survival data. Frailty models have been successfully used to model dependence in clustered survival models (Clayton 1991; Sastry 1997). The unavailability of information about the distribution of the random effects, and the possibility of bias in parameter estimation when the distribution is mis-specified, motivates nonparametric or semi-parametric approaches in frailty survival modelling (Zhang and Steele 2004; Manda 2011).

The basic proportional hazards model will be formulated using the counting process approach as in Andersen and Gill (1982) and Clayton (1991). We suppose there are I areas and each has n_i subjects. For subject ij $(i = 1, \ldots, I; j = 1, \ldots n_i)$, a process $N_{ij}(t)$ is observed, which counts the number of events which have occurred for the subject by time t. In addition, a process $Y_{ij}(t)$, which indicates whether or not the subject was at risk for the event of death at time t, is also observed. The intensity process $\lambda_{ij}(t)$ for subject ij is a product of the risk indicator and the hazard function $h_{ij}(t)$; ie $\lambda_{ij}(t) = Y_{ij}(t)h_{ij}(t)$. We also measure a possibly time-varying $p -$ dimensional vector of risk factors $x_{ij}(t)$, where p is the number of risk factors being investigated. Thus, for subject ij, the observed data are $D = \{N_{ij}(t),\ Y_{ij}(t),\ x_{ij}(t);\ t \geq 0\}$ and are assumed independent. Let $dN_{ij}(t)$ be the increment of $N_{ij}(t)$ in the infinitesimal interval $[t,\ t + dt]$ and F_t- be the available data just before time t. Since the increment $dN_{ij}(t)$ can take a value 1 or 0, we have $\lambda_{ij}(t)dt = \Pr\left(dN_{ij}(t) = 1|F_t-\right)$ as the mean increase in $N_{ij}(t)$ during the infinitesimal interval $[t,\ t + dt]$.

The effect of the risk factors on the baseline intensity function for subject ij at time t is given by the Cox proportional hazards model

$$\lambda_{ij}\left(t|\lambda_0(t),\ \beta,\ x_{ij}(t),\ w_i\right) = Y_{ij}(t)\lambda_0(t)\ \exp\ \left(\beta^T x_{ij}(t) + w_i\right)$$

Where β is a $p -$ dimensional parameter vector of regression coefficients; w_i is the area-specific unobserved frailty, which captures the risk of the unobserved or unmeasured risk variables; and λ_0 is the baseline intensity, which is unspecified and to be modeled non-parametrically. In the present study, the frailty effect w_i is assumed to be time-invariant, but this can be relaxed in certain situations (Manda and Meyer 2005). Under non-informative censoring, the (conditional) likelihood of the observed data D is proportional to

$$\prod_{i=1}^{I}\prod_{j=1}^{n_i}\prod_{t\geq 0}^{T}\left(\lambda_{ij}(t|\lambda_0(t),\ \beta,\ x_{ij}(t),\ w_i\right)^{dN_{ij}(t)}\ \exp\left(-(\lambda_{ij}(t|\lambda_0(t),\ \beta,\ x_{ij}(t), w_i\right)dt)$$

This is just a Poisson likelihood taking increments $dN_{ij}(t)$ as independent Poisson random variables with means $\mu_{ij}(t) = \lambda_{ij}\left(t|\lambda_0(t),\ \beta,\ x_{ij}(t),\ w_i\right)\ dt = Y_{ij}(t)\ \exp\left(\beta^T x_{ij}(t) + w_i\right)\ d\Lambda_0(t)$, where $d\Lambda_0(t)$ is the increment in the integrated baseline hazard function in interval $[t,\ t + dt]$. We conveniently model the baseline hazard function as piecewise constant, where in each interval increment $d\Lambda_0(t) = \mathrm{d}t\lambda_{0t} = \exp\ (\theta_{0t})$ In this way, the baseline hazard can be estimated with the fixed effects β as constants. In situations where the assumptions of time-constant hazards may not hold, the baseline hazard function is modeled using a random walk prior (Manda and Meyer 2005) or nonparametric approaches as in

Chap. 12. For computational purposes, the basic assumption has been that the area frailty effects are independently and identically distributed normal or log-gamma random variables with a mean of 0 and unknown variance.

However, in many epidemiological studies involving mortality and morbidity mapping, this assumption is overly simplistic and it becomes problematic as it is very unlikely that disease risks are independent across geographical areas, a concept which is difficult to justify when there may be significant evidence of clustering of mortality. For any given area i say, all neighbouring areas are likely to share similar environment exposures and therefore one would expect mortality rate estimates for the area i to resemble those of all adjacent areas. Statistically, it creates analytical problems in that observational units are not independent, and consequently, statistical analyses such as standard Cox regression model that rely upon the assumption of independence may no longer be valid.

8.3.2 *Modelling Spatially Correlated Area Frailty Effects*

The basic model for the frailty effect that has been considered so far allows for over dispersion in the distribution of subjects survival time t_{ij} by the use of random effects w_i. This may partially account for unmeasured covariates that induce dependence in the t_{ij}, but as discussed in the preceding subsection, it does not allow for explicit spatial dependence between the outcomes. The latter may arise, for example, through "lesser variation" in hazard rates in neighbouring densely urban populated areas as opposed to sparsely populated rural areas or through a putative infectious aetiology for the disease(s) under investigation. Such explicit spatial dependence may be incorporated into the model by including an additional spatially structured random effect term. The model is then extended to

$$\log u_{ij}(t) = \log d\Lambda_0(t) + \beta^T x_{ij}(t) + w_i + v_i$$

so that the log-hazards ratios are now given by $w_i + v_i$. The priors relating to w_i are specified as before, however, the v_i are taken to have a spatially structured prior of which. By writing, $\omega = (v_1, \ldots, v_I)$ the most common prior specification has the conditional intrinsic Gaussian autoregressive (CAR Normal) (Besag et al. 1991) given by the joint distribution

$$\begin{aligned}\Psi|\sigma_v^2 &\sim CAR\left(\sigma_v^2\right) \propto \sigma_v^{-1} \exp\left[-\frac{1}{2\sigma_v^2}\sum_{i\approx i'} (v_i - v_{i'})^2\right] \\ &\propto \sigma_v^{-1}\left[-\frac{1}{2\sigma_v^2}\sum m_i v_i (v_i - v_i)\right] \qquad (8.1)\end{aligned}$$

where $i \approx i$ means that regions i and i are adjacent, $\bar{v}$ is the average of the $v's$ that are adjacent to v_i, and m_i is the number of these neighbouring regions. The sum-to-zero constraint $\sum_{i=1} v_i = 0$ is added for identification purposes.

In a more familiar form, the prior specification in (8.1) appears as conditional distributions (Besag et al. 1991) as

$$v_i | v_{k \neq i} \sim N \left(\frac{\sum_{k \neq i} w_{ik} v_k}{\sum_{k \neq i} w_{ik}}, \frac{\sigma_v^2}{\sum_{k \neq i} w_{ik}} \right)$$

where w_{ik} are suitably chosen proximity weights for the areas (often simply 1 if two areas are adjacent, 0 otherwise) and the new hyperparameter σ_v^2 controls the strength of local spatial dependence. Typically a vague gamma hyperprior is assumed for the inverse of σ_v^2. An advantage of spatial smoothing technique is the ability to remove or reduce the effect of arbitrary geographical boundaries, since geo-political areas are unlikely to be related to the disease of interest. Thus, any artefactual variation exhibited in the data by methods of data aggregation is ameliorated.

However, information about the exact distribution of the spatial random effects is unavailable. Thus, it is not incorrect to make assumptions that the random frailty effects arise from a known parametric distribution, which might have a restrictive shape. This has led to choosing a frailty distribution that is flexible enough to account for arbitrary multimodality and unpredictable skewness. The use of nonparametric models such as those based on a Dirichlet process prior offer infinite possibilities for random effects distribution (Manda 2011). However, a Dirichlet process prior is not widely used in practice. A simpler approach to reducing the impact of parametric distributional assumptions on random effects is the use of finite mixture models (but problems remain in the choice of the number of mixture components) or random walk prior (Manda and Meyer 2005; Kandala and Ghilagaber 2006).

In this chapter, we follow the simpler approach where the conditional spatial random effect $v|v_{i=i'}$ is assumed to be drawn from one of two distributions, the conditional intrinsic autoregressive normal (ICAR Normal) and the ICAR double exponential. The latter, with its wider tails, offers a robust alternative to the normal distribution whose random effect estimates and inferences can be susceptible to district effect outliers. We assume that the conditional spatial effect has probability π_i of being drawn from ICAR Normal, and probability $1 - \pi_i$ of being drawn from ICAR double exponential. Thus,

$$v_i | v_{k \neq i} \sim \pi_i N \left(\frac{\sum_{k \neq i} w_{ik} v_{k1}}{\sum_{k \neq i} w_{ik}}, \frac{\sigma_{v1}^2}{\sum_{k \neq i} w_{ik}} \right) + (1 - \pi_i) DEXP \left(\frac{\sum_{k \neq i} w_{ik} v_{k2}}{\sum_{k \neq i} w_{ik}}, \frac{2\sigma_{v2}^2 \sigma_{v2}^2}{\sum_{k \neq i} w_{ik}} \right)$$

$y \sim DEXP(\mu, \sigma^2) = 1/2\sigma^2 \exp\,(-1/\sigma^2 |y - \mu|)$, with mean μ and variance $2\sigma^2\sigma^2$. We could follow outright membership of the conditional spatial effect to either component mixture based on its posterior membership probability π_i. Thus, if the probability exceeds 0.5, then a draw from the ICAR Normal is the value of the area-specific conditional spatial effect, otherwise the conditional spatial effect is assigned a value drawn from the ICAR double exponential. However, for the purpose of this study, we assign it the weighted draws from each of the two components using posterior estimates of π_i and $1 - \pi_i$ as weights.

8.4 Analysis of South Africa Under-Five Mortality

8.4.1 Data Source

The 1998 South African Demographic and Health Survey (SADHS) was a nationally representative probability sample of nearly 12,000 women between the ages of 15 and 49 years. The main report contains the full design, sampling procedures and various descriptive statistics (Department of Health 2002). Briefly, the women were selected using a two-stage sampling design. Firstly, the survey selected 976 primary units, which corresponded to the enumeration areas (EAs) using a sampling frame 86,000 EAs that were created for the Census 1996. The EAs were stratified by province, urban and non-urban residence. For a second stage sampling, a systematic sample of households was undertaken within each of the selected EAs. All the women between the ages of 15 and 49 in the household were identified and interviewed about information for all their births in the previous 5 years. In this study, we used only singleton births in this period, and the total number of births came to 4,903 after data cleaning and validations.

We used most of the individual and household variables discussed in Sect. 8.2. Three related variables: preceding birth interval, survival status of the preceding birth and birth order share the category of first birth, so the design matrix would be singular. Combining birth order and the preceding birth interval into a single variable avoids the problem of preceding birth interval, status of preceding birth and birth order sharing the same category. We also included child's age as a predictor of child mortality where a series of child age intervals are specified to capture trends in the risk of death within 5 years (Bolstad and Manda 2001); the intervals are less than 1 month, 1–5 months, 6–11 months, 12–23 months, and 24–59 months. We also included child's sex because there is some evidence that male infants and children have a higher mortality risk than do females in the sub-Saharan African region (Manda 1999). The survival status of the child preceding the index child was also included to account for familial genetic predisposition to child health or shared household environment or to measure changes in parenting skills since parents might change their behaviour or environment after child death, thereby increasing the index child's survival probability (Manda 1999; Bolstad and Manda 2001).

Several background measures of socio-economic status are included in the analyses; these include maternal level of formal education. In addition, measures of urban–rural residence and province are used as proxies for measures of development

Table 8.1 Descriptive statistics of individual and household explanatory variables used in the analyses, South African Demographic and Health Survey 1998

Variable	Frequency	Percent
Gender of child		
Male	2,481	50.60
Female	2,422	40.40
Mother's ethnicity		
Black African	4,006	81.71
Coloured	581	11.85
White	208	4.24
Asian/Indian	108	2.20
Place of residence		
Urban	2,181	44.48
Rural	2,722	55.52
	Mean	Std Dev
Birth order	2.72	1.94
Mother's age	26.87	6.89
Mother's years of education	8.15	3.89
Preceding birth interval (months)	55.25	35.21

and customs which were not directly measured. However, in many developing countries, especially in rural areas, measuring income may be problematic since many people work in agriculture and informal sectors. Even though, Demographic and Health Surveys do not collect adequate data on household income and expenditure, they, nonetheless, provide information on household assets. This has prompted many researchers to use the information on household assets to calculate a composite measurement of household-level poverty (Booysen 2001). In particular, DHS data sets provide a wealth index which indirectly measures long-term economic status of a household. As mentioned earlier, in South Africa the mother's race is the key differential marker of child mortality as race is the major axis of differential health, social-economic and educational advantage. The distribution of some explanatory variables over the total sample at risk in the overall age interval 0–59 months is presented in Table 8.1.

In addition to modelling individual and household predictors of under-five morality, we performed an ecological investigation of the mortality at the level of health district. The District Health System (DHS) is the basic channel through which the delivery of Primary Health Care is undertaken in South Africa (Hall 2009). Thus, the individual level bio-demographic and socioeconomic and household data in the SADHS 1998 were enriched with the spatially-relevant health district contextual factors: district-level material and social deprivation level and district-level HIV prevalence among pregnant women. The deprivation score is a measure of relative deprivation across districts and sub-districts within South Africa, and is a composite measure derived from a set of variables that are considered to be indicators of material and social deprivation (Noble et al. 2006). The districts with higher values are relatively more deprived, and as a measure of socio-economic status, it is particularly helpful in identifying more deprived districts which potentially have a greater need for primary health care service (Hall 2009). Differentials in HIV prevalence rates among pregnant women are an indication of inequalities in health deprivation, which may impact on vertical HIV transmission and PMTCT programmes (Bradshaw et al. 2004; Hall 2009).

8.4.2 Implementation of the Models

In the implementation of a Bayesian fit and estimation of the various models to the child survival data, all the fixed effect parameters were assigned independent Normal $(0,\ 10^3)$ prior distributions. The precision parameters were independently assigned a hyper-prior Gamma (0.5, 0.0005) distribution, where a $Gamma\ (a,\ b)$ distribution has mean a/b and variance a/b^2. A Gamma (0.5, 0.0005) prior distribution on the precision parameter implies that the random effects variance falls between 0.0002 and 1.02 with 95 % probability; a variance of 0.0002 implies a 1.06-fold increase in the mortality hazard between a district at the 2.5th percentile of hazard and a district at the 97.5th percentile of risk; this is quite conservative; while a variance of 1.02 implies a 54.41 fold increase in risk; this is overly optimistic. However, the modal variance is 0.00033, implying a 1.07-fold increase in hazard risk; thus the prior concentrated hazard ratios towards unity.

We did not set out to perform prediction analyses, but rather to use a best model that describes the child mortality in South Africa. Thus, we did not embark on diagnostic tools to detect unusual observations, but to choose the best model among a number of possible candidates. Their performances were compared using model Deviance Information Criterion (DIC), which is a sum of model fit and complexity (Spiegelhalter et al. 2002). The fit of the model is given by the posterior mean of the deviance $\bar{D}$, whereas the model complexity is given by the effective number of parameters, p_D. The quantity p_D is defined as $p_D = D(\bar{\Omega}) - \bar{D}$, where $D(\bar{\Omega})$ is the deviance evaluated at the posterior expectations of the model parameters, Ω. Thus, $DIC = \bar{D} + p_D$ and a model with the smaller DIC is better supported by the data.

The computation of the parameter estimates was accomplished in *WinBUGS* software (Spiegelhalter et al. 2004). For each model considered, two parallel Gibbs sampler chains from independent starting positions were ran for 30,000 iterations. All fixed effects and covariance parameters were monitored for convergence. Trace plots of sample values of each of these parameters showed that they were converging to the same distribution. We formally assessed convergence of the three chains using the German-Rubin reduction factor, and it stabilised to 1.0 by 5,000 iterations. For posterior inference, we used a combined sample of the last 25,000 iterations from the respective chains.

8.5 Results

There was considerable variation with respect to sample size and the under-five mortality rate among the 52 districts. The district-level sample size ranged from 1 to 573 children, with a median sample size of 78; the under-five mortality ranged from 0 to 129, with a median rate of 39. This is reflected in the observed under-five mortality rate map in Fig. 8.1, which shows a large amount of noise; which makes it difficult to discern any geographical trends in under-five mortality rate. Nonetheless, some of the highest rates of under-five mortality are indicated in the districts of KwaZulu-Natal, Eastern Cape and Mpumalanga and Limpopo provinces, while the provinces of the Western Cape and Northern Cape have some of the lowest under-five mortality rates. Figures 8.2 and 8.3 show, respectively, levels of deprivation and pregnant-woman HIV prevalence for all of the 52 health districts in South Africa. It is clearly seen that most of the deprived districts are in the Eastern Cape and Kwazulu-Natal provinces, and the least deprived districts are in the Western Cape Province. A further investigation (results not shown), revealed most rural districts are among the most deprived districts, while districts in the metropolitan areas are the least deprived. In regards to HIV prevalence among pregnant women, discernable trends are that ddistricts in the provinces of Kwazulu-Natal, Mpumalanga, Free State and south-eastern parts of the Eastern Cape Province have some of the highest prevalence, while the lowest HIV prevalence is shown in districts of the Western Cape and Northern Cape provinces. Thus, districts that have higher under-five mortality rates are more likely to be more deprived and have higher rate of HIV among pregnant women.

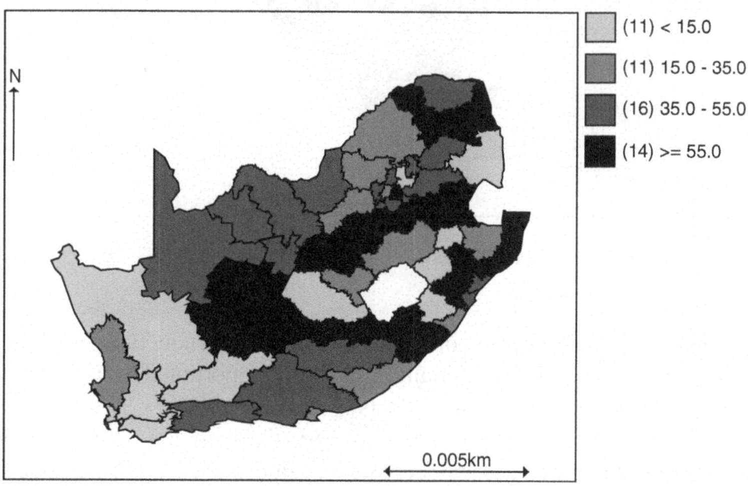

Fig. 8.1 Under-five mortality rate distribution by health district in South Africa, 1983–1998

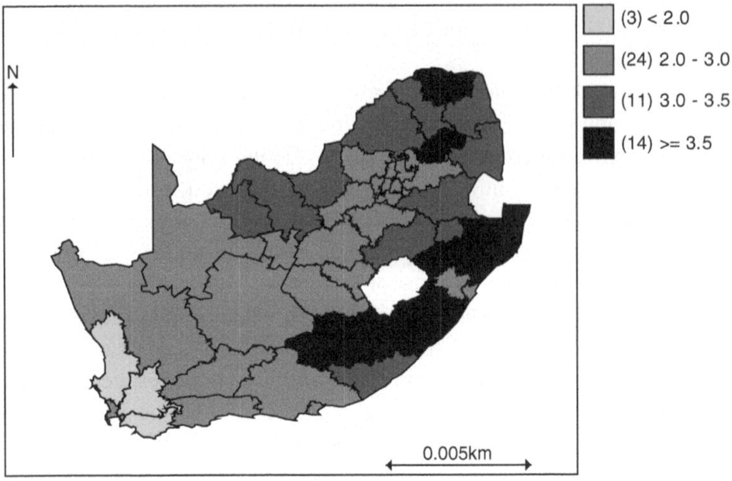

Fig. 8.2 Level of material and social deprivation by health district in South Africa, 2001

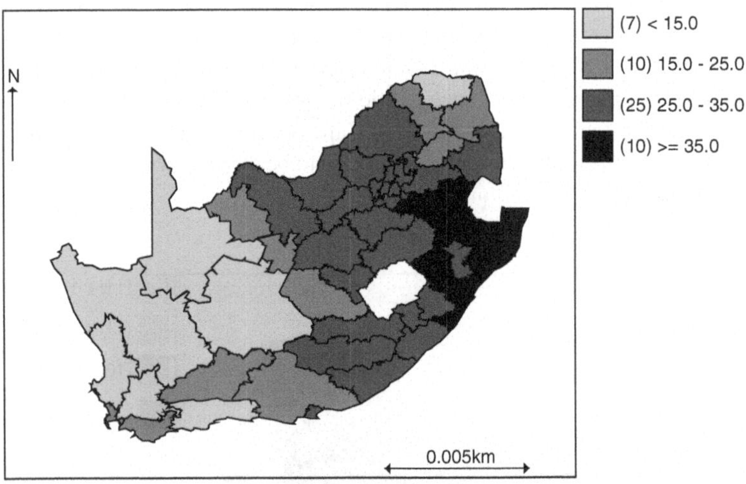

Fig. 8.3 Antenatal HIV prevalence by health district in South Africa, 2006–2007

A comparison of a number of competing models is shown in Table 8.2, where all the DIC components are shown. Initially, a standard proportional hazards regression model was fitted without any frailty effects (*NonFrailty Model*). This has effective number of parameters as 23.49, which is very close to the actual number of parameters, 24 (19 fixed effects and 5 constant hazards). We also fitted models with only the unstructured frailty effects (*NonSpatial Frailty Model*). Then, we fitted a number of spatial models with or without the covariates using the conventional unstructured and spatially structured frailty effects (*Convolution Model*) or the convolution model where the spatially structured random effect is a mixture of the

Table 8.2 Comparison of the fitted models using DIC components

Model	$\overline{D}$	$D(\overline{\Omega})$	p_D	DIC
NonFrailty	2,504.69	2,481.19	23.49	2,528.18
NonSpatial frailty, noncovariates	2,516.08	2,495.6	20.484	2,536.56
Convolution spatial frailty, nocovariates	2,514.85	2,494.32	20.53	2,535.38
Spatial mixture frailty, nocovariates	2,514.76	2,501.04	13.717	2,528.48
Nonspatial frailty	2,497.87	2,468.90	28.97	2,526.84
Convolution frailty	2,498.61	2,470.65	27.96	2,526.57
Spatial mixture frailty	2,486.30	2,452.15	34.191	2,520.53

ICAR Normal and ICAR double exponential (*Spatial Mixture Frailty Model*). As expected, the models without the inclusion of the covariates have lower effective number of parameters, but with substantially larger DIC values. The DIC values favour Mixture Spatial Frailty models over the Convolution models. The best fitting model is the Mixture Spatial Frailty Model, with the smallest DIC value of 2520.53, at least 5 lower than the other models.

Across all the fitted models, it was shown that the under-five mortality hazard depended on age of the child, which declined with increasing age (results not shown). For instance, the mortality hazard in the first month was about 1.11 times that in the months 1–5, 17. 86 times that in the months 6–11, and 20.07 and 28.55 times that in the months 12–23 and 24–59 months, respectively. In Table 8.3, we present the posterior summaries for the fixed effect parameters from only four models; two basic models: the NonFrailty Model and the NonSpatial Model and two spatial models: the *Spatial Mixture Frailty Model (A)* which only included the individual and households covariates, and the *Spatial Mixture Frailty Model (B)* which is an extension of the *Spatial Mixture Frailty Model (A)* with the inclusion of two district level factors: deprivation and HIV prevalence among pregnant women. The results are shown on the logarithm scale where no risk is represented by 0.

In all of the four models shown, there is general consistency in the estimate for the predictor effect, and that the individual and household estimates are unaffected by the inclusion of district-level factors. Using the nonspatial model analysis, and on the basis of the 95 % CI, not all of the fixed effects are significant; however, the median estimated effects support the findings in previous studies on child mortality in Sub-Saharan Africa and other less developed countries (Sastry 1997; Manda 1999). In particular, the under-five mortality hazard for boys is consistently slightly higher than that for girls. First births or lower birth orders combined with short preceding birth interval have high mortality hazards. The coefficient of the quadratic part of the age of the mother is significant, and it indicates a child born to a younger or older mother has higher under-five mortality hazard. As expected, maternal education inversely and significantly affects under-five mortality hazard. It is also evidently clear that the mother's ethnicity affects the hazard of under-five mortality; the fully adjusted hazard for White or Indian children is about $e^{-1,206} = 0.300$, a third of that for Black African children. Furthermore, children born in the rural areas have higher hazard of death in the first 5 years of life than children born in the urban areas (Table 8.3).

Table 8.3 Posterior median (95 % CI) log-hazards of the individual and household fixed effects for various models

Coefficient	Nonfrailty model	Nonspatial frailty model	Spatial mixture frailty model (A)	Spatial mixture frailty model (B)
Male child (0: no; 1: yes)	0.188 (−0.067, 0.443)	0.189 (−0.060, 0.452)	0.175 (−0.080, 0.436)	0.178 (−0.081, 0.438)
Birth order/preceding birth interval				
First birth	0.129 (−0.288, 0.589)	0.136 (−0.299, 0.609)	0.138 (−0.324, 0.590)	0.130 (−0.323, 0.599)
2–3 & < =36 months	0.267 (−0.185, 0.739)	0.270 (−0.191, 0.728)	0.264 (−0.200, 0.716)	0.254 (−0.209, 0.711)
2–3 & > 36 months	0 (–, –)	0 (–, –)	0 (–, –)	0 (–, –)
4+ & < =36 months	0.382 (−0.096, 0.871)	0.364 (−0.125, 0.857)	0.378 (0.104, 0.856)	0.350 (−0.137, 0.830)
4+ & >36 months	−0.069 (−0.603, 0.475)	−0.070 (−0.609, 0.466)	−0.050 (−0.573, 0.469)	−0.073 (−0.604, 0.441)
Mother's age				
Age linear	−0.264 (−0.566, 0.043)	−0.254 (−0.561, 0.046)	−0.257 (−0.581, 0.045)	−0.256 (−0.572, 0.059)
((Age- 26)/10)^2	0.276 (0.020, 0.508)	0.274 (0.028, 0.509)	0.281 (0.32, 0.524)	0.280 (0.033, 0.521)
Mother's education (years)	−0.046 (−0.082, -0.009)	−0.046 (−0.084, −0.010)	−0.048 (−0.085, −0.009)	−0.047 (−0.084, −0.009)
Mother's race				
Black African	0 (–, –)	0 (–, –)	0 (–, –)	0 (–, –)
Coloured	−0.093(−0.786, 0.597)	−0.047 (−0.746, 0.597)	−0.160 (−0.771, 0.418)	−0.125 (−0.856, 0.577)
White/Indian	−1.204 (−2.442, −0.284)	−1.185 (−2.397, −0.250)	−1.187 (−2.437, −0.262)	−1.206 (−2.435, −0.275)
Rural residence (0: no; 1: yes	0.221 (−0.144, 0.571)	0.230 (−0.133, 0.607)	0.241 (−0.090, 0.581)	0.282 (−0.104, 0.674)
District deprivation				
I (Least deprived)	0 (–, –)	0 (–, –)		0 (–, –)
II	0.361 (−0.306, 0.867)	0.330 (−0.305, 0.982)		0.304 (−0.503, 1.108)
III	−0.329 (−0.966, 0.326)	−0.299 (−0.982, 0.426)		−0.320 (−1.224, 0.619)
IV	−0.026 (−0.686, 0.642)	0.041 (−0.632, 0.779)		−0.019 (−0.929, 0.891)
V (Most deprived)	0.382 (−0.275, 1.060)	0.414 (−0.299, 1.120)		0.195 (−0.746, 1.157)
District HIV rate				
I (Least affected)	0 (–, –)	0 (–, –)		0 (–, –)
II	0.372 (−0.097, 0.893)	0.376 (−0.154, 0.894)		0.167 (−0.657, 0.950)
III	0.233 (−0.210, 0.682)	0.190 (−0.407, 0.695)		−0.037 (−0.094, 0.804)
IV	0.113 (−0.458, 0.721)	0.148 (−0.440, 0.740)		−0.007 (0.0890, 0.863)
V (Most affect)	0.430 (−0.036, 0.930)	0.436 (−0.095, 0.955)		0.201 (−0.757, 1.087)

There is evidence that under-five mortality hazard is related to deprivation level of a district, but the relationship is not linear, it is a U-shaped relationship. In both nonfrailty and nonspatial frailty models, higher levels of HIV consistently have elevated under-five mortality hazard; however, after taking into account the spatial dependence in the mortality, the relationship is U-shaped.

8.6 Mapping the Fitted District-Level Mortality Hazard

Figures 8.4, 8.5, and 8.6 display the unadjusted posterior means of the log-hazards from different models for the under-five mortality across the 52 health districts. Under the nonspatial frailty model (Fig. 8.4); the rate of childhood mortality appears to be relatively higher in the central, south-eastern and north-eastern parts of South Africa. However, a clear discernable picture emerges when considering spatial models (Figs. 8.5 and 8.6) that reveal excess mortality in the central, south-eastern and the northern parts of the country; covering districts in the Eastern Cape, Free State, Kwazulu-Natal and Limpopo provinces. The maps of excess mortality risk not explained by the individual, household and district-level covariates, under both the nonspatial and mixture models shows the distribution of the mortality risk has become more evenly distributed across the country with fewer districts having excess log-hazard mortality above 0.2 or below −0.2 (Figs. 8.7 and 8.8). Thus, the factors included, some of which vary spatially, may have explained some of the observed differential geographical patterns in the under-five mortality hazards.

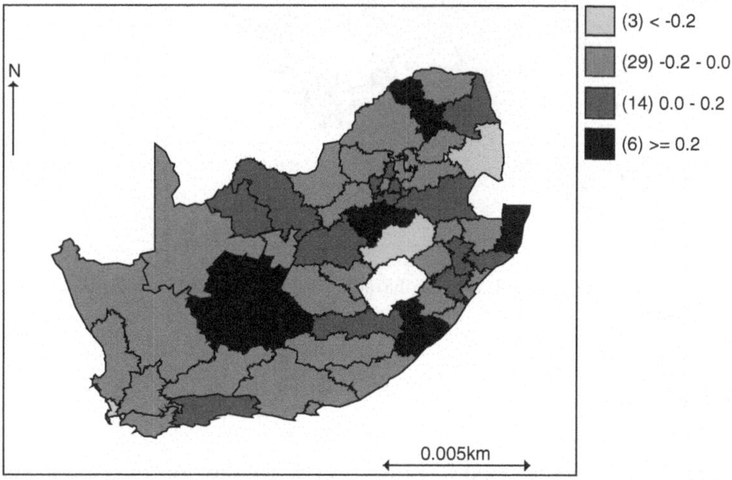

Fig. 8.4 Estimated under-five mortality log-hazards based on the Nonspatial Frailty Model without covariates

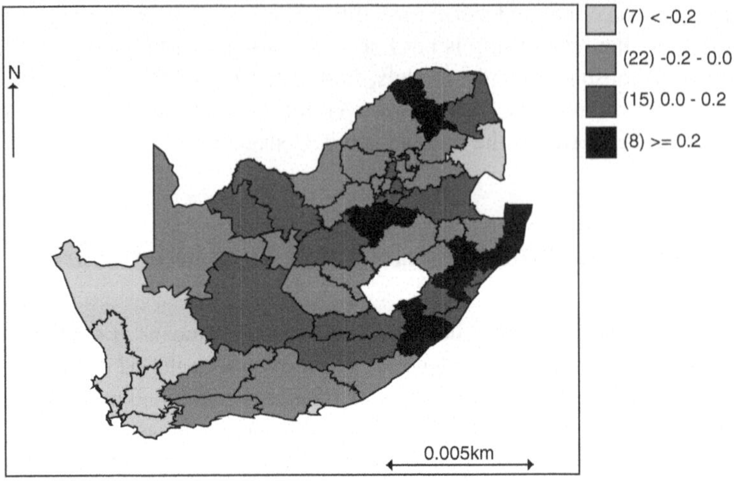

Fig. 8.5 Estimated under-five mortality log-hazards based on the Convolution Frailty Model without covariates

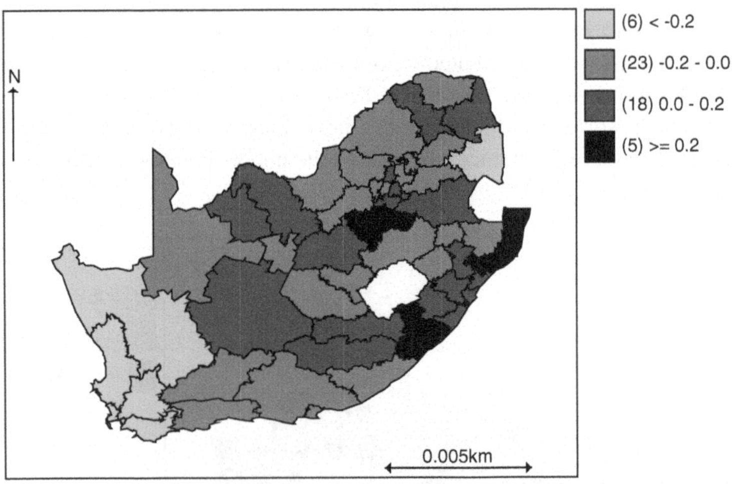

Fig. 8.6 Estimated under-five mortality log-hazards based on the Robust Mixture Frailty Model without covariates

8.7 Discussion

This chapter has demonstrated the use and feasibility of modelling spatially correlated maternal and child health data, where the outcomes are time to event; in our application, we investigated under-five mortality in South Africa. Spatial smoothing allowed us to discern the inherent spatial patterns of the mortality hazard

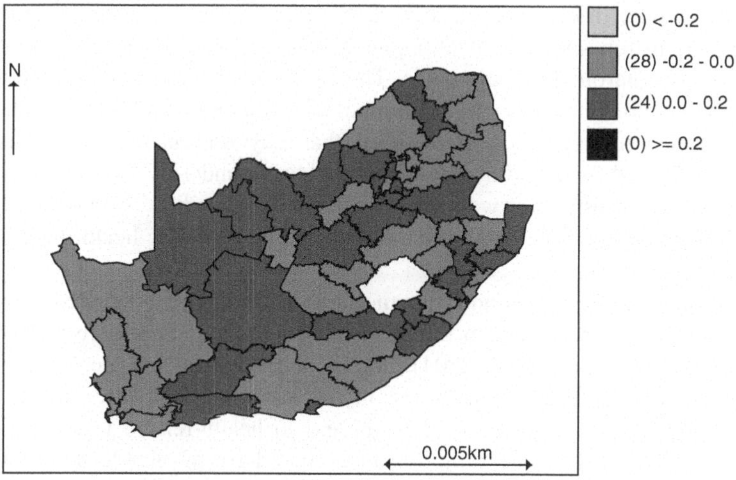

Fig. 8.7 Estimated under-five mortality log-hazards based on the Covariate-adjusted Nonspatial Frailty model

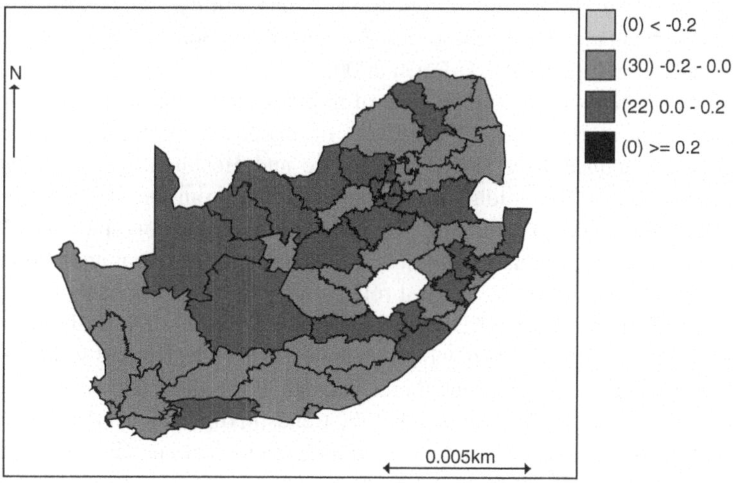

Fig. 8.8 Estimated under-five mortality log-hazards based on the Covariate-adjusted Robust Mixture Frailty model

of childhood mortality across the country. We were able, by using our methods, to show general trends in childhood mortality hazards attributed to measured individual and district-level covariates. Increasing district deprivation and HIV prevalence among pregnant women were associated with excess hazard for under-five mortality. Adjusting for these ecological factors and individual and household covariates weakened the association, but there was still a cluster of high mortality risk in the country. These excess district-level variations may indication a number of confounding factors such urbanization, health care and nutritional differentials that were directly controlled in the models. Thus, the models described here go a long way in maintaining parsimony in the number of predictor variables to include. This application has revealed probable districts that may warrant further examination to find out how they fall into the highest or lowest under-five mortality hazards categories. This investigation would then lead into the identification of other relevant spatially varying covariates within the broad context of public health intervention efforts.

The estimated effects on under-five mortality hazards of the included individual and household covariates are in the expected direction and they are well known (Manda 1999; Gemperli et al. 2004). For instance, due to biological differences, boys are more vulnerable to infection in the early years of life. Mothers with increased formal education have better access to health-related information and may be more efficient at using the resources they have to raise healthy children. Furthermore, young mothers have less experience in childbearing and their reproductive systems have not sufficiently developed compared to older mothers whose children are more likely to be in later birth orders. The clear ethnical differential in the hazard of under-five death, which is exceedingly lower for children born to White or Asian children, is a reflection of institutionalized racial social and material disadvantage among the Black African population in the country during the apartheid era (Burgard and Treiman 2006).

There are some issues around the use of mortality outcomes and some covariate factors as used in this study. The levels of under-five mortality used in this chapter were obtained from the Demographic and Health Survey conducted in 1998. The most reliable childhood mortality data are from the Demographic and Health Surveys (DHS) programme. The South African Demographic and Health Survey of 2003 had data quality problems, especially for maternal and child health (Department of Health 2007). The last reliable data to base estimates of childhood mortality are from the 1998 SADHS (Burgard and Treiman 2006; Hall 2009). The district-level district deprivation and antenatal HIV prevalence used were for 2001 and 2006–2007, respectively; thus there were some misalignment of the outcome measure and risk factors. We believe that the trends in district level deprivation and antenatal HIV prevalence have not changed much in to the trends in 1998; only that magnitudes may have gone up or down.

Analysis of survey data with complex sampling design needs to account for the design. The SADHS 1998 used weighted, stratified and clustered sampling procedure to draw the ultimate sample of women respondents. Any DHS data contains the sampling weights for each sample subjects, and in estimation of national effects, the weights correct for the unequal sampling probabilities (under/oversampled groups may influence results). However, the use of sampling weights to correct for unequal sampling probabilities is controversial (Pfeffermann 1993; Korn and Graubard 1995). A model-based approach includes variables used for determining weights in the regression model and a design-based approach uses individual weights accordingly in the analyses. We opted for former where we have urban or rural residence, variables that contributed to the weights and stratification, as repressor variables.

A second concern relates to measures of district-level deprivation and HIV prevalence, and the geography. The social and material deprivation used here is for the whole population, rather than specific to children. Attempts have been made to produce deprivation indices that directly affect children, but these are yet to be available at the district level (Noble et al. 2006; Barnes et al. 2008). The HIV prevalence was estimated for pregnant women in 2006–2007, attending in public hospitals. This is not a representative sample of the total population in the country; the antenatal HIV prevalence estimate might be biased upwards compared to the general population's HIV prevalence (Manda et al. 2012). However, in a generalised epidemic like HIV, these estimates are adequate and reliable, and they can be used as proxies for health deprivation, especially in accessing primary health care for PMTCT of HIV (Bradshaw et al. 2004). There also has been a change in the names and number of health districts over the years. Even though the geography that was sampled from 1998 was automatically linked to the current districts, there were some very few that were manually linked. This might have created spatial uncertainties in the definitions of locations over time. Although a better resolution of the analysis can be done at the municipality level, the geography below the district level, most of the important contextual factors related to childhood mortality are not yet available at this lower level.

Perhaps, a main limitation of the results in this chapter may concern the overall quality of the data used. The retrospective nature of data collection in these surveys renders the data to many biases resulting from missing data and nonresponse. For birth histories, women may provide an incorrect recall on birth and death dates for their children or even deaths omission especially for infants (Fotso et al. 2007). Even fieldworkers can introduce bias, especially when they transfer births out of the interest period to avoid lengthier questionnaires. The SADHS 1998 had a very high response rate of 92 %, and only 89 cases (0.15 %) had missing information. There was very high completeness of reporting of dates of birth and death, and very little evidence of transfer of child births (Department of Health 2002).

Even though there were some imputations of ages at death of dead siblings, DHS datasets are of high quality to directly estimate childhood mortality (Fotso et al. 2007). Thus, the substantive conclusions are less likely to be affected are sufficiently robust for decision-making are indicated in this discussion.

8.8 Conclusions

In conclusion, our methods and analysis offer valuable tools for producing robust and flexible covariate-adjusted maps of under-five morality that may indicate underlying latent risk profiles. We have also indicated how the otherwise limited data in most survey data can be enriched with external sources using the geographical information system tools. Such an integration methods and data sources will increase the relevance of statistical models for many problems, including epidemiology and medicine.

The generated maps may help the search for possible persistent spatial correlation, which may suggest links with district-specific covariates. Therefore this study has shown a novel methodology that could help to identify groups of children and places to be targeted with relevant and effective interventions. Such a process will help stakeholders to prioritise the available resources to places and sub-groups that are in greater need.

8.9 Further Reading

The current trends in child mortality rates in the sub-Saharan African region and the progress toward Millennium Development Goal 4 of two-third reduction in the mortality by 2015 is found in Fotso et al. (2007). The overall world-wide state of child mortality is contained in United National (UNICEF) report (UNICEF 2010, which shows that the SSA region, despite declines in child mortality, still lags far behind the rest of the world.

The idea of using frailty effects for child survival modelling in the developing countries can be found in Sastry and Bolstad and Manda, to name a few. The general theoretical ideas of frailty effects can be found in Hougaard (2000), who presents an excellent treatise on the various specification of the shared frailty model using independent and identically distributed assumptions. Theoretical extensions to modelling spatially structured shared frailty effects can be found in Banerjee and Carlin (2003) and Banerjee et al. (2004) using the CAR model. Nonparametric frailties have recently appeared in the literation (Manda 2011; Naskar 2008). However, methodological developments for nonparametric spatially structured models are still being investigated, even though methodology is typically computationally intensive.

Acknowledgments I wish to acknowledge the help I received from Statistics South Africa on linking the current geography of health districts with the data collected in the 1998 SADHS. The shape files for the mapping the districts were obtained from Demarcation Board of South Africa.

References

African Population and Health Research Center. (2008). *2008 African population data sheet*. Washington, DC/Nairobi.

Amouzou, A., & Hill, K. (2004). Child mortality and socioeconomic status in sub-Saharan Africa. *African Population Studies/Etude de la Population Africaine, 19*, 1–11.

Andersen, P. K., & Gill, R. D. (1982). Cox's regression models for counting processes. *The Annals of Statistics, 10*, 1100–1120.

Balk, D., Pullum, T., Storeygard, A., Greenwell, F., & Neuman, M. (2004). A spatial analysis of childhood mortality in West Africa. *Population, Space and Place, 10*, 175–216.

Banerjee, S., & Carlin, B. P. (2003). Semiparametric spatio-temporal frailty modeling. *Environmetrics, 14*, 523–535.

Banerjee, S., Carlin, B. P., Alan, E., & Gelfand, A. E. (2004). *Hierarchical modeling and analysis for spatial data*. Boca Raton: Chapman & Hall.

Banerjee, S., Wall, M. M., & Carlin, B. P. (2003). Frailty modelling for spatially correlated survival data, with application to infant mortality in Minnesota. *Biostatistics, 4*, 123–142.

Barnes, H., Noble, M., Wright, G., & Dawes, A. (2008). Geographical profile of child deprivation in South Africa. *Child Indicators Research, 2*, 181–199.

Besag, J., York, J., & Mollie, A. (1991). Bayesian image restoration, with two applications in spatial statistics (with discussion). *Annals of the Institute of Statistical Mathematics, 43*, 1–75.

Bolstad, W. M., & Manda, S. O. M. (2001). Investigation child mortality in Malawi using family and community random effects: A Bayesian analysis. *Journal of the American Statistical Association, 96*, 12–19.

Booysen, F. (2001). The measurement of poverty. In: D. Bradshaw & K. Steyn (Eds.), *Poverty and chronic disease in South Africa* (Technical Report, pp. 15–38). Cape Town: Medical Research Council.

Bradshaw, D., Nannan, N., Laubscher, R., Groenewald, P., Joubert, J., Nojilana, B., Norman, R., Desiree, P., & Schneider, M. (2004). *South African national burden of disease study 2000 – Estimates of provincial mortality*. Cape Town: Medical Research Council, Burden of Disease Unit.

Burgard, S., & Treiman, D. J. (2006). Trends and racial differences in infant mortality in South Africa. *Social Science & Medicine, 62*(5), 1126–1137.

Clayton, D. G. (1991). A Monte Carlo method for Bayesian inference in frailty models. *Biometrics, 47*, 467–485.

Department of Health. (2002). *South Africa demographic and health survey 1998, full report*. Pretoria: National Department of Health, Republic of South Africa.

Department of Health. (2007). *South African demographic and health survey 2003*. Pretoria: Department of Health South Africa.

Forste, R. (1994). The effects of breastfeeding and child mortality in Bolivia. *Population Studies, 48*, 397–511.

Fotso, J. C., Ezeh, A., Madise, N. J., & Ciera, J. (2007). Progress towards the child mortality millennium development goal in urban Sub-Saharan Africa: The dynamics of population growth, immunization, and access to clean water. *BMC Public Health, 7*, 218.

Gemperli, A., Vounatsou, P., Kleinschmidt, I., Bagayako, M., Lengeler, C., & Smith, T. (2004). Spatial patterns of infant mortality in Mali: The effect of malaria endemicity. *American Journal of Epidemiology, 159*, 64–72.

Hall, K. (2009). *Statistics on children in South Africa: HIV and health- child mortality (IMR & U5MR)*. Cape Town: Children's Institute, University of Cape Town.

Heaton, T. B., & Amoateng, A. Y. (2007). The family context for racial differences in child mortality in South Africa. In A. Y. Amoateng & T. B. Heaton (Eds.), *Families and households in post-apartheid South Africa: Socio-demographic perspectives*. Cape Town: Human Sciences Research Council Press.

Hougaard, P. (2000). *Analysis of multivariate survival data*. New York: Springer.

Huang, W., Yu, H., Wang, F., & Li, G. (1997). Infant mortality among various nationalities in the middle part of Guizghou, China. *Social Science & Medicine, 45*, 1031–1040.

Kalipeni, E. (1993). Determinants of infant mortality in Malawi: A spatial perspective. *Social Science & Medicine, 37*, 183–198.

Kandala, N.-B., & Ghilagaber, G. (2006). A Geo-additive Bayesian discrete-time survival model and its application to spatial analysis of childhood mortality in Malawi. *Quality and Quantity, 40*(6), 935–957.

Korn, E. L., & Graubard, B. I. (1995). Analysis of large health surveys: Accounting for the sampling design. *Journal of the Royal Statistical Society A, 158*, 263–295.
Manda, S. O. M. (1999). Birth intervals, breastfeeding and determinants of childhood mortality in Malawi. *Social Science & Medicine, 48*, 301–312.
Manda, S. O. M. (2011). A nonparametric frailty model for clustered survival data. *Communications in Statistics: Methods and Theory, 40*(5), 863–875.
Manda, S. O. M., & Meyer, R. (2005). Bayesian inference for recurrent events data using time-dependent frailty. *Statistics in Medicine, 24*, 1263–1274.
Manda, S. O. M., Lombard, C. L., & Mosala, T. (2012). Divergent spatial patterns in the prevalence of the human immunodeficiency virus (HIV) and syphilis in South African pregnant women. *Geospatial Health, 6*(2), 221–231.
Naskar, N. (2008). Semiparametric analysis of clustered survival data under nonparametric frailty. *Statistica Neerlandica, 62*, 155–172.
Noble, M., Babita, M., Barnes, H., Dibben, C., Magasela, W., Noble, S., Ntshongwana, P., Phillips, H., Rama, S., Roberts, B., Wright, G., & Zungu, S. (2006). *The provincial indices of multiple deprivation for South Africa 2001* (Technical Report), University of Oxford, UK.
Pfeffermann, D. (1993). The role of sampling weights when modelling survey data. *International Statistical Review, 61*, 317–337.
Romani, J. H., & Anderson, B. A. (2002). *Development, health, and the environment: Factors influencing infant and child survival in South Africa*. Cape Town: Human Sciences Research Council Press.
Root, G. (1997). Population density and spatial differentials in child mortality in Zimbabwe. *Social Science & Medicine, 44*, 413–421.
Sastry, N. (1997). A nested frailty model for survival data, with an application to the study of child survival in northeast Brazil. *Journal of the American Statistical Association, 92*, 426–435.
Spiegelhalter, D. J., Best, N. G., Carlin, B. P., & Van der Linde, A. (2002). Bayesian measures of model complexity and fit (with Discussion). *Journal of the Royal Statistical Societ, B, 64*, 583–616.
Spiegelhalter, D. J., Thomas, A., Best, N. G., & Lunn, D. (2004). *BUGS: Bayesian inference Using Gibbs Sampling*, Version 1.4.1. Medical Research Council Biostatistics Unit, Cambridge University.
UNICEF. (2010). *ChildInfo: Monitoring the situation of children and woman*. http://www.childinfo.org/mortality.html
United Nations. (2012). *The millennium development goals report 2012*. New York: United Nations.
Zhang, W., & Steele, F. (2004). A semiparametric multilevel survival model. *Journal of the Royal Statistical Society, Series C, 53*, 387–404.

Chapter 9
Socio-Demographic Determinants of Anaemia in Children in Uganda: A Multilevel Analysis

Ngianga II Kandala (Shadrack)

9.1 Introduction

Anaemia is the most common nutritional problem in both developed and developing countries. In developing countries between one and two-thirds of children are affected (Levin 1986). Currently it affects two billion people throughout the world (WHO 2008). This includes pre-school and school aged children. It appears to be not only a major cause of pre and post-partum morbidity and mortalitity in developing countries but also it affects the physical development of children.

Many researchers suspect that anaemia may increase children's susceptibility to infection (Stoltzfus et al. 2006). There is a growing body of evidence, based on animal studies, which suggests that iron deficiency adversely affects the immune system (Abouzahr and Royston 1991). Anaemia can also affect a person's learning ability. It has adverse effects on cognition and the effect is most probably located at the level of information reception (Pollitt 1982). In pre-school and school aged children, anaemia impaired motor development and administration, language development and scholastic achievement, and it develops in children psychological and behavioural effects such as inattention, fatigue, insecurity and it decreases children's physical activity (DeMaeyer 1990). It was estimated that globally, 200 million under 5 year olds fail to reach their cognitive and socio-emotional development, because of under nutrition, including anaemia (Badham 2007).

Children are the future of a nation, and there is no single effort more radical in its potential for saving the nation's future than optimising children's wellbeing. Although the biological immediate causes of anaemia are documented, its

N.II. Kandala (Shadrack) (✉)
Division of Social Statistics, University of Southampton, Southampton SO17 1BJ, UK
e-mail: N.Kandala@southampton.ac.uk

N.-B. Kandala and G. Ghilagaber (eds.), *Advanced Techniques for Modelling Maternal and Child Health in Africa*, The Springer Series on Demographic Methods and Population Analysis 34, DOI 10.1007/978-94-007-6778-2_9,

socioeconomic and demographic related factors and the fact that anaemia differs markedly between individuals within households and communities have rarely been explored.

This study aims to explore socio-demographic determinants of anaemia among children in Uganda after accounting for some proximate determinants and use multilevel modelling to quantify the effects due to individual, household and community levels. Multilevel modelling will be used because simple logistic regressions assume that errors are binomially distributed and outcomes are independent. However, due to unmeasured factors such as traditional beliefs or cultures, this might not be the case (Madise et al. 1999). Since observations within communities are not independent, the fixed effects model underestimates the standard errors and overestimates the significance of some variables (Snijders and Boker 1999).

Knowing the determinants of the disease and understanding its relationship with individuals, households and community factors are important for policy makers to plan and develop anaemia intervention at appropriate level and achieve Millennium Development Goals (MGD 1,2, 4, 5, & 6).

9.1.1 The Study Area

Uganda is one of the world's less developed countries. Agriculture is the most important sector of the economy and it employs over 80 % of the work force. Coffee is the main source of foreign trade. The country poses substantial natural resources like fertile soils and regular rainfalls. Uganda's climate is equatorial climate with a mean annual temperature ranging from about 16 °C in the Southwestern highland to 25 °C in the Northwest, but in the northeast, temperature exceed 30 °C. Except in the Northeastern region, rainfall is well distributed across the country. Uganda is faced with a number of environmental and socioeconomic problems. Almost every year heavy rains have triggered flooding that displaces thousands of peoples and sweeps away crops and livestock thereby creating food insecurity responsible for malnutrition to many children.

9.2 Data and Methods

9.2.1 Data

Data used in this study is from the 2006 Uganda Demographic Health Survey. The sample design involved a probabilistic two-stage sampling. It is a representative probabilistic sample where the country was divided into 368 clusters. 9,864 households were selected based on a completed sample frame of households. 15–20 households were randomly selected from each cluster. An additional 10 households from each cluster were selected from the 2005 Uganda National Health Services (UNHS) list. All women aged 15–49 (permanent resident or not) present in the household on the night before the 2006 survey were eligible to be interviewed. In addition, 2,110 children aged less than 5 years present in the selected households were tested for anaemia. It should be noted that the 2006 UDHS is the first UDHS which includes the entire country (UDHS 2007). In the previous surveys some groups or districts were excluded for security problems. A detailed sampling methodology can be found in the 2006 Uganda Demographic Health survey final report (UDHS 2007).

9.2.2 Socio-Demographic Information and Potential Risk Factors of Anaemia

This analysis is based on a binary outcome (anaemic/not anaemic) and categorical variables grouped as individual, household, maternal, nutritional and community related factors.

Individual factors included gender (male/female), birth order categorised (first birth, 2–3 and 6+), preceding birth interval in months (<24, 24–35 and 36+), diarrhoeal infections (yes/no), and birth weight (low, normal and overweight). Bed net use (yes/no), maternal education (uneducated, primary and secondary +), partner education (no partner, primary and secondary +), maternal occupation (not working, agricultural, non-agricultural), toilet facility (none, flush and pit/bucket), wealth quintiles (lowest, lower, middle, higher and highest) and religion (Catholics, Muslim, Pentecostal, protestant, Seven Days Adventist and other) were classified as household related factors. Maternal factors comprised maternal age (<20 years, 20–34 years and 35+), maternal smoking habit (yes/no) and mother's anaemia status (yes/no). The place of residence (rural/urban), the place of delivery (home, hospital or other), and the nine region of Uganda and water source (other, piped) were considered as community related factors. Additional nutritional factors included breastfeeding (yes/no), breastfeeding time during the day (2–4, 4–8, 8+), whether the child ate meat (yes/no) and whether the child was given green leafy vegetables (yes/no). Also contextual variables such as the proportion of children from households with piped water and from the lowest and highest wealth quintiles by community were computed and included as continuous variables.

9.2.3 Statistical Analysis

SPSS 17 (SPSS corp., Tx, USA) enabled to acquire the data and recode some variables. Stata/SE10 (Stata Corp., College Station, TX, USA) was used for the initial analysis. In the bivariate analysis, cross-tabulation was made between each of the above potential risk factors and the presence of anaemia. Chi-square test was used to test the significance of each of the selected potential risk factors in the model. A p-value of 0.05 served as a cut off point.

In the multivariate analysis, MLwIn 2.11 was used to fit multilevel logistic regression models, to account and quantify the variability due to individual, household and community levels. Forward model selection (Rabe-Hesketh and Everitt 2004) was used for the model specification. The Wald test was used to test the joint significance for each of the selected categorical factors. Adjusted Odds ratio and their associated 95 % confidence intervals (C.I) were computed and are presented.

Multilevel Models

Most data collected in human or biological sciences have a hierarchical structure. For example, children with the same parents tend to be more alike in their physical and mental characteristics than random individuals from a population (Goldstein 2010). Individuals may be further nested within geographical areas such as communities. Multilevel model recognises the existence of such data hierarchies by allowing for residual components at each level in the hierarchy. For example, a two-level model, which allows for grouping of child outcomes within households would include residuals at child and household level. Thus the residual variance is partitioned into between-household component (the variance of household level residuals) and within household component (the variance of the child-level residuals). Household residual, often called "household effects", represent unobserved characteristics that affect child outcomes. These unobserved variables lead to correlation between outcomes for children from the same household. Multilevel models are useful for a number of reasons (1) correct inferences, standard regression approaches assume that the units of analysis are independent observations. One consequence of failing to recognise hierarchical structures is that standard errors of regression coefficients will be underestimated resulting to an overstatement of statistical significance. The standard error for the coefficient of higher-level predictor variables might be the most affected if grouping or clustering is ignored. (2) Interest in group effects: in many situations, research question concerns the extend of grouping in individual outcomes, and the identification of "outlying" groups in evaluation of household effect, for example, the investigators are interested to see the household effects on children risk of having anaemia. Such effects correspond to household residual in multilevel model. (3) Inferences to a population of groups: in a multilevel model the grouping in the sample is treated as a random sample from a population of groups. Using a fixed effects model, inferences cannot be made beyond the groups in the sample.

Multilevel Logistics Model Specification

In situation with clustered data where observations in the same group are related, for example, children nested within households it is possible to find out by using a random effect model how much of an effect household has on children after controlling for children background characteristics.

Let $\pi_{ijk} = p(y_{ijk} = 1)$ be the probability that a child (i) in the household j, from the community k, is anaemic. Where y_{ijk} is equal to 1 if a child is anaemic and 0 if not. We define this probability as a function of an intercept and the exploratory variables as follows:

$$\log it(\pi_{ijk}) = \log\left(\frac{\pi_{ijk}}{1-\pi_{ijk}}\right) = \beta_{0jk} + \beta_1 x_{1ijk} + \beta_2 x_{2ijk} + \beta_3 x_{3ijk} + \ldots + \beta_n x_{nijk}$$

With $\beta_{0jk} = \beta_0 + \mu_{0jk}$.

In this equation, β_{0jk} indicates that we are modelling the intercept in this relationship as random at j^{th} (household) and k^{th} (community) levels. The variables x_{1ijk} to x_{nijk} are the exploratory variables and their coefficients are fixed effects. The logit link function is assumed in the above equation, however other software allow also to use a probit or a complementary log-log function (McCullagh and Neder 1989). The intercept consists of two terms, a fixed term β_0 and a random term μ_{0jk}. The standard assumption is that the response y_{ijk} is distributed as Binomial $(1,\ \pi_{ijk})$. We may write this distributional assumption in a general form as: π_{ijk} – Binomial $(n_{ijk},\ \pi_{ijk})$ where in our case n_{ijk} are all equal to 1. This standard distributional form is also used to model proportions, where each proportion y_{ijk} is based on n_{ijk} observations and has a denominator n_{ijk} and is a special case where the denominator is everywhere 1 (Rasbash et al. 2005).

Using MLwiN, the estimates procedures were implemented. These procedures use a linearization methods, based on a Taylor series expansion, that transforms a discrete response model to continuous response model (Rasbash et al. 2005). After applying the linearization, the model is estimated using the Restricted Iterative Generalized Least squares (RIGLS) and quasi-likelihood methods to convert estimates into Predictive quasi-likelihood (PQL), where the level 2 residual are added to the linear element of the model at each stage. The transformation to linear model requires an approximation to be used and the type of approximation available in MLwiN are: marginal quasi-likelihood (MQL) and predictive quasi-likelihood (PQL). There are two orders in both of these methods, 1st and 2nd order terms of the Taylor series expansion. Both orders can be used, however the second is preferable because it is an improved approximation procedure (Rasbash et al. 2005). However it is less stable. The first order MQL is also useful, but when the sample sizes within the level 2 units are small or the response proportion is extern, the estimates may be biased. Further details can be found in Goldstein (2009).

9.3 Results

9.3.1 Characteristics of the Study Population

Among the 2,110 children who were included in this study, 51 % were males and 49 % were females, most of children (56 %) were between 2 and 5 birth and 22 % were respectively the first birth and 6th birth of their mothers, the majority (33 %) had a preceding birth interval between 24 and 35 months, 26 % less than 20 months, and 20 % with 36 months or plus. Few (12 %) were delivered at the hospital, 17 % at home and the majority (71 %) at others places, 55 % were breastfeed and 45 % were not.

9.3.2 Bivariate Analysis and Prevalence of Anaemia

Of the 2,110 children tested for anaemia, 73 % are anaemic. Anaemia was cross-tabulated with each of the selected potential risk factors and the prevalence of anaemia by the study characteristics was examined. The results indicate that maternal education (Chi-square =44.73, $p < 0.001$), paternal education (Chi-square =35.43, $p < 0.001$), maternal occupation (Chi-square =71.37, $p < 0.001$), wealth quintiles (Chi-square =133.65, $p < 0.001$), religion (Chi-square =65.21, $p < 0.001$), mother's anaemia status (Chi-square = 98.65, $p < 0.001$), the place of residence (Chi-square =181.93, $p < 0.001$), the place of delivery (Chi-square =22.51, $p < 0.001$), region (Chi-square =373.20, $p < 0.001$), water source (Chi-square =15.88, $p < 0.001$), breastfeeding (Chi-square = 5.02, $p = 0.025$), breastfeeding times per day (Chi-square =15.55, $p = 0.004$), whether the child was given meat (Chi-square = 4.55, $p = 0.033$) and whether the child ate green leafy vegetables (Chi-square = 10.20, $p < 0.001$) are factors associated with anaemia in children in Uganda (Table 9.1).

The bivariate analysis suggests that the prevalence of anaemia decreases with an increased maternal and father's level of education and wealth quintiles. Anaemia is much more prevalent among children of uneducated women (56 %) or fathers (59 %) than it is among those whose mothers are educated (46 %), 43 % among children from households in the highest wealth quintiles and 58 % among those form the lowest wealth quintiles (see Figs. 9.1 and 9.2). Anaemia is much more prevalent (65 %) among Pentecostal children, followed by Catholics (52 %), and Protestant (50 %). However it is less prevalent among Seven Day Adventist (SDA) children (see Fig. 9.3). 54 % of children of women working in the agriculture sector are anaemic, while it is 46 % among those whose mothers work in other sectors. Maternal anaemia status is another risk factor of anaemia among children; children of anaemic women are associated with a higher prevalence (64 %) than those of no anaemic women (34 %). Anaemia is highly prevalent in rural areas (54 %) while it is 32 % in urban, lower among children from households connected with piped water (40 %) than among those from households which use others sources.

Table 9.1 Potential socioeconomic and demographic risk factors associated with anaemia in children

Variable	Chi-square	P-value
Maternal education	44.73	<0.001
Maternal occupation	35.43	<0.001
Paternal education	71.37	<0.001
Wealth quintiles	133.65	<0.001
Mother's anaemia status	98.65	<0.001
Urban/Rural residence	181.93	<0.001
Place of delivery	22.51	<0.001
Source of drinking water	15.88	<0.001
Breastfeeding	5.02	0.025
Breastfeeding times	15.55	0.004
Child ate meat	4.55	0.033
Child ate green vegetables	10.22	<0.001
Region	375.2	<0.001
Religion	65.21	<0.001

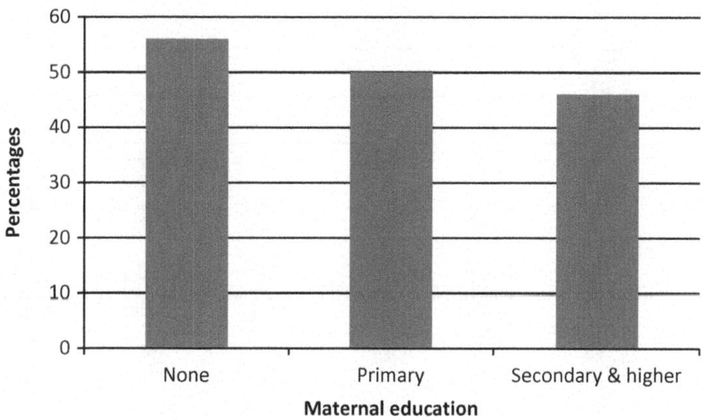

Fig. 9.1 The prevalence of anaemia by maternal education

9.3.3 Multivariate Analysis

This study suggests that beside other unknown risk factors of anaemia among children, in Uganda, age, gender, maternal occupation, and whether or not the mother is anaemic are factors significantly associated with anaemia (see Table 9.2). Younger children (below the age of 2 years old) and male are associated with an increased risk of having anaemia compared with their counterparts who are 2 years old or female.

With regards to maternal anaemia status, children of anaemic mothers are associated with two folds increased risk of anaemia compared with those whose mothers are not anaemic.

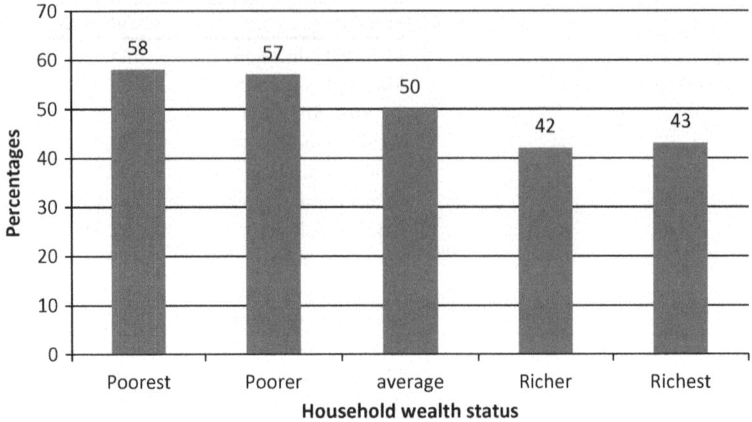

Fig. 9.2 The prevalence of anaemia by wealth quintiles

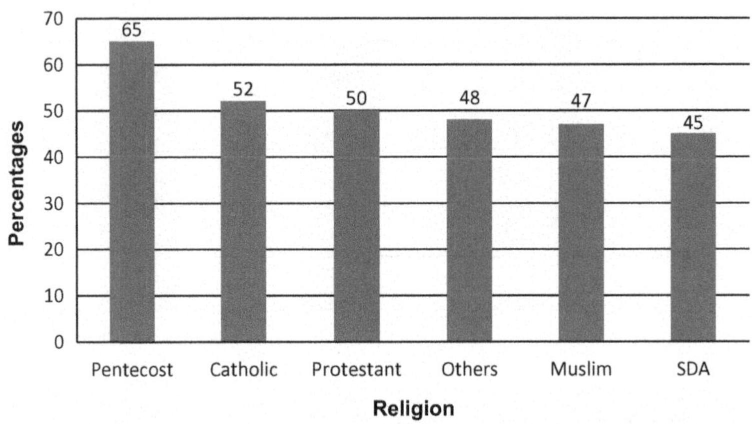

Fig. 9.3 The prevalence of anaemia by religion

Maternal occupation is another risk factor of anaemia in children in Uganda. Compared with children whose mothers work in other sectors or are not working, children of skilled mothers or of those who work in services sector have 81 % decreased risk of anaemia.

In addition, the results from this study support those from previous studies which suggest that anaemia intervention is much more needed at community level followed by individual level and that the variability due to community effects are fewer.

However, no association was found between anaemia and maternal level of education, household wealth status, maternal smoking habit, the place of residence, region, the source of drinking water, whether the child was given meat or green leafy vegetables, maternal age and breastfeeding.

Table 9.2 Estimates and odds ratios of multilevel logistic and simple logistic regression models

	Multilevel logistic regression model						Simple logistic regression model		
Variables	Category	Estimates	SE	OR	95 % CI		Estimates	SE	OR
	Cons	3.325	1.410				3.077	0.726	
Age	> 2 years (Ref.)			1.00					1.00
	2–5 years	−1.025	0.211	**0.36**	0.24	0.54	**−0.997**	0.211	**0.37**
Gender	Male (Ref)			1.00					1.00
	Female	−0.505	0.204	**0.60**	0.40	0.90	**0.508**	0.201	**1.66**
Maternal education	None (Ref.)			1.00					1.00
	Primary	−0.115	0.276	0.89	0.52	1.53	−0.136	0.257	0.87
	Secondary +	−0.241	0.450	0.79	0.33	1.90	−0.246	0.402	0.78
Maternal occupation	Not working (Ref.)			1.00					1.00
	Prof tech & management	−0.974	0.843	0.38	0.07	1.97	−0.920	0.789	0.40
	Clerical & sales	−1.026	0.549	0.36	0.12	1.05	**−0.993**	0.511	0.37
	Agriculture	−0.720	0.515	0.49	0.18	1.34	−0.666	0.497	0.51
	Household & domestic	−1.095	1.496	0.33	0.02	6.28	−1.051	1.088	0.35
	Services/skilled	−1.228	0.579	**0.29**	0.09	0.91	**−1.163**	0.561	0.31
	others	−2.580	1.676	0.08	0.01	2.02	**−2.548**	1.205	0.08
Wealth quintiles	Average (Ref.)			1.00					1.00
	Poorer	0.227	0.357	1.25	0.62	2.53	−0.222	0.325	0.80
	Poorest	0.017	0.309	1.02	0.56	1.86	−0.274	0.346	0.76
	Richer	0.214	0.329	1.24	0.65	2.36	−0.058	0.361	0.94
	Richest	−0.003	0.415	1.00	0.44	2.25	−0.230	0.463	0.79
Mother's smoking status	Non-smoker (Ref.)			1.00					1.00
	Smoker	0.302	0.538	1.35	0.47	3.88	0.309	0.505	1.36
Mother's health status	Not anaemic			1.00					1.00
	Anaemic	0.731	0.208	**2.08**	1.38	3.12	**0.748**	0.198	**2.11**

(continued)

Table 9.2 (continued)

Variables	Multilevel logistic regression model						Simple logistic regression model		
	Category	Estimates	SE	OR	95 % CI		Estimates	SE	OR
Place of residence	Rural (Ref.)			1.00					1.00
	Urban	0.317	0.612	1.37	0.41	4.56	0.331	0.587	1.39
Region	Kampala (Ref.)			1.00					1.00
	Central 1	0.946	0.759	2.58	0.58	11.40	0.199	0.595	1.22
	Central 2	1.159	0.777	3.19	0.69	14.61	−0.960	0.669	0.38
	East Central	1.060	0.756	2.89	0.66	12.70	0.125	0.551	1.13
	Eastern	0.512	0.733	1.67	0.40	7.02	−0.450	0.510	0.64
	North	0.299	0.708	1.35	0.34	5.40	−0.660	0.501	0.52
	Southwest	0.288	0.727	1.33	0.32	5.55	−0.667	0.509	0.51
	West Nile	−0.397	0.686	0.67	0.18	2.58	**−1.336**	0.477	**0.26**
	Western	−0.605	0.688	0.55	0.14	2.10	**−1.551**	0.486	**0.21**
Gave child meat	No			1.00					1.00
	Yes	0.020	0.343	1.02	0.52	2.00	−0.010	0.318	0.99
Gave child vegetable	No			1.00					1.00
	Yes	−0.302	0.208	0.74	0.49	1.11	−0.305	0.212	0.74
Contextual variables	Proportion with piped water	−0.669	0.356	0.51	0.25	1.03	**−0.715**	0.348	**0.49**

S.E standard error, *C.I* confidence Interval, *O.R* Odds Ratios, *Bold* indicates a significant difference with the reference category

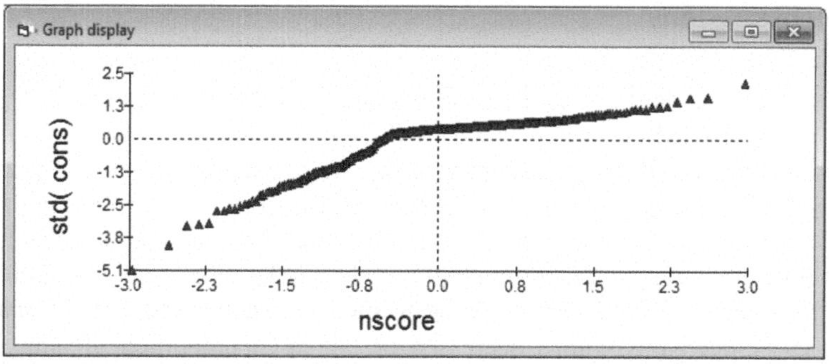

Fig. 9.4 Residual diagnostic

9.3.4 Multilevel Logistic Regression Model Versus Simple Logistic Regression

Table 9.2 presents both, results from multilevel logistics regression and simple logistic regression model. Simple logistic model estimates and standard errors are presented just for comparison reasons. In Sect. 9.3.2 it was mentioned that one consequence of failing to recognise hierarchical structures of the data is the standard errors of regression coefficients are underestimated resulting to an overstatement of statistical significance of some variables in the model. Table 9.2 confirms this indicating that if we ignore the hierarchical nature of the data, age, gender, maternal occupation, whether the mother is anaemic, the region and the proportion of household connected with piped water in communities are all factors associated with the risk of anaemia in children in Uganda. The standard errors of all the variables in the model are biased downward. Multilevel logistic model, however, suggests that the differences in children's risk of having anaemia observed between the nine regions of Uganda are not statistically significant, the proportion of household connected with piped water is not significantly associated with the risk of having anaemia among these children. Children's risk of having anaemia differs significantly between communities in which children's live.

Model Assumption and Diagnostics

Residual were analysed using graphical display to check the plausible model assumptions of normally distributed errors. The results suggest that the residuals are normally distributed at community level (see Fig. 9.4).

9.4 Discussions

A cross sectional study of 2,110 children aged less than 5 years old in Uganda in 2006 was carried out and potential risk factors of anaemia were examined at individual, household and community levels. The first aim of this study was to explore the risk factors of anaemia in children at each level and then use multilevel logistic regression model to quantify variability due to individual, household and community effects in order to inform policy makers in Uganda and in other countries with the same characteristics. Hypothesis such as whether the risk of anaemia increases or decreases with a decreased or increased proportion of households connected to a piped water or within the lower or highest wealth quintiles by community were tested. Individual, household and community effects were quantified.

This study suggests a higher prevalence of anaemia in children in Uganda. The overall prevalence of anaemia in children is 73 %. There are important and significant relationships between anaemia and some of the selected potential risk factors. These included age, gender, maternal occupation and whether the mother is anaemic. It suggests that maternal health plays a significant role in children's risk of anaemia and that children of anaemic mothers are more likely to have anaemia and this was consistent even after accounting for the place of residence, region, and mother's smoking habit.

The results also suggest that children of mothers who are skilled and work in services sector are less likely to have anaemia compared with children of those women who don't work at all or who work in others economic sectors. It is argued that in Uganda, over 75 % of skilled women work in government services such as those in medical (nurses and midwives) and teaching fields. Significant lower risk of anaemia associated with children of those women who are skilled or who work in services could indirectly be attributed to women's education or income although women's education is not directly related with anaemia in children in this study. Educated women have better job opportunity with reasonable income than uneducated women and they can make a good choice for their household diet for their children's health in order to protect them from some preventable diseases. The other reason might be the fact that in least developed countries the access to health facilities is limited. In areas with health facilities, the quality of services provided is poor and women who are not educated might not overcome these obstacles (Caldwell 2000; Hobcraft 1993; Mensch 1986; Cleland and van Ginneken 1988).

Although there has been little investigation of socioeconomic factors associated with anaemia in children, these finding are consistent with few studies that have analysed the overall nutritional status of children in the region (Smith et al. 2004; Fotso 2006).

In addition, it indicates that more variability in children's risk of anaemia is due to community level, followed by individual factors and there is few variability due to household level factors. This study brings to light that anaemia intervention in Uganda needs to be targeted at community, which could help spread the relevant information. The results from this study indicate that if the individuals are nested within households and households are nested within communities (data are hierarchical), ignoring the hierarchical nature of the data could result in over statement of the significance of some of the variables included in the model. Most importantly, the standard errors are biased downward.

Anaemia is a widespread health problem in Uganda. The study findings have some important and relevant policy messages. Policy makers should place more emphasis on the role of remoteness as well as environmental or climatic factors on diseases. The links between the age, gender, the differences between maternal occupations need to be addressed in order to achieve the Millennium Development Goals (MDG 1,2, 4, 5, & 6) as well as fostering human development.

9.5 Limitations

There are some limitations. As for many questionnaire-based data, the limitations for the UDHS included reporting and recall bias, particularly for age or other retrospective data relying on memory of a past event. Therefore, individual level data required more careful interpretation. Nevertheless, these results are important in guiding the assessment of current evidence and the definition of future research strategies.

9.6 Conclusions

This analysis suggests that anaemia in children is highly prevalent in Uganda. This higher prevalence in Africa in general and in Uganda in particular may be due to diverse factors. However, in this study children's age, gender, maternal occupation and whether the mother is anaemic are factors significantly associated with anaemia in children. Children aged below 2 years old, male, those whose mothers work in other sectors or are not working at all and children's of anaemic mothers are associated with a higher risk of anaemia. These differences need to be well scrutinised in future studies. The results also suggest that the hierarchical nature of the data need to be accounted for, otherwise, the standard errors of some factors are underestimated and some factors might seem significant while in reality they are not. This study throws light on the fact that anaemia intervention needs to focus more at community level followed by individual level.

References

Abouzahr, C., & Royston, E. (1991). *Maternal mortality: A global factbook*. Geneva: World Health Organisation.

Badham, J. (2007). *The guidebook of nutritional anaemia*. Basel: Sight and Life Press.

Caldwell, J. A. C. W. P. (2000). *The link between health and Education for Indigenous Australian Children. Approching Indigenous Health through Eduaction*. Barton: Australian Medical Association Limited.
Cleland, J. G., & van Ginneken J. K. (1988). Maternal education and child survival in developed countries: The search for pathways of influence. *Social Sciences and Medicine, 27*, 1357–1368.
Demaeyer, E. M. (1990). *Preventing and controlling iron deficiency anaemia through primary health care: A guide for health administrators and programme managers*. Geneva: World Health Organisation.
Fotso, J. C. (2006). Child health inequities in developing countries: Differences across urban and rural areas. *International Journal for Equity in Health, 5*, 9.
Goldstein, H. (2010). *Multilevel statistical models*. Chichester: Wiley.
Goldstein, H., & Browne, W. J. (2009). *A user's guide to MLwiN*. Bristol: Centre for Multilevel Modelling, University of Bristol.
Hobcraft, J. (1993). Women's education, child welfare and child survival: A review of the evidence. *Health Transition Review, 3*(2), 159–175.
Levin, H. M. (1986). *A benefit-cost analysis of nutritional programs for anaemia reduction*. Washington, DC: World Bank.
Madise, N. J., Matthews, Z., & Margetts, B. (1999). Heterogeneity of child nutritional status between households: A comparison of six sub-saharan countries. *Population Studies, 53*, 331–343.
McCullagh, P., & Neder, L. (1989). *Generalized linear models*. London: Chapman and hall.
Mensch, B. (1986). Age differences between spouses in first marriages. *Socity of Biology, 33*(3–4), 229–240.
Pollitt, E. (1982). Behavioural effects of iron deficiency anaemia in children. In E. Pollitt et al. (Eds.), *Iron deficiency: Brain biochemistry and behaviour*. New York: New York Press.
Rabe-Hesketh, S., & Everitt, B. (2004). *A handbook of statistical analysis using stata*. Washington, DC: Chapman &Hall/CRC.
Rasbash, J. S. F., Browne, W., & Prosser, B. (2005). *A user's guide to MLwiN*. Bristol: Centre for Multilevel Modelling, University of Bristol.
Smith, L. C., Ruel, M. T., & Ndiaye, A. (2004). Why is child malnutrition lower in urban than rural areas?. FCND discussion papers.Ruta.org. http://ruta.org:8180/xmlui/handle/123456789/676
Snijders, T. A., & Boker, R. J. (1999). *Multilevel analysis: An introduction to basic and advanced multilevel Modelling*. London: Sage.
Stoltzfus, R. J., Ayoya, A. M., Spiekermann-Brouwer, G. M., Traore, A. K., & Garza, C. (2006). Determinants of aneamia among pregnant women in Mali. *Food and Nutritional Bulletin, 27*, 3–11.
UDHS. (2007). Uganda Demographic Health Survey general report. In U. B. O. (Ed.), *Statistics*. Calverton: Macro International.
WHO. (2008). *Worldwide prevalence of anaemia 1993–2005, WHO Global database*. Geneva: World Health Organisation.

Part II
Maternal Health

Chapter 10
A Family of Flexible Parametric Duration Functions and Their Applications to Modeling Child-Spacing in Sub-Saharan Africa

Gebrenegus Ghilagaber, Woldeyesus Elisa, and Stephen Obeng Gyimah[†]

10.1 Introduction

Examining the dynamics of child spacing is of interest for several reasons. First, several inferences are consistent with the view that in much of the developing world, women with large families have shorter birth intervals than those with smaller families. There is thus an indication of an inverse relationship between spacing and completed or cumulative fertility. The spacing of births also has a significant bearing on maternal and child health through the dynamics of *sibling competition, maternal depletion* and *interval effect* hypotheses (Gribble 1993; Gyimah in press; Hobcraft et al. 1985; Majumder et al. 1997; Palloni & Millman 1986; Pederson 2000; Rafalimanana and Westoff 2000; Rodriguez et al. 1984).

According to the competition hypothesis, the birth of each successive child generates competition for scarce resources among siblings in the household which subsequently leads to a lower quality of care and attention to each child. The family resources may also be stretched to the limit, increasing the probability of children in such households becoming malnourished (Gribble 1993). The maternal depletion syndrome contends that births in rapid succession physiologically deplete the mother of energy and nutrition which may lead to premature births or pregnancy complications; thus increase the risk of infant or maternal death or impairing the

[†] deceased

G. Ghilagaber (✉)
Department of Statistics, Stockholm University, SE-106 91 Stockholm, Sweden
e-mail: Gebre@stat.su.se

W. Elisa
Statistics and Evaluation Office, Asmara, Eritrea

N.-B. Kandala and G. Ghilagaber (eds.), *Advanced Techniques for Modelling Maternal and Child Health in Africa*, The Springer Series on Demographic Methods and Population Analysis 34, DOI 10.1007/978-94-007-6778-2_10,

mother's ability to nurture her children. Additionally, women with closely spaced births may still have very young children and, as such, are less likely to attend prenatal care services which may increase maternal and child mortality risks.

Further, the early arrival of a new child often necessitates the premature weaning of the previous child, exposing the weaned one to malnutrition and increasing the child's vulnerability to infectious and parasitic diseases. Invariably, longer birth spacing has been found to increase profoundly the probability of infant survival (Bicego and Ahmad 1996; Defo 1997; Pederson 2000). Understanding the timing and spacing of births thus provides a thorough view of attitudes toward family size as well as differentials in fertility and childhood mortality levels.

The birth interval approach to studying fertility views the family building process as consisting of a series of stages, where women move successively from marriage to first birth, from first to second birth, and so on, until they reach their completed family size (Rodriguez et al. 1984). The point of entry into the process may be defined either as marriage or as entry into motherhood, but the main focus of this analysis is on the process of transition from one stage to the next, or the intervals between successive births. The transition process is studied in terms of the birth function,[1] defined as the cumulative proportion of women having a birth by successive duration since the previous birth (or marriage in the case of first birth). This function reflects two aspects of the process of reproduction. The first is *the quantum of fertility* indicated by the proportion of women progressing to the next higher parity (parity progression ratio), and the second is *the tempo of fertility* measured by the time it takes to make the transition for those women who continue reproduction.

In most empirical analyses of birth interval data, the focus has been on the quantum of fertility using proportional hazard models for the intensity of birth. That is, the rates at which children are born to a defined set of women within a specified unit of time. The proportional hazards model (Cox 1972) specifies the intensity of birth as a function of an unspecified time dependent baseline hazard, $\lambda\ O(t)$, and the covariates,

$$\lambda(\mathrm{t}, \mathbf{z}) = \lambda_0(\mathrm{t}) \exp(\mathbf{z}\boldsymbol{\beta}) \tag{10.1}$$

where, z is a vector of covariates and $\boldsymbol{\beta}$ is a vector of unknown regression parameters.

While the nuisance baseline specification makes the Cox model attractive particularly in contexts where the focus is not on the timing function, the model may be too restrictive because the assumption of proportional hazards is often unrealistic

[1]In mortality analysis, interest is usually focussed on survival probability. The proportion surviving up to time t, is commonly denoted by $S(t)$, and is defined as $S(t) = P(T > t)$. In fertility analysis, however, interest is focused on the proportion having a subsequent child (partial parity progression ratio). Thus, the birth function is simply the complementary function, $B(t) = 1 - S(t) = F(t) = P(T \leq t)$. It is simply the cumulative proportion of women having a subsequent birth by single months of duration since previous birth (or marriage).

in many real life situations. Also, there are instances where one's research interest centers on the distributional shape of the timing function and thus calling for alternative models.

In this chapter, we present a second class of models, more akin to ordinary linear regression, that specifies the covariates to act multiplicatively on tempo of fertility (or linearly on log-tempo) rather than on the quantum (intensity of birth). We demonstrate how a number of common parametric duration models like the Weibull and log-normal may be embedded in a single parametric framework, and how each special-case model may be assessed relative to a more comprehensive one. This class of models is then applied on birth interval data from three African countries (Eritrea, Ghana, & Kenya) with a view to examining the distributional shape of birth intervals and the sensitivity of inferences to the choice of a model.

The chapter thus has both methodological and substantive objectives. The methodological objective centres on the application of a flexible family of parametric survival models to the analysis of birth interval data. The second set of objectives, of a substantive nature, relate to examining correlates of birth spacing in sub-Saharan Africa using Demographic and Health Surveys data from Eritrea, Ghana, and Kenya. In the next section, we introduce the class of flexible parametric duration models and describe how covariates effects are estimated in such models. In Sect. 10.3, we fit this family of models to birth interval data from the three African countries and discuss the results, while Sect. 10.4 provides a summary.

10.2 A Family of Flexible Parametric Duration Functions

10.2.1 Accelerated Failure-Time Models for the Tempo of Fertility

Suppose we denote by *To* the time (birth interval in months) associated with the baseline level corresponding to zero values for the covariates ($z = \boldsymbol{0}$). Such baseline levels may, for example, be women with no education (to be later compared with those having some primary- or secondary-level education) or urban residents (to be compared with rural residents). Then, the accelerated tempo model specifies that if the vector of covariates had been z ($z \neq \boldsymbol{0}$), the event time (time to birth) would have been

$$\mathrm{T} = \mathrm{T_o}\exp(\mathbf{z}\boldsymbol{\beta}), \tag{10.2}$$

or equivalently, that

$$\ln\ \mathrm{T} = \ln\ \mathrm{T_o} + \mathbf{z}\boldsymbol{\beta} \tag{10.3}$$

where, as before, T is the vector of failure times, z is a vector of covariates, $\boldsymbol{\beta}$ is a vector of unknown regression parameters. Since covariates alter, by a scale factor, the rate at which an individual woman traverses the time axis, (10.2) may be referred to as the *accelerated failure time model* (*accelerated tempo of fertility* in the context of this chapter). Thus, for proportional hazards model (10.1), the explanatory variables act multiplicatively on the baseline intensity so that their effect is to increase or decrease the intensity of birth relative to λ0(t). For accelerated tempo models, on the other hand, the explanatory variables act multiplicatively on time to the event (birth in our case) so that their effect is to accelerate or decelerate transition time to birth relative to *T0*.

The model in (10.3) is a linear model with ln*To* playing the role of an error term with an underlying baseline distribution. Usually, an intercept term α and a scale parameter δ are allowed in the model to give

$$\ln \mathrm{T} = \alpha + \mathbf{z}\boldsymbol{\beta} + \delta \ln \mathrm{T}_o \tag{10.4}$$

In terms of the original (untransformed) times to birth, the effect of the intercept term and the scale factor are to scale and power the time to birth, respectively:

$$\mathrm{T} = \exp(\alpha + \mathbf{z}\boldsymbol{\beta} + \delta \ln \mathrm{T}_o) = \mathrm{T}_o{}^{\delta} \exp(\alpha) \exp(\mathbf{z}\boldsymbol{\beta}) \tag{10.5}$$

In other words, the effect of covariates in an accelerated tempo model is to change the scale, but not the location, of a baseline distribution of birth times. A point worth noting at this stage is that the parameterizations in (10.1) and (10.2) are different. A positive coefficient in (10.1) implies an increased birth intensity (shorter interval) while in (10.2) it implies longer interval (decreased intensity) relative to that of the baseline level.

10.2.2 The Choice Between Alternative Baseline Distributions

As we saw above, the model for the response variable (10.4) consists of a linear effect composed of the covariates together with a random disturbance term. Such models may be rewritten more explicitly as

$$\ln \mathrm{T} = \mathbf{z}\boldsymbol{\beta} + \delta\boldsymbol{\varepsilon} \tag{10.6}$$

in which the intercept is incorporated in the coefficient vector $\boldsymbol{\beta}$ and a more conventional notation is used for the random error term. The distribution of the random error term can be taken from a class of distributions that includes the extreme-value, normal, and logistic distributions, and by using a log-transformation, exponential, Weibull, log-normal, log-logistic and gamma distributions. In general, the distribution may depend on additional shape parameter *k*.

Embedding competing models in a single parametric framework allows the methods of ordinary parametric inference to be used for discrimination and leads to an assessment of each competing model relative to a more comprehensive one. Stacey (1962) showed that the *generalized gamma* model could be useful in this regard. The generalized-gamma model is the distribution of T such that $\ln T = \mathbf{z\beta}+\delta\boldsymbol{\varepsilon}$, where the random error term $\boldsymbol{\varepsilon}$ has the density;

$$\mathrm{f(k,\varepsilon)} = \frac{1}{\Gamma(k)} \exp\left\{k\varepsilon - \exp(\varepsilon)\right\}, -\infty < \mathbf{z\beta} < \infty, -\infty < \boldsymbol{\varepsilon} < \infty, \text{ and } \delta, \mathrm{k} > 0. \tag{10.7}$$

Prentice (1974) showed that a transformation of the form $w = k^{1/2}(\varepsilon - \ln k)$ leads to a *standard normal* distribution for w as $k \to \infty$. Further, he extended the generalized gamma distribution by setting $q = k^{-1/2}$ and by allowing the error density at $-q$ to be a reflection, about the origin, of that of q. The parameter $q = k^{-1/2}$ was chosen as the unique power of k that leads to finite, nonzero likelihood derivatives at the log-normal model for T.

The final model with parameters $-\infty < z\beta < \infty$, $-\infty < q < \infty$, and $\delta > 0$, can be written as $\ln T = \mathbf{z\beta} + \delta\boldsymbol{\varepsilon}$ where the error density function $\mathrm{f}(q,\varepsilon)$ is

$$f(q,\varepsilon) = \begin{cases} \dfrac{|q|}{\Gamma(q^{-2})}\left(q^{-2}\right)^{q^{-2}} \exp\left[q^{-2}\left\{q\varepsilon - \exp(q\varepsilon)\right\}\right], & q \neq 0 \\ (2\pi)^{-1/2} \exp\left(-\dfrac{\varepsilon^2}{2}\right), & q = 0 \end{cases} \tag{10.8}$$

The distribution of T, when the error term has the density (10.8) will henceforth be called the *Extended Generalized Gamma (EGG)* distribution. As can be seen from the lower part of (10.8), the EGG model reduces to the *standard normal* distribution for ε when the shape parameter q is equal to zero. Accordingly, T will have a *log-normal* distribution. When the shape parameter q equals 1, (10.8) reduces to $\mathrm{f}(1,\varepsilon) = \mathrm{f}(\varepsilon) = \exp\{\varepsilon - \exp(\varepsilon)\}$, $-\infty < \varepsilon < \infty$, which is the standard (type 1) extreme-value distribution. As $\ln T$ is a linear function of ε, it has the same (extreme-value) distribution as ε. Hence $T = \exp(\mathbf{z\beta}+\delta\boldsymbol{\varepsilon})$ will have a *Weibull* distribution. If $q = 1$ and $\delta = 1$, then T has the *exponential* distribution as a special case of the Weibull distribution. The case of $q = -1$ corresponds to *extreme maximum-value* distribution for $\ln T$. This, in turn, corresponds to *reciprocal Weibull* distribution for T. The case of $\delta = 1$ and $q > 0$ is also of interest. Farewell and Prentice (1977) argue that this gives the ordinary gamma distribution for T, though, in accordance with Bergström and Edin (1992), this does not hold in our case illustration. Consequently, we shall label this special case ($\delta = 1$, $q > 0$) the '*gamma*' distribution in our illustrative example.

Thus, five models for T are included as special cases of the EGG model. Since each of these five models is nested within the EGG model, its goodness of fit to the data, in relation to the more comprehensive EGG model, may be assessed through standard likelihood ratio tests. Another model of interest, though not a special case of the EGG model, is the *log-logistic* model. A log-logistic distribution is the distribution of T such that $\log T$ follows a logistic distribution. Description and applications of the log-logistic model may be found in Diekmann (1992), Little et al. (1994), Nandram (1989), Shoukri et al. (1988), and Singh et al. (1988).

10.2.3 Estimation

The practical estimation of (10.6) proceeds as follows. Consider survival times of n individuals $t_1, t_2, \ldots, t_n$ and p covariates $z_1, z_2, \ldots, z_p$. Let di take value 0 if ti is a censoring time and value 1 if ti represents an event time. The log-likelihood function $\ln(\ln t;\, \mathbf{z\beta},\, \delta,\, q)$, assuming a noninformative censoring mechanism, will then be proportional to

$$\sum_{i=1}^{n} d_i \{\ln f(\varepsilon; q) - \ln \delta\} + \sum_{i=1}^{n} (1 - d_i) \ln S(\varepsilon_i; q), \tag{10.9}$$

where $f(\varepsilon;q)$ is given by the EGG model (10.8), $S(\varepsilon;q)$ is the corresponding survivor function, and $\varepsilon_i = (y_i - z_i\beta)/\delta$. At each of several q-values the maximum likelihood estimates $(\hat{\beta}(q),\ \hat{\delta}(q))$ are obtained by using the Newton–Raphson method to solve the normal equations arising from (10.9). Standard errors of coefficients may be obtained from the information matrix as usual.

10.3 Illustration: Analysis of Birth-Interval Data in Eritrea, Ghana, and Kenya

10.3.1 Background

The aim of the present illustration is to fit the models discussed above to birth interval data to study the distributional shape and discriminate among special-case models. Related questions concern identifying correlates of child spacing and, more importantly, the dependence of inference about these correlates on the distributional shape of the duration variable (birth intervals).

The data sets come from the Demographic and Health Survey (DHS) data for Ghana (1998) and Kenya (1998) and Eritrea (1995). The DHS are funded by the United States Agency for International Development (USAID) and administered by Macro International in conjunction with reputable host institutions in selected developing countries. These are national representative self-weighting samples of women in the reproductive ages of 15–49 years. The respondents for the interview were women who had spent the previous night in the selected households. The quality of DHS data has been extensively discussed in the literature and will not be highlighted here. Although there are non sampling errors on some age-related variables, evaluation studies suggest the DHS compares favorably with other large scale surveys such as the World Fertility Survey (Gage, 1995).

The dependent variable for this illustrative analysis is transition time between successive births measured in months. For comparison purposes, we shall also fit the Cox model (10.1) in which the dependent variable is the birth intensity at a given time. Generally, differences in birth intervals can be explained through demographic, socio-economic and socio-cultural factors. On the basis of previous work, we have selected an array of theoretically relevant variables as likely covariates of birth intervals. These include mother's birth cohort, age at first marriage and at first birth, residence, maternal education, and the survival status of the index child.

A cohort is indicative of structural factors that have shaped the life of individuals. At the macro level, similar life experiences can be detected among women belonging to the same cohort despite subtle micro level differences. Given the changing contextual factors affecting reproduction in sub-Saharan Africa, we expect the younger cohorts, who became adolescents in a period of a more egalitarian gender role, efficient contraceptives, and higher female enrolments in formal education, to have wider intervals than earlier cohorts.

Age at first marriage and age at first birth are also of tremendous importance in fertility studies because of their inverse relation to the exposure to the risk of conception (see, e.g., Gyimah, 2003; Westoff, 1992). They also represent a number of unmeasured factors that predispose women to differential timing of births and, thus, overall fertility. Women who marry at younger ages or have first births earlier are likely to come from disadvantaged socio-economic backgrounds and are thus more likely to be associated with the higher risks of births than their counterparts whose first marriages or first birth occurs late (Gyimah, 2001). Consequently, we expect women who marry or have birth early to be associated with shorter intervals.

Also significant in determining the length of the inter-birth interval is the survival status of the index child (Montgomery and Cohen 1998; Preston 1978). In both Ghana and Kenya, it has been demonstrated that intervals following the death of the index child tend to be significantly shorter than intervals where the child survived, a result of biological and behavioral processes (Gyimah and Fernando 2002). We thus expect the death of the index child to be associated with shorter intervals.

There is also a considerable empirical evidence that associates urban residence and high levels of maternal education with low fertility. The pathways through which these happen have been explained through an array of mechanisms including late age at marriage, greater knowledge and access to contraception, high labor force participation and alternative values regarding family size (Cochrane 1979, 1983; Martin 1995; Ware 1984). Previous work in Ghana has found a positive linear effect of education on the intervals between successive births (Ghana Statistical Service and Macro International 1999). Consistent with previous research, we expect the intervals between births to be longer among urban residents and highly educated women.

10.3.2 Descriptive Results

Summary statistics for the data are given in Tables 10.1, 10.2 and 10.3 for Eritrea, Ghana, and Kenya respectively. It is worth noting, right at the outset, that while the datasets for Eritrea and Kenya refer to the totality of children born by all women

Table 10.1 Frequency distribution and summary statistics, Eritrea, 1995

Variables	Sub sample (#of children)	Number with closed intervals	% with closed intervals	Exposure (months)	Case/exposure (per 1,000)	Relative hazards
Mother's birth cohort						
1946–1950	2,997	2,523	84.18	140,164	18.00	1.00
1951–1960	6,176	5,060	81.93	231,022	21.90	1.22
1961–1970	4,067	2,841	69.85	126,450	22.47	1.25
1971–1980	1,028	376	36.58	23,500	16.00	0.89
Birth period of index child						
1960–1964	1,510	1,469	97.28	62,886	23.36	1.00
1975–1990	8,962	8,005	89.32	369,943	21.64	0.93
1991–1995	3,796	1,326	34.93	88,307	15.02	0.64
Mother's education						
None	10,898	8,458	77.61	393,508	21.49	
Primary	2,339	1,697	72.55	88,444	19.19	0.89
Secondary+	1,031	645	62.56	39,184	16.46	0.77
Residence						
Urban	5,943	4,454	74.95	236,086	18.87	1.00
Rural	8,320	6,343	76.24	284,895	22.26	1.18
Death status of index child						
Alive	11,692	8,536	73.01	431,832	19.77	1.00
Dead	2,576	2,264	87.89	89,304	25.35	1.28
Age at first marriage						
Under 20 years	11,721	9,016	76.92	429,433	21.00	
20–24 years	1,941	1,387	71.46	67,876	20.43	0.97
25–29 years	438	293	66.89	17,326	16.91	0.81
30 + years	126	84	66.67	4,505	18.65	0.89
Age at first birth						
Under 20 years	7,274	5,602	77.01	276,886	20.23	
20–24 years	5,004	3,778	75.50	175,613	21.51	1.06
25–29 years	1,581	1,150	72.74	54,180	21.23	1.05
30 + years	409	270	66.01	14,457	18.68	0.92
Total	14,268	10,800	75.69	521,136	20.72	

interviewed (and ranging from birth order 1 to birth order 14), those from Ghana refer to children born in the five years before the survey and thus range between birth orders 1 and 5. Thus, 14,268, 3,176, and 22,493 index children were analyzed for Eritrea, Ghana and Kenya, respectively.

The columns labeled 'closed intervals' (and % closed intervals) in these Tables (10.1, 10.2, 10.3) relate to children with at least one younger sibling at the time of

Table 10.2 Frequency distribution and summary statistics, Ghana, 1998

Variables	Sub sample (#of children)	Number with closed intervals	% with closed intervals	Exposure (months)	Case/exposure (per 1,000)	Relative hazards
Mother's current age						
15–24	739	174	23.55	15,790	11.02	1.00
25–34	1,482	440	29.69	37,562	11.71	1.06
35–49	955	233	24.40	27,327	8.53	0.77
Mother's education						
None	1,506	449	29.81	38,404	11.69	1.00
Primary	567	150	26.46	14,176	10.58	0.91
Secondary+	1,103	248	22.48	28,099	8.83	0.75
Residence						
Urban	687	144	20.96	17,793	8.09	1.00
Rural	2,489	703	28.24	62,886	11.18	1.38
Death status of index child						
Alive	2,941	718	24.41	75,241	9.54	1.00
Dead	235	129	54.89	5,438	23.72	2.49
Age at first marriage						
Under 20 years	2,131	565	26.51	54,744	10.32	1.00
20–24 years	817	219	26.81	20,203	10.84	1.05
25 + years	228	63	27.63	5,732	10.99	1.07
Age at first birth						
Under 20 years	1,641	434	26.45	42,508	10.21	1.00
20–24 years	1,169	309	26.43	29,298	10.55	1.03
25 + years	366	104	28.42	8,873	11.72	1.15
Length of succeding interval (months)						
Under 18 months	1,063	85	8.00	9,582	8.87	1.00
18–29 months	888	307	34.57	20,888	14.70	1.66
30–47 months	940	406	43.19	35,237	11.52	1.30
48 + months	285	49	17.19	14,972	3.27	0.37
Total	3,176	847	26.67	80,679	10.50	

the survey. The next column 'exposure' refers to the exposure months contributed by each sub-sample, including those children who were censored (did not get a younger sibling) by the survey time. The 'case/exposure' column is just the crude birth intensity (births per 1,000 person months) while the last column gives ratios of the birth intensities to that of the baseline level of each variables. These are unstandardized versions of the relative intensities in proportional hazards models.

Table 10.3 Frequency distribution and summary statistics, Kenya, 1998

Variables	Sub sample (#of children)	Number with closed intervals	% with closed intervals	Exposure (months)	Case/exposure (per 1,000)	Relative hazards
Mother's birth cohort						
1946–1950	1,180	1,614	136.78	91,989	17.55	1.00
1951–1960	8,826	7,434	84.23	370,059	20.09	14.00
1961–1970	8,496	6,476	76.22	300,847	21.53	1.23
1971–1980	3,291	1,699	51.63	86,929	19.54	1.11
Birth period of index child						
1960–1974	1,841	1,800	97.77	70,083	25.68	1.00
1975–1990	12,895	11,776	91.32	545,277	21.60	0.84
1991–1995	1,157	3,647	315.21	234,464	15.55	0.61
Mother's education						
None	5,375	4,461	83.00	214,927	20.76	
Primary	13,010	9,916	76.22	474,999	20.88	1.01
Secondary+	4,108	2,846	69.28	159,898	17.80	0.86
Residence						
Urban	2,712	1,817	67.00	120,038	15.14	1.00
Rural	19,781	15,406	77.88	729,786	21.11	1.39
Death status of index child						
Alive	20,466	15,589	76.17	776,073	20.09	1.00
Dead	2,027	1,634	80.61	73,751	22.16	1.10
Age at first marriage						
Under 20 years	16,404	12,887	78.56	612,783	21.03	1.00
20–24 years	5,108	3,652	71.50	195,065	18.72	0.89
25–29 years	806	564	69.98	32,574	17.31	0.82
30 + years	175	120	68.57	9,402	12.76	0.69
Age at first birth						
Under 20 years	15,559	12,230	78.60	591,033	20.69	1.00
20–24 years	6,162	4,488	72.83	229,826	19.53	0.94
25–29 years	665	443	66.62	25,216	17.57	0.85
30 + years	107	62	57.94	749	82.78	4.00
Total	22,493	17,223	76.57	849,824	20.27	–

From Table 10.1, we note that 10,800 (75.7 %) of the Eritrean children in the study had younger siblings (the birth intervals were closed) while the rest were censored as at the survey time (the birth intervals were still open). Of the 10,800 with younger siblings, the majority (8,536) were alive when their next younger siblings were born while in the rest (2,264) cases the index child has died before the birth of the younger sibling. Thus, as shown in the last column of Table 10.1, a crude estimate of birth intensity of women who lost their index child is 1.28 times (about 28 % higher) that of women with a living index child. Similar patterns are noticeable in Tables 10.2 and 10.3 for Ghana and Kenya, respectively.

10.3.3 Covariate Effects

In Tables 10.4, 10.5, and 10.6, we report results of fitting models (10.1) and (10.8) to data for Eritrea, Ghana and Kenya, respectively. The estimated coefficients in the first seven columns under 'parametric models' come from fitting the model in (10.8) and, hence, represent effects of the respective levels of a factor on log-birth interval (that of baseline level is set to 0 by design). These were obtained using the LifeReg procedure in SAS by including some options that restrict the shape and/or scale parameter whenever the need arises. Estimates given in the column labeled Cox were obtaine using the PhReg procedure in SAS and are related to model (10.1) and, as such, measure the effect of the covariates on the log-intensity of transition to the next higher parity (birth intensity). The last column is just relative intensities (intensity ratios, or hazard ratios) obtained by exponentiating the estimates in the Cox model.

As we pointed out earlier, the two classes of models follow slightly different parameterizations. A positive coefficient in any of the seven columns under parametric models implies an extended birth interval (decreased birth intensity) while a positive coefficient in column under Cox implies increased birth intensity (shorter birth interval) relative to that of the baseline. Further, it may be worth noting that the shape and scale parameters are free (estimated from the data) in the more comprehensive EGG model, while in the five special case-models one or both of these parameters are set to some fixed value(s) as discussed in Sect. 10.2.

According to Table 10.4, for example, the factors that considerably shorten the birth interval (increase the birth intensity) are belonging to a younger birth cohort, death of index child, and a delayed age at first birth. Having the birth in recent periods seem to have the opposite effect while residence, education, and age at first marriage seem to have only marginal effects. Such results are reported by most models though the Weibull and Exponential models show stronger effects of Education (increase of birth intervals with increase in education) and Residence (shorter birth intervals in rural areas). In the next section, we shall examine if these models have adequate goodness of fit.

10.3.4 Discrimination Among Parametric Models

When parametric models are nested, the likelihood ratio tests can be used to assess the best fit model (Heckman and Walker 1991; Allison 2010). The likelihood-ratio statistics corresponding to various tests for special cases of the EGG model (10.8) are presented in Table 10.7. These are used to test whether the corresponding

Table 10.4 Estimated coefficients for various parametric models, Eritrea, 1995

	Parametric models							Cox model	
Covariates	Extended Generalized Gamma	Reciprocal Weibull	Log normal	Weibull	Gamma	Exponential	Log logistic	Coefficient	Hazard ratio
Intercept	3.243	3.261	3.587	4.125	3.463	3.993	3.492	–	–
Scale	0.558	0.563	0.667	0.739	1.000	1.000	0.364	–	–
Shape	−1.068	−1.000	0.000	1.000	−0.576	1.000	–	–	–
Mother's birth cohort									
1946–1950 (reference)	0.000	0.000	0.000	0.000	0.000	0.000	0.000	0.000	1.000
1951–1955	−0.078	−0.081	−0.163	−0.322	−0.134	−0.312	−0.118	0.251	1.285
1961–1970	−0.136	−0.140	−0.254	−0.490	−0.217	−0.473	−0.181	−0.376	1.456
1971–1980	−0.131	−0.135	−0.238	−0.447	−0.179	−0.374	−0.172	0.331	1.392
Birth period of index child									
1960–1964 (reference)	0.000	0.000	0.000	0.000	0.000	0.000	0.000	0.000	1.000
1975–1990	0.076	0.080	0.182	0.225	0.159	0.282	0.145	−0.335	0.715
1991–1995	0.273	0.279	0.387	0.437	0.507	0.744	0.350	−0.741	0.477
Mother's education									
None (reference)	0.000	0.000	0.000	0.000	0.000	0.000	0.000	0.000	1.000
Primary	−0.020	−0.019	0.013	0.043	0.001	0.044	0.008	−0.038	0.963
Secondary+	0.048	0.050	0.109	0.151	0.096	0.177	0.099	−0.191	0.826
Residence									
Urban (reference)	0.000	0.000	0.000	0.000	0.000	0.000	0.000	0.000	1.000
Rural	0.033	0.029	−0.041	−0.143	−0.015	−0.130	−0.022	0.091	1.095

Death status of index child									
Alive (reference)	0.000	0.000	0.000	0.000	0.000	0.000	0.000	0.000	1.000
Dead	−0.207	−0.207	−0.196	−0.165	−0.216	−0.194	−0.191	0.263	1.301
Age at first marriage									
under 20 years (reference)	0.000	0.000	0.000	0.000	0.000	0.000	0.000	0.000	1.000
20–24 years	−0.005	−0.004	0.025	0.084	0.013	0.074	0.012	−0.037	0.964
25–29 years	0.105	0.106	0.153	0.233	0.137	0.237	0.121	−0.193	0.824
30+years	0.023	0.022	−0.102	−0.096	0.021	−0.068	0.012	0.043	1.044
Age at first birth									
under 20 years (reference)	0.000	0.000	0.000	0.000	0.000	0.000	0.000	0.000	1.000
20–24 years	−0.046	−0.047	−0.083	−0.147	−0.069	−0.140	−0.065	0.124	1.132
25–29 years	−0.118	−0.119	−0.153	−0.250	−0.146	−0.242	−0.133	0.214	1.239
30+years	−0.176	−0.174	−0.157	−0.230	−0.165	−0.205	−0.139	0.160	1.174
−2 Log likelihood	23,796	23,805	26,034	30,979	28,028	32,590	25,315	1,87,003	

Table 10.5 Estimated coefficients for various parametric models, Ghana, 1998

	Parametric models							Cox model	
Covariates	Extended Generalized Gamma	Reciprocal Weibull	Log normal	Weibull	Gamma	Exponential	Log logistic	Coefficient	Hazard ratio
Intercept	3.796	3.657	3.806	3.920	3.876	4.335	3.791	–	–
Scale	0.482	0.561	0.474	0.328	1.000	1.000	0.264	–	–
Shape	−0.069	−1.000	0.000	1.000	−0.903	1.000	–	–	–
Mother's current age									
Under 25 (reference)	0.000	0.000	0.000	0.000	0.000	0.000	0.000	0.000	1.000
25–34	0.061	0.037	0.062	0.076	0.058	0.112	0.074	−0.186	0.830
35–49	0.220	0.133	0.226	0.279	0.248	0.585	0.257	−0.759	0.468
Mother's education									
None (reference)	0.000	0.000	0.000	0.000	0.000	0.000	0.000	0.000	1.000
Primary	0.023	0.016	0.024	0.034	0.018	0.060	0.021	−0.092	0.912
Secondary+	0.065	0.055	0.066	0.079	0.089	0.201	0.064	−0.220	0.803
Residence									
Urban (reference)	0.000	0.000	0.000	0.000	0.000	0.000	0.000	0.000	1.000
Rural	−0.093	−0.079	−0.094	−0.109	−0.125	−0.267	−0.103	0.307	1.359
Death status of index child									
Alive (reference)	0.000	0.000	0.000	0.000	0.000	0.000	0.000	0.000	1.000
Dead	−0.527	−0.591	−0.519	−0.365	−0.704	−0.827	−0.491	1.086	2.962
Age at first marriage									
Under 20 years (reference)	0.000	0.000	0.000	0.000	0.000	0.000	0.000	0.000	1.000
20–24 years	−0.018	−0.140	−0.019	−0.037	−0.035	−0.091	−0.017	0.094	1.099
25 + years	−0.042	−0.135	−0.042	−0.051	−0.059	−0.125	−0.048	0.158	1.171
Age at first birth									
Under 20 years (reference)	0.000	0.000	0.000	0.000	0.000	0.000	0.000	0.000	1.000
20–24 years	−0.059	−0.470	−0.059	−0.058	−0.071	−0.124	−0.063	0.165	1.179
25 + years	−0.134	−0.114	−0.134	−0.119	−0.152	−0.253	−0.145	0.346	1.413
−2 Log likelihood	2,343	2,396	2,343	2,422	2,779	3,359	2,362	11,589	

Table 10.6 Estimated coefficients for various parametric models, Kenya, 1998

	Parametric models							Cox model	
Covariates	Extended Generalized Gamma	Reciprocal Weibull	Log normal	Weibull	Gamma	Exponential	Log logistic	Coefficient	Hazard ratio
Intercept	3.185	3.220	3.635	4.268	3.481	4.134	3.543	–	–
Scale	0.553	0.562	0.669	0.743	1.000	1.000	0.365	–	–
Shape	−1.106	−1.000	0.000	1.000	−0.584	1.000	–	–	–
Mother's birth cohort									
1946–1950 (reference)	0.000	0.000	0.000	0.000	0.000	0.000	0.000	0.000	1.000
1951–1960	−0.034	−0.039	−0.131	−0.280	−0.094	−0.267	−0.084	0.182	1.200
1961–1970	−0.073	−0.083	−0.254	−0.529	−0.193	−0.512	−0.171	0.381	1.464
1971–1980	−0.126	−0.141	−0.360	−0.661	−0.277	−0.630	−0.280	0.569	1.766
Birth period of index child									
1960–1964 (reference)	0.000	0.000	0.000	0.000	0.000	0.000	0.000	0.000	1.000
1975–1990	0.095	0.104	0.229	0.279	0.190	0.335	0.179	−0.392	0.676
1991–1995	0.311	0.328	0.514	0.560	0.568	0.810	0.477	−0.934	0.393
Mother's education									
None (reference)	0.000	0.000	0.000	0.000	0.000	0.000	0.000	0.000	1.000
Primary	0.026	0.024	0.008	−0.007	0.013	−0.002	0.003	−0.001	0.999
Secondary+	0.050	0.049	0.064	0.092	0.061	0.104	0.045	−0.097	0.908
Residence									
Urban (reference)	0.000	0.000	0.000	0.000	0.000	0.000	0.000	0.000	1.000
Rural	−0.045	−0.056	−0.188	−0.322	−0.146	−0.331	−0.170	0.308	1.361
Death status of index child									
Alive (reference)	0.000	0.000	0.000	0.000	0.000	0.000	0.000	0.000	1.000
Dead	−0.212	−0.212	−0.160	−0.043	−0.201	−0.082	−0.180	0.185	1.203

(continued)

Table 10.6 (continued)

	Parametric models							Cox model	
Covariates	Extended Generalized Gamma	Reciprocal Weibull	Log normal	Weibull	Gamma	Exponential	Log logistic	Coefficient	Hazard ratio
Age at first marriage									
Under 20 years (reference)	0.000	0.000	0.000	0.000	0.000	0.000	0.000	0.000	1.000
20–24 years	0.068	0.069	0.080	0.075	0.077	0.081	0.082	−0.109	0.897
25–29 years	0.105	0.109	0.145	0.129	0.136	0.141	0.167	−0.221	0.802
30 + years	0.110	0.133	0.311	0.465	0.241	0.479	0.293	−0.446	0.640
Age at first birth									
Under 20 years (reference)	0.000	0.000	0.000	0.000	0.000	0.000	0.000	0.000	1.000
20–24 years	−0.085	−0.085	−0.095	−0.108	−0.091	−0.108	−0.088	0.123	1.131
25–29 years	−0.153	−0.151	−0.178	−0.106	−0.170	−0.170	−0.186	0.222	1.249
30 + years		−0.195	−0.252	−0.296	−0.220	−0.291	−0.233	0.326	1.385
−2 Log likelihood	38,118	38,151	41,816	49,798	44,953	52,308	40,666	315,307	

Table 10.7 Hypotheses and corresponding likelihood ratio statistics for testing special cases (Null) against the more general (H1) within the parametric family of models for Eritrea, Ghana and Kenya

	Null hypothesis	Model under *null* hypothesis	Model under alternative hypothesis	Likelihood ratio statistic (p values)
Eritrea	Shape = −1	Reciprocal Weibull	Extended Generalized Gamma	9 (0.000)
	Shape = 0	Log-normal	Extended Generalized Gamma	2,238 (0.000)
	Shape = 1	Weibull	Extended Generalized Gamma	7,183 (0.000)
	Scale = 1, given Shape >0	Gamma'	Extended Generalized Gamma	4,232 (0.000)
	Scale = 1 and Shape =1	Exponential	Extended Generalized Gamma	8,794 (0.000)
	Scale =1, given Shape =1	Exponential	Weibull	1,611 (0.000)
Ghana	Shape = −1	Reciprocal Weibull	Extended Generalized Gamma	53 (0.000)
	Shape = 0	Log-normal	Extended Generalized Gamma	0.4 (0.472)
	Shape = 1	Weibull	Extended Generalized Gamma	79 (0.000)
	Scale = 1, given Shape >0	Gamma'	Extended Generalized Gamma	436 (0.000)
	Scale = 1 and Shape =1	Exponential	Extended Generalized Gamma	1,016 (0.000)
	Scale =1, given Shape =1	Exponential	Weibull	937 (0.000)
Kenya	Shape = −1	Reciprocal Weibull	Extended Generalized Gamma	33 (0.000)
	Shape = 0	Log-normal	Extended Generalized Gamma	3,666 (0.472)
	Shape = 1	Weibull	Extended Generalized Gamma	11,648 (0.000)
	Scale = 1, given Shape >0	Gamma'	Extended Generalized Gamma	6,803 (0.000)
	Scale = 1 and Shape =1	Exponential	Extended Generalized Gamma	14,158 (0.000)
	Scale =1, given Shape =1	Exponential	Weibull	2,510 (0.000)

special-case model is adequate enough relative to the more comprehensive EGG model. The results for Eritrea show that all special cases are rejected in favor of the more general EGG model, though the Reciprocal Weibull model is the closest to the EGG model. This is in accordance with the estimated value of the shape parameter under the EGG model. The estimate of the shape parameter, as reported in Table 10.4, is −1.068 (corresponding to the EGG model). This estimate is closer to the assertion of the Reciprocal Weibull where the shape parameter is fixed to −1 than to any other value set by the other alternative distributions. When compared to the Weibull model, the exponential model is also rejected as shown in the last row of Table 10.7.

The results for Kenya are also consistent with observations made on Eritrea – all special case distributions are rejected in favor of the EGG model. Again, the Reciprocal Weibull model is the closest to the EGG model, and this is consistent with the estimate of the shape parameter (−1.106) in Table 10.6, which is close to −1. The results for Ghana (Table 10.5) come from birth intervals of children born within five years before the survey as earlier mentioned and thus, are not directly comparable to those of Eritrea and Kenya where all children were included in the analyses. Not surprisingly, therefore, the results for Ghana show a different picture of the distributional shape of birth intervals. Here, the log-normal distribution fits the data as adequately as the more comprehensive EGG model. This is shown by the insignificant difference between the log-likelihoods of these models (difference = 0.4 with a p-value of 0.472 for a Chi-square with 1 degree of freedom).

The equivalence of the EGG and the log normal models for Ghana is clearly indicated by the estimated shape parameter in the EGG model (see Table 10.5). The estimated shape parameter of −0.069 is very close to 0 and the log-normal model is obtained as a special case of the EGG model when the shape parameter of the latter is constrained to 0. Another important point worth noting here is that the estimated effects of covariates on the log-interval corresponding to the EGG and the log-normal models are almost identical (see Table 10.5) while the estimates from the other models are far from those of these two models.

10.3.5 Determinants of Child-Spacing in the Three Countries

A summary of the results for the three countries is given in Table 10.8. The results for each country relate to the most suitable model in the respective countries. That is, the EGG model for Eritrea and Kenya, and the log-normal model for Ghana. Although the levels of some covariates in the three countries were not fully identical, it is clear from Table 10.8 that women from the younger birth cohort, those with delayed age at first birth, and those who have lost their index child tend to have shortened birth intervals. Rural residence is associated with longer birth intervals in Eritrea but with shorter birth intervals in Ghana and Kenya. Women with secondary level education (and in Kenya even those with primary level education) tend to have longer birth interval though the evidence is marginal in Ghana. Lastly, in Eritrea

Table 10.8 Comparison of estimated coefficients in the best fit models for Eritrea, Ghana and Kenya

	Eritrea	Ghana	Kenya
Covariates	Extended Generalized Gamma Model	Log normal Model	Extended Generalized Gamma Model
Intercept	3.243[c]	3.806[c]	3.185[c]
Shape	0.558	0.474	0.553
Scale	−1.068	0.000	−1.106
Mother's birth cohort, Ghana age at survey			
1946–1950 (reference), Ghana (under 25 reference)	0.000	0.000	0.000
1951–1960, Ghana 25–34 years	−0.078[c]	0.062[a]	−0.034[b]
1961–1970, Ghana 35–49 years	−0.136[c]	0.226[c]	−0.073[c]
1971–1980	−0.131[c]	–	−0.126[c]
Birth period of index child			
1960–1964 (reference)	0.000	–	0.000
1975–1990	0.076[c]	–	0.095[c]
1991–1995	0.273[c]	–	0.311[c]
Mother's education			
None (reference)	0.000	0.000	0.000
Primary	−0.020	0.024	0.026[c]
Secondary+	0.048[c]	0.066[a]	0.050[c]
Residence			
Urban (reference)	0.000	0.000	0.000
Rural	0.033[c]	−0.094[c]	−0.045[c]
Death Status of index child			
Alive (reference)	0.000	0.000	0.000
Dead	−0.207[c]	−0.519[c]	−0.212[c]
Age at first marriage			
Under 20 years (reference)	0.000	0.000	0.000
20–24 years	−0.005	−0.019	0.068[c]
25–29 years, Ghana 25 + years	0.105[c]	−0.042	0.105[c]
30 + years	0.023	–	0.11[b]
Age at first birth			
Under 20 years (reference)	0.000	0.000	0.000
20–24 years	−0.046[c]	−0.059[a]	−0.085[c]
25–29 years, Ghana 25 + years	−0.118[c]	−0.134[c]	−0.153[c]
30 + years	−0.176[c]	–	–

[a]Indicates the corresponding effect is statistically significant at 10 %
[b]Indicates significance at 5 %
[c]Indicates significance at 1 %

and Kenya, there is strong evidence that children born in more recent periods tend to have been spaced wider than those born earlier.

In an attempt to further our knowledge on these models, we also fitted them to data on first birth interval (interval between first marriage and first birth) for Eritrea. The results are presented in Table 10.9. Here, we note that the estimated scale

Table 10.9 Transition to parenthood (first birth interval), Eritrea, 1995

	Parametric models							Cox model	
Covariates	Extended Generalized Gamma	Reciprocal Weibull	Log normal	Weibull	Gamma	Exponential	Log logistic	Coefficient	Hazard ratio
Intercept	4.007	3.542	3.875	4.093	4.018	4.194	3.853	–	–
Shape	0.899	1.208	1.010	0.831	1.000	1.000	0.548	–	–
Scale	0.573	−1.000	0.000	1.000	0.437	1.000	–	–	–
Mother's birth cohort									
Before 1951 (reference)	0.000	0.000	0.000	0.000	0.000	0.000	0.000	0.000	1.000
1951–1955	−0.106	−0.248	−0.153	−0.087	−0.147	−0.178	−0.080	0.122	1.130
1956–1960	0.102	−0.258	−0.007	0.154	0.035	0.029	0.110	−0.129	0.879
1961–1965	0.179	−0.088	0.070	0.254	0.104	0.109	0.160	−0.216	0.806
1966–1970	0.314	−0.011	0.191	0.393	0.234	0.242	0.299	−0.371	0.690
1971–1975	0.461	0.046	0.299	0.575	0.370	0.414	0.406	−0.526	0.591
1976–1980	0.400	−0.167	0.214	0.513	0.304	0.348	0.353	−0.461	0.631
Birth period of index child									
1960–1964 (reference)	0.000	0.000	0.000	0.000	0.000	0.000	0.000	0.000	1.000
1975–1990	−0.037	−0.022	−0.041	−0.028	−0.040	−0.033	−0.054	0.040	1.041
1991–1995	−0.050	−0.064	−0.069	−0.030	−0.057	−0.037	−0.083	0.039	1.040
Mother's education									
None (reference)	0.000	0.000	0.000	0.000	0.000	0.000	0.000	0.000	1.000
Primary	−0.228	−0.063	−0.215	−0.204	−0.233	−0.233	−0.273	0.250	1.284
Secondary+	−0.556	−0.231	−0.499	−0.549	−0.555	−0.572	−0.571	0.650	1.916

Mother's occupation									
Not working (reference)	0.000	0.000	0.000	0.000	0.000	0.000	0.000	0.000	1.000
Professional	−0.027	−0.070	−0.061	0.020	−0.039	0.008	−0.099	−0.012	0.988
Agriculture	−0.123	0.073	−0.069	−0.140	−0.117	−0.151	−0.103	0.153	1.165
Household, service, unskilled	0.312	0.076	0.198	0.392	0.286	0.394	0.148	−0.428	0.652
Residence									
Urban (reference)	0.000	0.000	0.000	0.000	0.000	0.000	0.000	0.000	1.000
Rural	−0.003	0.029	0.005	−0.013	−0.001	−0.013	0.010	0.012	1.012
Age at first marriage									
Under 15 years (reference)	0.000	0.000	0.000	0.000	0.000	0.000	0.000	0.000	1.000
15–19 years	−0.319	−0.455	−0.353	−0.299	−0.326	−0.301	−0.344	0.333	1.000
20–24 years	−0.595	−0.625	−0.599	−0.593	−0.588	−0.575	−0.600	0.344	1.411
25 + years	−0.673	−0.620	−0.662	−0.669	−0.657	−0.631	−0.728	0.728	2.071
−2 Log likelihood	9,651	10,978	9,851	9,752	9,698	9,918	9,657	47,048	

Table 10.10 Hypotheses and corresponding likelihood ratio statistics for testing special cases (Null) against the more general (H1) within the parametric family of models for Eritrea: transition to parenthood

Null hypothesis	Model under null hypothesis	Model under alternative hypothesis	Likelihood ratio statistic (p values)
Shape = −1	Reciprocal Weibull	Extended generalized gamma	1,327 (0.000)
Shape = 0	Log-normal	Extended generalized gamma	200 (0.000)
Shape = 1	Weibull	Extended generalized gamma	101 (0.000)
Scale = 1, given Shape >0	**Gamma'**	**Extended generalized gamma**	**47 (0.000)**
Scale = 1 and Shape = 1	Exponential	Extended generalized gamma	267 (0.000)
Scale = 1, given Shape = 1	Exponential	Weibull	166 (0.000)

parameter of 0.899 of the EGG is very close to 1. From Sect. 10.2, we recall that if we constrain the scale parameter of the EGG model to 1, then we get the "Gamma" model as a special case. Accordingly, the Likelihood Ratio Test in Table 10.10 shows that while all special case models are rejected in favor of the EGG model, the closest model is the "Gamma" model. This is in contrast to the case with all birth intervals from Eritrea and Kenya (where the Reciprocal Weibull model was the closest) or in the case with the most recent birth intervals from Ghana (where the log-normal model was the closest).

10.4 Summary

A natural question arises as to which model to fit or which procedure to use when one is confronted with a specific data analysis problem. As with most statistical or demographic methods, it is rather difficult to codify the procedures involved in choosing a model. There are many factors, such as mathematical convenience, theoretical appropriateness, and empirical evidence that should legitimately enter the decision and none can be easily quantified.

Given the wide range of fertility models in the literature, it is worth asking whether conclusions are sensitive to the particular statistical model chosen. The answer to this question is unknown until results obtained with one method have been compared to those obtained by another method. Such comparisons have been one of the objectives of the present chapter. Our empirical results indicate that the distributional shape of birth intervals is different depending on whether we refer to the first or higher-order birth intervals. It also depends on the subset of birth intervals analyzed (analyzing all available birth intervals or restricting oneself to the most recent subset of birth intervals). More importantly, our results demonstrate that inferences concerning covariate effects on birth intervals are sensitive to the choice of the distributional shape.

In summary, our results indicate that the choice of the appropriate distribution of birth intervals is of crucial importance in order to make valid inference and, thereby, suggest sound and effective policy interventions. This chapter has outlined a statistically well grounded, theoretically appropriate, and empirically evident procedure on how to identify the most appropriate distribution for a given dataset.

This study is, however, not without limitations. The units of analysis in this chapter have been the records on birth intervals of individual children. However, many of these children belong to the same mother. Children of the same mother are more alike than those selected at random from the population. Thus, using mothers as units of analysis and treating children of the same mother as clustered cases (multi-levels) of the same unit (mother) would be a more appropriate procedure. Such a formulation would allow investigators to examine unobserved heterogeneity at the cluster (mother) level and partition the variability into the contributions of the individual child (level 1) and the mother (level 2).

Further, unlike death, the event studied in this chapter (childbearing) is not a certain event to all individuals – there may be long-term survivors in the sense of Maller and Zhou (1996). Accordingly, alternative models that allow for this feature, such as Li and Choe (1997), Yamaguchi (2003), or Land et al. (2001), could be appropriate. We have also not attempted to relate our findings to theories like rational choice theory (Yamaguchi and Ferguson 1995).

It is our ambition to address this issue in the near future. Meanwhile, it is also our hope that the findings in this chapter bring the importance of how to specify duration phenomena into the surface, and motivate researchers to look for stronger links between the underlying reality and the models we present and investigate what behavioural or biological processes are better represented by one model than another and what sorts of bias would one expect to observe in estimated effects if those processes are not appropriately modelled.

References

Allison, P. D. (2010). *Survival analysis using the SAS system* (2nd ed.). Cary: SAS Institute Inc.

Bergström, R., & Edin, P. A. (1992). Time aggregation and the distributional shape of unemployement duration. *Journal of Applied Econometrics, 7*, 5–30.

Bicego, G., & Ahmad O. B. (1996). Infant and child mortality (DHS Comparative Studies No. 20). Calverton: Macro International, Demographic and Health Surveys.

Cochrane, S. (1979). *Fertility and education: What do we really know?* Baltimore: John Hopkins University Press.

Cochrane, S. (1983). Effects of education and urbanization on fertility. In R. A. Bulatao & R. D. Lee (Eds.), *Determinants of fertility in developing countries. A summary of knowledge, part B*. New York: Academic.

Cox, D. R. (1972). Regression models and life-tables (with discussion). *Journal of the Royal Statistical Society – Series B, 34*, 187–220.

Defo, K. B. (1997). Effects of infant feeding practices and birth spacing on infant and child survival: A reassessment from retrospective and prospective data. *Journal of Biosocial Science, 29*, 303–323.

Diekmann, A. (1992). The log-logistic distribution as a model for social diffusion processes. *Journal of Scientific and Industrial Research, 51*, 285.

Farewell, V. T., & Prentice, R. L. (1977). A study of distributional shape in life testing. *Technometrics, 19*, 69–75.

Gage, A. (1995). *An assessment of the quality of data on age at first union, first birth and the first sexual intercourse for Phase II of the demographic and health surveys program* (DHS Occasional Papers No. 4). Calverton: Macro International, Demographic and Health Surveys.

Ghana Statistical Service (GSS), & Macro International (MI). (1999). *Ghana demographic and health survey 1998*. Calverton: GSS and MI.

Gribble, J. N. (1993). Birth intervals, gestational age and low birth weight: Are the relationships confounded? *Population Studies, 47*, 133–146.

Gyimah, S. O. (2001). *Childhood mortality and reproductive behavior in Ghana and Kenya: An Examination of Frailty and Non-frailty Models*. Ph.D Dissertation, Faculty of Graduate Studies, The University of Western Ontario, London.

Gyimah, S. O. (2003). A cohort analysis of timing of the first birth and cumulative fertility in Ghana. *Population Research and Policy Review, 22*(3), 251–266.

Gyimah, S. O. (in press). The dynamics of timing and spacing of births in Ghana. *Journal of Comparative Family Studies*.

Gyimah, S. O., & Fernando, R. (2002). The physiological effects of infant death on fertility: A comparative analysis of DHS data from Ghana and Kenya. *Social Biology, 49*(1–2), 44–57.

Heckman, J., & Walker, J. (1991). Economic models of fertility dynamics: A case study of Swedish fertility. *Research in Population Economics, 7*, 3–91.

Hobcraft, J., McDonald, J., & Rustein, S. (1985). Demographic determinants of early infant and early child mortality: A comparative analysis. *Population Studies, 39*, 363–385.

Land, K. C., Nagin, D. S., & McCall, P. L. (2001). Discrete-time hazard regression models with hidden heterogeneity – The semiparametric mixed Poisson regression approach. *Sociological Methods & Research, 29*, 342–373.

Li, L., & Choe, M. K. (1997). A mixture model for duration data: Analysis of second births in China. *Demography, 34*, 189–197.

Little, C. L., Adams, M. R. & Anderson, W. A. (1994). Application of a log-logistic model to describe the survival of Yersinia enterocolitica at sub-optimal pH and temperature. *International Journal of Food Microbiology, 22*, 63–71.

Majumder, A. H., May, M., & Pant, P. D. (1997). Infant and child mortality determinants in Bangladesh: Are they changing? *Journal of Biosocial Science, 29*, 385–399.

Maller, R. A., & Zhou, S. (1996). *Survival analysis with long-term survivors*. New York: Wiley.

Martin, T. (1995). Women's education and fertility: Results from 26 Demographic and Health Surveys. *Studies in Family Planning, 26*, 187–202.

Montgomery, M., & Cohen, B. (Eds.). (1998). *From death to Birth: Mortality decline and reproductive change*. Washington, DC: National Academy Press.

Nandram, B. (1989). Discrimination between the complimentary log-log and logistic model for ordinal data. *Communications in Statistics: Theory and Applications, 18*, 2155.

Palloni, A., & Millman, S. (1986). Effects of inter-births intervals and breastfeeding on infant and early age mortality. *Population Studies, 40*, 215–236.

Pederson, J. (2000). Determinants of infant and child mortality in the West Bank and Gaza strip. *Journal of Biosocial Science, 32*, 527–546.

Prentice, R. L. (1974). A log-gamma model and its maximum likelihood estimation. *Biometrika, 61*, 539–544.

Preston, S. H. (Ed.). (1978). *The effects of infant and child mortality on fertility*. New York: Academic.

Rafalimanana, H., & Westoff, C. E. (2000). Potential effects on fertility and child health and survival of birth-spacing preferences in sub-Saharan Africa. *Studies in Family Planning, 31*, 99–110.

Rodriguez, G., Hobcraft, J., Menken, J., & Trussell, J. (1984). *Analysis of the determinants of birth intervals*. Comparative Studies No. 30. London: World Fertility Survey.

Shoukri, M. M., Mian, I. U. H., & Tracy, D. S. (1988). Sampling properties of estimators of the log-logistic distribution with application to Canadian precipitation data. *The Canadian Journal of Statistics, 16*, 223.

Singh, K. P., Lee, C. M.-S., & George, E. O. (1988). On generalized log-logistic model for censored survival data. *Biometrical Journal, 7*, 843.

Stacey, E. W. (1962). A generalization of the gamma distribution. *Annals of Mathematical Statistics, 33*, 1187–1192.

Ware, H. (1984). Effects of maternal education, women's roles and child care on child mortality. In H. Mosley & L. C. Chen (Eds.), *Child survival: Strategies for research*. New York: The Population Council.

Westoff, C. F. (1992). *Age at marriage, age at first birth, and fertility in Africa* (World Bank Technical Paper No. 169). Washington, DC: World Bank.

Yamaguchi, K. (2003). Accelerated failure-time mover-stayer regression models for the analysis of last-episode data. *Sociological Methodology, 33*, 81–110.

Yamaguchi, K., & Ferguson, L. (1995). The Stopping and spacing of childbirths and their birth-history predictors: Rational-choice theory and event-history analysis. *American Sociological Review, 60*, 272–298.

Chapter 11
Spatial Variation of Predictors of Prevalent Hypertension in Sub-Saharan Africa: A Case Study of South-Africa

Ngianga-Bakwin Kandala

11.1 Introduction

Sub-Saharan Africa (SSA) is a region of striking socio-economic and demographic diversities. There are enormous variations between and within countries in the epidemiologic transition, basic socio-economic and demographic indicators. For instance, rural sub-Saharan Africa is at an earlier stage of economic and health transition than the urban settings.

In a recent systematic review of hypertension in SSA, Addo et al. (2007) note that hypertension is of public health importance in SSA, particularly in urban areas with evidence of considerable under-diagnosis, lack of treatment and control. The authors also point to the lack of strategies to prevent, detect, treat and control hypertension effectively in the African region.

While much attention in the region has been focused on communicable and infectious diseases such as diarrhoea, malaria, tuberculosis etc. and the pandemic of HIV/AIDS, it is predicted that the twenty-first century will see a serious added health and economic burden from non-communicable diseases including vascular disease as SSA progresses through the epidemiologic transition.

The stage of vascular disease in a population is thought to result from the prevalence of vascular risk factors. Already hypertension and stroke are common in adults in SSA. In South Africa (SA) for instance, the prevalence of people with high blood pressure (HBP) was estimated to be 14 % and 25.1 % based on

N.-B. Kandala (✉)
Warwick Medical School, Division of Health Sciences, University of Warwick, Coventry, UK
e-mail: n-b.kandala@warwick.ac.uk

N.-B. Kandala and G. Ghilagaber (eds.), *Advanced Techniques for Modelling Maternal and Child Health in Africa*, The Springer Series on Demographic Methods and Population Analysis 34, DOI 10.1007/978-94-007-6778-2_11,

measured blood pressure (BP) available on data from the 1998 Adult health module of the 1998 South Africa Demographic and Health Survey data (SADHS) (MRC 2006; Cappuccio 2004; Steyn et al. 2001). The overall prevalence is so low for two reasons:

1. They used the definition of high blood pressure based on the cut-off of (160/95 mmHg) and of BP ≥140/90 mmHg without including people with diagnosed hypertension and
2. The prevalence was not age adjusted and the age structure is heavily weighted to the younger ages, while the prevalence of HBP increases sharply with age (for example they reported 34.4 % in women aged 65+). The same data suggest that only 29 % of men and 55 % of women who had hypertension reported that they had hypertension. Therefore, most of hypertensive participants had undiagnosed hypertension.

From cross-sectional surveys in SSA it is estimated that the true prevalence of hypertension could be as high as 40 % in urban areas and in some rural areas it already approaches 25 % (Thorogood et al. 2007a, b; MRC 2006; Cappuccio 2004; Steyn et al. 2001).

The objective of this chapter is to apply the new cut off of HBP (BP ≥140/90 mmHg) to the SADHS data including also people with diagnosed hypertension and examine the spatial distribution of hypertension including a number of socio-demographic, household and community characteristics that could confound or mediate the observed variation in the prevalence of hypertension in South Africa. It further seeks to highlight patterns that exist within the data, after multiple adjustments of proximate variables. Such estimates illustrate how much can be learned by detailed exploratory analyses and suggest how these data can be used to strategically inform policy.

The epidemiologic transition from low to high levels of chronic diseases is associated with advancing acculturation, urbanization and affluence with a progressive increase in salt intake, smoking habit and saturated fat intake. The appearance of hypertension (and associated stroke) as the predominant form of cardiovascular disease being observed in SSA is also a by-product of eco-biological (interaction between biology and environment), psychological, medical (bio-technology and public health) advances, economic growth and rising incomes.

South Africa is characterized by a marked socio-cultural, economic and environmental diversity likely to cause variations in chronic diseases. Although the prevalence of chronic diseases is well documented in some communities in South Africa, the fact that chronic diseases differ markedly between individuals, households and communities has rarely been explored. Further, the chronic diseases risk factors included in these studies were all at the level of household, without the inclusion of community characteristics such as the province of residence. For the above reasons, the ethnic diversity and the inter-province variations of the prevalence of hypertension in South Africa provide a unique opportunity to study the determinants of HBP in this diverse society. Using a Bayesian approach we wish to assess the spatial variation of the prevalence of hypertension risk factors (socio-economic status, BP, BMI, waist circumference, Hip circumference, co-morbidities (diabetes, asthma, and chronic bronchitis), lifestyle (alcohol, smoking, diet, and quality of sleep)) in South Africa, using a cross-sectional population based survey on adult health. We will identify the extent of province-level variations in the prevalence of hypertension, the link with ethnicity, urbanization and other risk factors and the amount of residual geographic variation due to unobserved factors, which may include environmental causes. As the epidemiological transition in South Africa is faster than anticipated, by identifying groups or settings, in which chronic illness is high, preventive actions can be targeted more effectively.

11.2 Background of the Study Area (South Africa)

South Africa is located in the Sub-Saharan African (SSA) region of the world. It shares borders with Zimbabwe, Botswana, Namibia, Lesotho, Swaziland and Mozambique. Demographically, it is the most populous country in the southern region with an estimated population of 49, 99 million according to Statistics South Africa's mid-2010 estimates (Statistics South Africa 2010). About half of the population are women and an increasing number of people in the older age group (7.3 %); hence the burden of chronic diseases, which affect mostly older people, should not be ignored. Economically, South Africa is very buoyant. South Africa combines a developed first-world infrastructure with a vibrant emerging market economy to create huge investment potential. With the real gross domestic product (GDP) growth expected to come in at 3 % in 2010/11 and high per capita income, but with high HIV/AIDS prevalence, the country would find it difficult to bear the cost implications of the health burden arising from the complications of chronic diseases. Therefore, there is strong economic and public health justification to tackle hypertension.

Moreover, SA is multicultural because of its different ethnic groups, races, languages, dialects and cultures. Few countries in Sub-Saharan African have been exposed to such diversity. The SADHS reports the following ethnic composition: Black 79.6 %, White 9.1 %, Coloured 8.9 %, Asian 2.5 %. The Multi-cultural population is distributed in 9 provinces with an estimated urban population of 57 % in 2007. Since the end of apartheid in 1994, most South Africans have high expectations and hopes for their future.

However, life expectancy at birth for men and women was estimated in 2009 at 49.8 (53.3 in 2010) and 48.1 years (55.2 in 2010) and the infant mortality per 1,000 live births was 44.4 (46.9 in 2010) coupled with a maternal mortality rate of 551 per 100 000 live births.

According to Statistics South African mid-year population estimates, in 2011, the HIV prevalence rate among age 2 and over was estimated at 17 % and 5.24 million people living with HIV/AIDS were reported. The total number of new HIV infections for 2010 is estimated at 410,000. Of these, an estimated 40,000 will be among children. Total fertility rate was estimated at 2.38 children per woman of reproductive health (Stats South Africa 2010; UNDP Report 2009, World Bank 2008).

In terms of per capita South Africa is considered an emerging economy (upper-middle-income country), but notwithstanding this relative wealth, most households in South Africa are poor or continue to be vulnerable to being poor. In addition, the distribution of income and wealth in South Africa is among the most unequal in the world, and many households still have unsatisfactory access to education, health care, energy and clean water (Woolard 2002; Schwabe 2004).

Looking at a wide range of poverty measures, recent data from South Africa indicates that poverty has remained stagnant but for less optimistic South Africans, poverty has deepened, inequality has increased and the benefits of growth have not reached the poorest of the poor (Woolard 2002; Schwabe 2004).

The assessment of SA by some of the key social indicators of deprivation, a decade after the end of apartheid shows the extent and depth of poverty and inequality. These indicators also reflect on how serious the income distribution and poverty is skewed in South Africa. However, it is important to note that some measures also have been taken to address these issues and the benefits of these measures are yet to be seen.

For instance, in 2010, South Africa has a per capita GNP of USD 7,158 per annum, yet about 18 % of adults are illiterate, 9.2 % of children under-five are malnourished and life expectancy has fallen from 62 years in 1990 to 48 in 2007 as a consequence of AIDS.

Of the estimated 47 million people in the country in 2009, about 8 million were surviving on less than the international dollar a day poverty line and 18 million were living on less than 2 dollars per day.

Also, 60 % of the poor get no social transfers and health expenditure is 7 % of the GNP, but less than half of this is public spending (Woolard 2002; Schwabe 2004).

The rural areas are the most affected by poverty, contain 50 % of the population of South Africa and they constitute 72 % of those members of the total population who are poor. The poverty gap (which is the annual amount needed to uplift the poor to the poverty line by means of a perfectly-targeted transfer of money, and which measures how deep or intense the poverty is) was about R28 billion in 1995, and 76 % of this was concentrated in the rural areas (Schwabe 2004, Landman 2003, p. 6).

11.2.1 Demographics and Spatial Dimension of Poverty in South Africa

For many decades, poverty in South Africa had racial, gender and spatial dimensions, as a direct consequence of the policies of the successive colonial, segregationist and apartheid regimes (May 1998). There is an unequal distribution of poverty among the 9 provinces. The distribution of provincial poverty rates are as follows: the rates are highest for the Eastern Cape (71 %), Free State (63 %), North-West (62 %), Northern Province (59 %) and Mpumalanga (57 %), and lowest for Gauteng (17 %) and the Western Cape (28 %). The provinces most affected by poverty are the Eastern Cape, Free State and Northern Province, which together make up 36 % of the population but account for 51 % of the total poverty gap (May 1998). It is worth mentioning that while poverty is general, it is mostly concentrated among black Africans (61 %) followed by coloureds (38 %) compared with 5 % of Indians and 1 % of whites.

Following a household poverty line of US$220 per month in 1999, it was noted that 52 % of the South African population was poor while 95 % of poor people were African, though Africans were only 79 % of the population as a whole. 72 % of the poor live in rural areas and 60 % are female mostly without any social security transfers (Everatt 2005, p.78; Woolard 2002; Gelb 2003; Schwabe 2004).

As chronic diseases in later life have been shown to be linked to health behaviours in childhood, it is not surprising to note that three children in five live in poor households, and many children are exposed to public and domestic violence, malnutrition and inconsistent parenting and schooling. There is a huge spatial variation in the risk of childhood poverty by province varying from 78 % in Eastern Cape compared to 20 % in Gauteng (May 1998).

The above evidence in poverty indicators and inequality can explain in part the spatial variation of chronic diseases in South Africa within the different social groups of the 9 provinces. High mortality and disease prevalence are easily understood if discussed together with the environment and location where they are occurring, since they almost always interact, but this chapter appreciates that at times there can be a high disease prevalence inequality resulting from biological factors, though rarely.

Looking at the 2010 Human Development Index (HDI), an indicator developed to determine the degree to which people live long, informed and comfortable lives, and which combines measures of life expectancy at birth, education levels, and standard of living, South Africa ranks 113th out of 172 countries. It is not surprising that these indicators also show a wider discrepancy by race group, gender and geographical location within the country confirming low measures already observed in human development, such as life expectancy, infant mortality and adult illiteracy (Gelb 2003, p. 18).

11.3 Current Challenges for Africa

The epidemiology of chronic diseases in Africa differs across certain groups of the population, probably due to different exposure to known and unknown risk factors, like unhealthy lifestyles, access to health care and environmental conditions including traditional customs. It should be noted that diseases linked to poverty and famine are still highly prevalent.

A major challenge for Africa is to increase knowledge on the epidemiology and pathogenesis of neglected conditions to allow improvements in management and prevention.

However, research-funding sources are rare because there are few industries and trusts. On the other hand, policymakers are concerned that investment in research into the conditions will interfere with efforts to control communicable diseases.

As in many countries around the world, some of the African population is undergoing a demographic transition from higher to lower levels of fertility and mortality. Although initially experienced by the more developed countries, population ageing is now a global phenomenon, experienced in virtually all countries of the world. As South Africa's population is also undergoing demographic transition from higher to lower levels of fertility and mortality, population ageing has become a matter of public concern because of health consequences in South Africa (MRC 2006). A prominent feature in almost all countries of population ageing is the onset of chronic disease among older people.

The 2001 population census of South Africa found that 7.3 % of the total population were 60 years or older. This proportion may be perceived as low, or at least considerably lower than the 2000 proportions of some developed nations, such as Italy (24.1 %), Greece (23.4 %) and Japan (23.2 %), but it is higher than the proportions of almost all other African nations in 2000, with the exception of the two island populations of Mauritius (9 %) and Reunion (9.9 %). South Africa's 7.3 % was noticeably higher than the 5.1 % for the African continent as a whole, but displayed similar levels of ageing as those in such nations as Brazil (7.8 %), India (7.6 %), Mexico (6.9 %), Samoa (6.8 %) and Vietnam (7.5 %). The average proportion for the Southern African region in 2000 was 5.7 %, and neighbouring countries' proportions ranged from 4.5 % in Angola and Botswana to 6.5 % in Lesotho. Moreover, this older proportion of South Africa is projected to increase over the next decades, and that by 2025 more than one person in ten will be 60 years or older (MRC 2006; Steyn et al. 2001; Dennison et al. 2007; Seedat 1999).

According to the 2006 South Africa Medical Research Council (MRC) report, High blood pressure (BP) or hypertension is a common condition in South Africa and is a risk factor for heart attacks, stroke, left ventricular hypertrophy, renal disease and blindness. It is believed that people who have hypertension are usually unaware that they have the condition, unless the BP has been measured at health-care facilities. It is therefore frequently referred to as a 'silent epidemic' in South Africa. Consequently, hypertension is universally under reported and/or inadequately treated resulting in extensive target-organ damage and premature death. The report suggested that hypertension frequently co-exists with other risk factors for chronic diseases of lifestyle (CDL), such as diabetes and obesity.

This study is part of the effort to compliment work of many South African experts by introducing the impact environmental dimension on health has (i.e. impact of environment, geographic location on health). Since lifestyle and location has an impact on health, we examine how the prevalence of hypertension varies across space (provinces) and the role that individual factors play in this relationship.

11.4 Measures

11.4.1 The Spatial Determinants of Hypertension

The spatial risk factors of hypertension refer to both specific features and pathways by which societal conditions affect health status and that potentially can be altered by informed action. These risk factors include the lack of health infrastructures adequately equipped for diagnosis and care and the absence of research to deliver the required scientific advances in a reasonable timescale. Rapid urbanization, lack of physical activity, obesity, high-salt and high-cholesterol content diets, tobacco, diabetes and increase in life expectancy are all lifestyle factors that can be associated with chronic diseases.

South Africa is divided into 9 provinces. Hypertension prevalence is aggregated and known at a national level. We went a step further and accounted, simultaneously, for geographic location effects on hypertension at the disaggregated level of provinces, thereby highlighting the spatial distribution of hypertension. We recognise that the province is still a large unit but disaggregating to this level represents a considerable advance over the use of national averages and our analysis provides adjusted province-level estimates of hypertension.

We used geo-additive Bayesian modelling, with dynamic and spatial effects, to assess temporal and geographical variation in hypertension. The model used also allows for non-linear effects of covariates on hypertension. The modelling approach is described in more detail in the next section.

11.4.2 Dependent Variable

For the present analyses, the outcome or dependent variable we considered hypertension defined as systolic or diastolic blood pressure $\geq$140 or $\geq$90 mmHg, respectively, or self-report of a health professional diagnosis, a binary outcome. We choose the binary outcome instead of the continuous blood pressure because of interpretability reasons since with the binary outcome one can estimate posterior odds ratios (POR) of hypertension comparing high risk hypertension provinces to the relative low risk provinces, while accounting for a number of potential confounders.

Blood pressure was measured three times using a standard mercury manometer by trained and certified technicians in both examinations. The onsets of the first-phase (systolic) and fifth-phase (diastolic) Korotkoff sounds were recorded. The mean of the second and third measures were used in the analyses.

Using the above definition, the 1998 SADHS sample nationwide produces a prevalence of 30.4 %. The geographic distribution of the prevalence of hypertension by provinces of South Africa is shown in Table 11.1. The data indicates the

Table 11.1 Baseline characteristics of the study population (SADHS 1998)[a]

Variable	N = 13,596
Mean age[b] (SD)	38.5(17.9)
Women (%)	58.2
Ethnicity (%)	
Black/African	75.8
Coloured	13.0
White	7.8
Asian/Indian	3.3
Education (%)	
No education	14.1
Primary education	77.3
Secondary education	4.7
Higher education	3.9
Urban population (%)	56.0
Mean BMI, kg/m^2 (SD)	25.2(6.2)
Mean Waist (SD)	83.7(15.2)
Smoking status (%)	
Non-current smoker	63.3
Current smoker	36.7
Drinking status (%)	
Non-current drinker	38.9
Current drinker	61.1
Sleep problems (%)	
Yes	16.2
No	83.8
Diabetes (%)	
Yes	3.0
No	97.0
High blood cholesterol (%)	
Yes	1.3
No	98.7
Heart attack or angina (%)	
Yes	4.8
No	95.2
Stroke in the 12 months (%)	
Yes	0.9
No	99.1
Salty foods (%)	
Yes	13.5
No	86.5
Hypertension[c] (%)	
Yes	30.4
No	69.6
Hypertension by province of residence (%)	
Northern Cape	36.0
Free State	33.5
Western Cape	32.4
North West	32.2

(continued)

Table 11.1 (continued)

Variable	N = 13,596
Eastern Cape	31.6
Gauteng	31.2
Kwazulu Natal	30.8
Mpumalanga	23.0
Northern province	20.8

[a]Data are expressed as mean (standard deviation) or as percentages
[b]Age ranges from 15 to 95 years of age
[c]Defined as blood pressure ≥ 140/90 mmHg or self-report

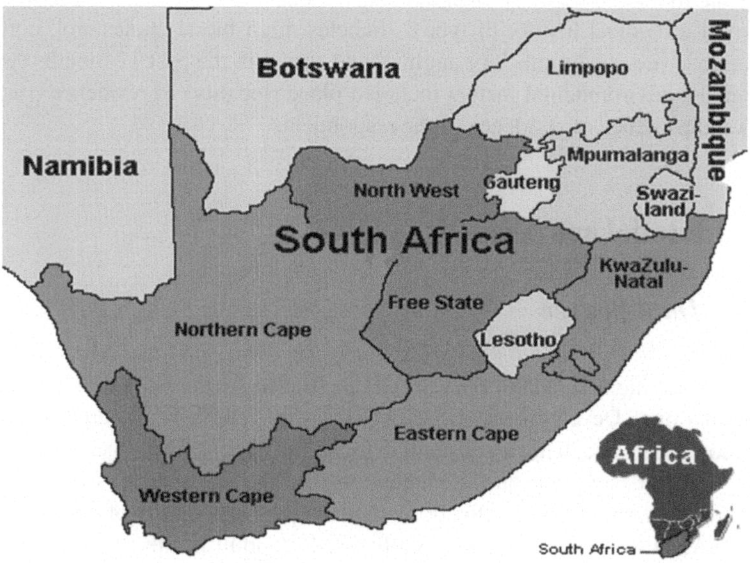

Fig. 11.1 Map of South Africa showing the 9 administrative provinces

following distribution of hypertension ranked by provinces: Northern Cape (36.0), Free State (33.5 %), Western Cape (32.4 %), North West (32.2 %), Eastern Cape (31.6 %), Gauteng (31.2 %), Kwazulu Natal (30.8 %), Mpumalanga (23.0 %), and Northern Province (20.8 %). However, the actual incidence may be much higher than the reported figures according to some South African experts in the field.

11.4.3 Independent Variables

The main exposure variable investigated was the respondent geographic location (province of residence: see Fig. 11.1) in addition to various individual-level control variables such as socio-demographics, lifestyle, and cardiovascular co-morbidities known to be associated with hypertension. The respondent's age at the time of survey was also included as an indicator of the birth cohort of the participant. Other socio-demographic covariates were gender, ethnicity (black/African vs. coloured, white and Asian/Indian), and education of the respondent (no education vs. primary, secondary and higher education). Anthropometric measures were taken, including height, weight, and waist circumference; body mass index (BMI) was calculated as weight in kilograms divided by height in meters squared and categorized as follows: <25, 25–29.9, ≥ 30. Lifestyle factors included smoking (non-current smoker vs. current smoker), drinking status (non-current alcohol drinker vs. current alcohol drinker), sleep quality (trouble sleeping vs. no trouble sleeping), and self-reported dietary habits including usual intake of salty foods. Cardiovascular co-morbidities comprised a medical history of type 2 diabetes, high blood cholesterol, coronary heart disease (i.e., heart attack or angina), and stroke in the past 12 months (yes vs. no). Finally, environmental factors included place (locality) of residence (rural vs. urban) and province of residence of the respondents.

11.5 Material and Methods

11.5.1 Data Source

The Demographic and Health Survey (DHS), funded by the United States Agency for International Development (USAID), is a well-established source of reliable population level data with a substantial focus on health. The objectives, organisation, sample design and questionnaires used in the DHS surveys are described elsewhere (Department of Health 2002). One unique particularity of the 1998 South Africa (SADHS) survey was a module focused on adult health. Briefly, a random probability sample of women and men aged 15 and over were selected in this cross-sectional survey, which used hypertension as an indicator condition to assess the prevalence, determinants and quality of care provided for hypertensive patients.

Data was collected on self-reported lifestyle habits that influence health and on commonly occurring chronic adult diseases. The blood pressure, height and weight of participants were measured and participants reported on any illness and injury suffered due to their workplace. A random sample of 13,827 persons 15 years and older was selected, their BP was measured electronically, some risk factors for hypertension and chronic prescribed medications were recorded, as were socio-demographic data and the province of residence. For this chapter, however, we use the individual records of 13,596 participants with complete information on measured systolic and diastolic blood pressure.

The DHS are known to be of good quality. The most comprehensive estimates of the prevalence of hypertension in South Africa are provided in the report of the SADHS that was conducted in the country in 1998 and in the SA MRC report 2006. In this study, we have linked hypertension status to the geographic location and a number of demographic, anthropometric, lifestyle and co-morbidity variables.

In the analysis of survey data, the commonly adopted models are probit or logit models and the standard measure of effect is the odds ratio. DHS data use cluster-sampling to draw upon respondents via multistage sampling. At the first stage, a stratified sample of enumeration areas (villages/communities) is taken; at the second stage, a sample of households within the selected communities is taken; and finally, at the third stage, all respondents (aged 15 and over) in the sample households are included. These households have at least one respondent. Although, cluster sampling is a cost-saving measure, without the need to list all the households, statistically, it creates analytical problems in that observational units are not independent. Thus, statistical analyses that rely upon the assumption of independence are no longer valid.

In the present study, however, the SADHS data contains geographic or spatial information, such as the province of individuals in the study and the presence of non-linear effects for some covariates means that strictly linear predictors cannot be assumed. Analysing and modelling geographical patterns for the prevalence of hypertension, in addition to the impact of other covariates, is of obvious interest in many studies. In a novel approach, the geographical patterns of hypertension and the possibly non-linear effects of other factors were therefore explored within a simultaneous, coherent regression framework, using a geo-additive, semi-parametric mixed model that simultaneously controlled spatial dependence and possibly nonlinear or time-varying effects of covariates and the complex sampling design (Kandala et al. 2011).

We use this nationally representative population household survey data (SADHS 1998) to quantify the provincial-level variation of prevalent hypertension risk among adults in South Africa. Previous research on cardiovascular diseases in South Africa did not account for geographic location, auto-correlation in the data, non-linear and time varying effects of covariates, and small samples, cast doubt on the generalizability of the findings. Specifically, these studies relied on the independence of random components at the contextual level (province). Most of these studies also based their conclusions on limited statistical analysis, neglecting to control for factors that may significantly affect adult health, such as physical environment where adults live and the potential impact of the geographic location where the adult lives. Finally, the findings represented in these studies provide national statistics; which cannot be extrapolated for a particular province. In this study we address these shortcomings by linking the prevalence of hypertension with geographic locations, by using all cases processed in each province of South Africa, and by accounting for the influence of such important factors as non-linear effects of covariates, dependence of random components and geographic location on case outcomes.

Our analysis aims also to document differences between provinces in the variations of the observed prevalence of hypertension risks by testing the bivariate and multivariate associations of well known lifestyle and socioeconomic correlates of cardiovascular disease risks. From this initial analysis, we expect to identify the association between lifestyle, socio-economic and demographic factors and hypertension while showing province related differences in the risks and variation across them in the correlates.

We use appropriate statistical techniques to explain differences across the provinces in prevalence of hypertension risks using the household socio-economic characteristics that are observed in our data. This allows us to see the degree to which the spatial variation in the raw data is reduced – or increased – when we take into account the differences in observed characteristics of households that are associated with the risk of hypertension.

Examples of issues we investigate in this chapter are: does prevalence of hypertension risk vary from province to province because of factors that are not measured by our survey data, where these factors could include environmental or biological factors? Are high risks for hypertension concentrated in poorer provinces? Does variation in prevalence of hypertension risk from province to province occur because of differences in household socioeconomic status, education, rural, race and ethnicity (Dennison et al. 2007; Seedat 1999).

In pursuing these aims, this chapter exhibits three key features. First, we re-analyze the 1998 SADHS. These data provide a representative cross-national sample of adults in South Africa.

Second, since SADHS data are hierarchical in nature at the family and community or province level, which are inter-related, we use flexible methods to model spatial determinants of hypertension and to allocate these spatial effects to structured and unstructured (random) components. This approach draws on Bayesian geo-additive methods of spatial statistics, taking advantage of advances in Geographic Information Systems. The modelling of the two components is done jointly in one estimation procedure that thereby simultaneously identifies lifestyle, socioeconomic determinants, and the spatial effects that are not explained by these determinants. In this way, we are able to identify province patterns of hypertension that are either related to left-out lifestyle and socioeconomic variables that have a clear spatial pattern or point to spatial (possibly epidemiological or environmental or biological) processes that account for these spatial patterns.

In so doing, this modeling approach identifies the extent of province-level variation in South Africa in the risk of hypertension, and the amount of residual variation due to unobserved factors, which may include environmental or biological factors. We anticipate that our study findings result in further research questions. In addition, our results should suggest avenues for further research to assess more directly the prevalence of cardiovascular disease risk in several SSA countries using a combination of data (for example: WHO Global Burden of disease and data from a collaborative network of disease prevalence from Gambia, Kenya, and Nigeria).

11.6 Statistical Analysis

To account for spatial autocorrelation of hypertension in South Africa, we applied a unified approach by exploring spatial patterns in the prevalence of hypertension and possible nonlinear effects within a simultaneous, coherent regression framework using a geo-additive semi-parametric mixed model. The model employed a fully Bayesian approach using Markov Chain Monte Carlo (MCMC) techniques for inference and model checking (Fahrmeir and Lang 2001; Kandala et al. 2011). The response variable is defined as $y_i = 1$ *if hypertensive and* $y_i = 0$ *otherwise.* The standard measure of effect is the posterior odds ratio (OR).

Epidemiological investigations of spatial variations of diseases are often confined to using province-specific dummy variables to capture the spatial dimension. The commonly adopted model for the analysis of these data is the logistic model, and the standard measure of effects is the odds ratio (OR). Because of the geographical nature of our data and the presence of non-linear effects for some covariates, the assumption of a strictly linear predictor may not be appropriate however.

In this analysis, we apply a novel approach by exploring provincial patterns of hypertension prevalence and possible non-linear effects of other factors within a simultaneous, coherent regression framework using a geo-additive semi-parametric mixed model. The model used for this investigation has been described elsewhere (Fahrmeir and Lang 2001; Kandala et al. 2011).

As the predictor contains usual linear terms, non-linear effects of metrical covariates and geographic effects in an additive form, such models are also called geo-additive models. Kammann and Wand 2003 proposed this type of model within an empirical Bayesian approach. Here, we apply a fully Bayesian approach as suggested in Fahrmeir and Lang 2001, which is based on Markov random field priors and uses Markov Chain Monte Carlo (MCMC) techniques for inference and model checking. Although the estimation process with this model is fully Bayesian, the estimated posterior odds ratios (OR) that are produced could be interpreted as similar to those of ordinary logistic models.

Consider regression situations, where observations (y_i; x_i; w_i); $i = 1; \ldots; N$, on a metrical response y, a vector $x = (x_i; \ldots; x_p)'$ of metrical covariates (age of participant), times scales or spatial covariates (province in South Africa) and a vector $w = (w_1; \ldots w_r)'$ of further covariates are made, in which categorical covariates are often given. The generalized additive modelling framework assumes that, given x_i and w_i, the distribution of the response y_i belongs to an exponential family, with mean $\mu_i = (y_i | x_{i,} w_i)$ linked to an additive semi-parametric predictor $\mu_i = h(\eta)$,where h is a known response function.

Traditionally, the effect of the covariates on the response is modelled by a linear predictor

$$\eta_\iota = x'_i \beta + w'_i \gamma \qquad (11.1)$$

The response variable in this application is defined as $Y_i = 1$, if individual *i* is hypertensive during the reference period *t* and $Y_i = 0$ otherwise. We have a logit link function $\Pr(y_i = 1 | \eta_\iota) = e^{\eta_\iota}/(1 + e^{\eta_\iota})$ for the probability of having hypertension at the reference period (i.e. we model the conditional probability of an individual having hypertension) given the individual's age in months, the province where the person lives, and X, with predictor (11.1).

In our application to chronic diseases prevalence and in many other regression situations, we are facing the following problems:

- For the continuous covariates in the data set, the assumption of a strictly linear effect on the response y may not be appropriate. In our study, such covariates are individual's age (*age*) at the time of the survey. Generally, it will be difficult to model the possibly non-linear effect of such covariates through a parametric functional form, which has to be linear in the parameters, prior to any data analysis.
- In addition to usual covariates, geographical small-area information is given in the form of a location variable s, indicating the province, district or community where individuals or units in the sample size live or come from. In our study, this geographical information is given by the provinces where the individual lives at the time of the survey. Attempts to include such small-area information using province-specific dummy-variables would in our case entail more than 50 dummy-variables and could not access spatial inter-dependence of provinces. The latter problem could not be solved through conventional multi-level modelling using uncorrelated random effects. It is reasonable to assume that areas close to each other are more similar than areas far apart, so that spatially correlated random effects are required.

To overcome these difficulties, we replace the strictly linear predictor with a *geo-additive predictor*, leading to the *geo-additive regression model:*

$$\eta_\iota = f_1(x_{i1}) + \ldots + f_p(x_{ip}) + f_{spat}(s_i) + w'_i\gamma \tag{11.2}$$

here, $f_1, \ldots, f_p$ are non-linear smooth effects of the metrical covariates, and $f_{spat}\ (s_i)$ is the effect of the spatial covariate $s_i \in \{1, \ldots, S\}$ labelling the province in South Africa. Regression models with predictors as in (11.2) are sometimes referred to as geo-additive models (Kammann and Wand 2003).

For our inference using the Bayesian approach, unknown functions f_j and parameters γ as well as the variance parameter σ^2 are considered as random variables and have to be supplemented with appropriate prior assumptions. In the absence of any prior knowledge we assume independent diffuse priors $\gamma_j \propto const$, $j = 1, \ldots, r$ for the parameters of fixed effects. Another common choice is highly dispersed Gaussian priors.

Several alternatives are available as *smoothness priors for the unknown functions* $f_j\ (x_j)$, (see Fahrmeir and Lang 2001). We use Bayesian P(enalized) – Splines (Eilers and Marx 1996), introduced by Eilers and Marx in a frequentist setting. For the spatially correlated effect f_{str} (s), s = 1,... S, we choose Markov random field priors common in spatial statistics (Fahrmeir and Lang 2001; Kandala et al. 2011). These priors reflect spatial neighbourhood relationships. For a spatially uncorrelated (unstructured) effect f_{unstr} a common assumption is that the parameters $f_{unstr}(s)$ are i.i.d. Gaussian. We also perform a sensitivity analysis using other priors for the spatial effect but results of the Markov random field priors outperformed other priors.

Although the estimation process with this model is fully Bayesian, the estimated posterior odds ratios (OR) that were produced could be interpreted as similar to those of ordinary logistic models.

For comparison with standard regression models such as ordinary logistic regression, the standard measure of effect is still the odds ratio (OR) and its 95 % confidence interval (CI) for a logistic model. However, because of the use of a fully Bayesian approach that relies on prior assumption to make posterior inference, instead of 'OR', we have 'posterior OR' and 95 % credible region (CR). For model choice and adequacy, we routinely use the Deviance Information Criterion (DIC) (Spiegelhalter et al. 2002) developed as a measure of model fit and complexity instead of tests for significance, linear trends and interactions. To account for possible departures from the assumed distribution, 95 % credible regions (CRs) for the posterior ORs and probability maps (the equivalent of CIs for the spatial effects) are calculated using robust standard errors estimated via MCMC simulation techniques.

11.7 Advantages of the Bayesian Geo-Additive Model Over Conventional Models

There are many potential advantages of the approach described above over more conventional approaches like regression models with fixed or random provinces effects; or standard 2-level multilevel modelling with unstructured spatial effects. In the conventional models, it is assumed that the random components at the contextual level (province in our case) are mutually independent. In practice, these approaches specify correlated random effects, which are contrary to that assumption. Further, the independence assumption has an inherent problem of inconsistency. If the location of the event matters, it makes sense to assume that areas close to each other are more similar than areas that are far apart. Moreover, treating groups (in our case provinces) as independent is unrealistic and leads to poor estimates of the standard errors. Standard errors for between-province factors are likely to be underestimated because we are treating observations from the same province as independent and thus increasing the apparent sample size. On the contrary, standard errors for within province factors are likely to be overestimated (Kandala and Ghilagaber 2006). On the other hand, Demographic and Health Survey data are based on a random sample of districts which, in turn, introduces a structured component. Such a component allows us to borrow strength from neighbours in order to cope with the posterior uncertainty of the district effect and obtain estimates for areas that may have inadequate sample sizes or are not represented in the sample.

In an attempt to highlight the advantages of our approach in a spatial context and examine the potential bias incurred when ignoring the dependence between aggregated spatial areas, we fitted several models with and without the structured and random components in this study.

Controlling for important risk factors such as geographical location (spatial auto-correlation) arising from environment impact on health and population mobility (migration) gives estimates of prevalence that are statistically robust.

The analysis was carried out using version 2.0.1 of the BayesX software package, which permits Bayesian inference based on Markov chain Monte Carlo (MCMC) simulation techniques. The statistical significances of apparent associations between potential risk factors and the prevalence of hypertension were first explored using chi-square and Mann–Whitney *U*-tests, as appropriate. Secondly, multivariate analysis was used to evaluate the significance of the posterior OR determined for the fixed, non-linear effects and spatial effects. A *P*-value of <0.05 was considered indicative of a statistically significant difference.

11.8 Results

Table 11.1 shows the overall prevalence of hypertension and baseline characteristics of the population, Table 11.2 indicates the prevalence of hypertension by some baseline characteristics and province and Table 11.3 the adjusted marginal odds ratios (MOR) using the traditional logistic regression model, and adjusted posterior odds ratios (POR) using the Bayesian approach. The overall hypertension prevalence was 30.4 % using the current recommended cut-off point of blood pressure (BP $\geq$140/90 mmHg) or diagnosed high BP. It is higher than the 14.0 % and 25.1 % suggested in the previous report using the 160/95 and 140/90 cut-offs only. Higher prevalence was observed among women, white and coloured compared to the national average and the prevalence was higher among people with no education, lower prevalence in rural areas, higher prevalence among obese people, higher prevalence among current smokers and current drinkers, higher prevalence among people with sleep problems, people with co-morbidities (diabetes, high blood cholesterol, heart attack, stroke), higher prevalence among people without salty food habits and lower prevalence in the northern province (now Limpopo) and Mpumalanga. The mean age of the participants in this study was older 38.5 (SD: 17.9) and 58.2 % of the sample was women. The results show distinct differences between urban and rural with higher proportion of hypertension in urban areas compared with rural areas (31.8 % vs. 28.7 %) and the difference persisted in terms of traditional hypertension risk factors, : smoking (33.8 % vs. 26.1 %), alcohol (34.6 % vs. 27.8 %) and obesity (49.5 % vs. 21.4 %). Adjusted marginal odds ratios indicate a large spatial variation of hypertension in 1998 with the highest prevalence of hypertension observed in North West [OR & 95 % CI: 2.06 (1.66, 2.56)], Free State [OR & 95 % CI: 2.02 (1.62, 2.53)], and Northern Cape [OR & 95 % CI: 1.95 (1.53, 2.47)] provinces, followed by Gauteng, Western Cape, Kwazulu Natal and Eastern Cape provinces, with the lowest prevalence in Northern province and Mpumalanga provinces (see Table 11.1). Adjustment of study characteristics and the province of residence without taking into account spatial auto-correlation in the data are shown in Table 11.3, first column (MOR). It is similar to the observed

Table 11.2 Baseline characteristics of the study population by hypertensive status[a] (SADHS 1998)[b]

Variable	Hypertensive (N = 4138)	Non-hypertensive (N = 9458)	P-value[c]
Mean age	50.3(17.2)	33.3(15.5)	<0.001
Gender (%)			
Male	1,560(37.7)	4,118(43.5)	
Female	2,578(62.3)	5,340(56.5)	<0.001
Ethnicity (%)			
Black/African	2,976(72.1)	7,321(77.5)	
Coloured	622(15.1)	1,148(12.2)	
White	397(9.6)	666(7.0)	
Asian/Indian	134(3.2)	312(3.3)	<0.001
Education (%)			
No education	907(22.1)	1,003(10.6)	
Primary education	2,862(69.7)	7,602(80.6)	
Secondary education	141(3.4)	496(5.3)	
Higher education	196(4.8)	332(3.5)	<0.001
Place of residence (%)			
Urban	2,422(58.5)	5,197(54.9)	
Rural	1,716(41.5)	4,261(45.1)	<0.001
BMI (kg/m^2) (%)			
< 25	1,639(40.3)	6,013(64.2)	
25–29.9	1,116(27.5)	2,021(21.6)	
≥ 30	1,306(32.2)	1,332(14.2)	<0.001
Waist (tertile) (%)			
1 (lowest)	717(17.6)	3,798(40.4)	
2	1,166(28.6)	3,301(35.2)	
3 (highest)	2,194(53.8)	2,287(24.4)	<0.001
Smoking status (%)			
Non-current smoker	2,301(55.6)	6,302(66.7)	
Current smoker	1,836(44.4)	3,150(33.3)	<0.001
Drinking status (%)			
Non-current drinker	2,309(55.9)	5,985(63.4)	
Current drinker	1,825(44.1)	3,450(36.6)	<0.001
Sleep problems (%)			
Yes	886(21.4)	1,317(13.9)	
No	3,252(78.6)	8,141(86.1)	<0.001
Diabetes (%)			
Yes	287(7.0)	113(1.2)	
No	3,823(93.0)	9,310(98.4)	<0.001
High blood cholesterol (%)			
Yes	100(2.5)	69(0.7)	
No	3,965(97.5)	9,290(99.3)	<0.001
Heart attack or angina (%)			
Yes	430(10.4)	225(2.4)	
No	3,687(89.6)	9,211(97.6)	<0.001

(continued)

Table 11.2 (continued)

Variable	Hypertensive (N = 4138)	Non-hypertensive (N = 9458)	P-value[c]
Stroke in the 12 months (%)			
Yes	87(2.1)	37(0.4)	
No	4,039(97.9)	9,410(99.6)	<0.001
Salty foods (%)			
Yes	495(12.0)	1,335(14.1)	
No	3,633(88.0)	8,111(85.9)	<0.001
Region of residence (%)			
Northern Cape	450(10.9)	801(8.5)	
Free State	397(9.6)	787(8.3)	
Western Cape	367(8.9)	765(8.1)	
North West	395(9.6)	832(8.8)	
Eastern Cape	1,049(25.3)	2,273(24.0)	
Gauteng	337(8.1)	742(7.9)	
Kwazulu Natal	619(14.9)	1,392(14.7)	
Mpumalanga	281(6.8)	940(9.9)	
Northern province	243(5.9)	926(9.8)	<0.001

[a]Defined as blood pressure ≥ 140/90 mmHg or self-report
[b]Data are expressed as mean (standard deviation) or as percentages
[c]*P*-values for comparison between hypertensive and non-hypertensive subjects

Table 11.3 Marginal and posterior odds ratios of hypertension across selected covariates (SADHS 1998)

Variable	Marginal OR & 95% CI[a]	Posterior OR & 95 % CI[b]
Age groups		*See* Fig. 11.2
<=30	1.00	
31–40	1.86(1.63, 2.12)	
41–60	4.68(4.16, 5.28)	
60+	10.5(9.07, 12.1)	
Gender		
Male	0.97(0.88, 1.08)	1.02 (0.71, 1.24)
Female	1.00	1.00
Ethnicity		
Black/African	1.00	1.00
Coloured	1.14(0.96, 1.34)	1.16 (0.99, 1.36)
White	0.85(0.71, 1.01)	0.81 (0.68, 0.95)
Asian/Indian	0.85(0.65, 1.11)	0.90 (0.69, 1.20)
Education		
No education	0.98(0.86, 1.12)	0.97 (0.77, 1.20)
Primary education	0.77(0.60, 1.00)	1.05 (0.88, 1.27)
Secondary education	0.99(0.79, 1.25)	0.83 (0.62, 1.11)
Higher education	1.00	1.00

(continued)

Table 11.3 (continued)

Variable	Marginal OR & 95% CI[a]	Posterior OR & 95 % CI[b]
Place of residence		
Urban	1.09(0.99, 1.21)	1.08 (0.99, 1.19)
Rural	1.00	1.00
BMI (kg/m^2)		
< 25	1.00	
25–29.9	1.59(1.43, 1.77)	
≥30	2.53(2.25, 2.84)	*See* Fig.11.2
Smoking status		
Non-current smoker	1.00	1.00
Current smoker	1.12(1.01, 1.24)	1.14 (1.03, 1.26)
Drinking status		
Non-current drinker	1.00	1.00
Current drinker	1.17(1.05, 1.30)	1.17 (1.05, 1.29)
Sleep problems		
Yes	1.13(1.00, 1.27)	1.16 (1.02, 1.31)
No	1.00	1.00
Diabetes		
Yes	2.57(2.00, 3.30)	2.49(1.92, 3.13)
No	1.00	1.00
High blood cholesterol		
Yes	1.47(1.01, 2.14)	1.38(0.99, 1.90)
No	1.00	1.00
Heart attack or angina		
Yes	2.47(2.03, 3.01)	2.41(2.01, 2.86)
No	1.00	1.00
Stroke in the 12 months		
Yes	2.09(1.31, 3.35)	2.11(1.36, 3.16)
No	1.00	1.00
Salty foods		
Yes	0.90(0.79, 1.02)	0.99 (0.81, 1.03)
No	1.00	1.00
Region of residence		*See also* Figs. 11.3 and 11.4
Northern Cape	1.95(1.53, 2.47)	1.30(1.02, 1.55)
Free State	2.02(1.62, 2.53)	1.32(1.08, 1.68)
Western Cape	1.49(1.15, 1.91)	0.93(0.73, 1.10)
North West	2.06(1.66, 2.56)	1.33(1.14, 1.61)
Eastern Cape	1.43(1.18,1.72)	0.93(0.79, 0.91)
Gauteng	1.55(1.22, 1.97)	1.00(0.81, 1.23)
Kwazulu Natal	1.46(1.19, 1.80)	0.94(0.81, 1.13)
Mpumalanga	1.11(0.89, 1.39)	0.77(0.63, 0.92)
Northern province	1.00	0.68(0.56, 0.84)

[a]Adjusted marginal odds ratio (OR) from standard logistic regression models. The Northern Province was used as the reference category because of the lowest crude hypertension prevalence (see Table 11.1)

[b]Spatially adjusted posterior odds ratio (OR) from Bayesian geo-additive regression models after controlling for nonlinear effect of age, categorical variables and the province of residence (spatial effects)

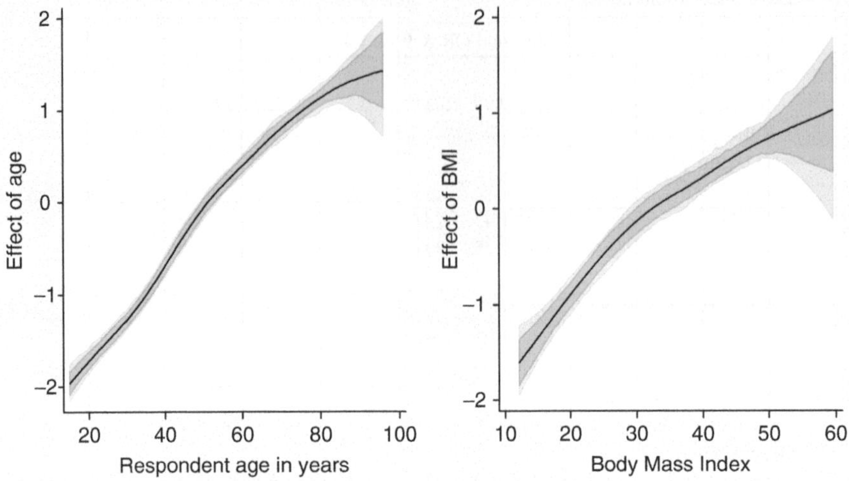

Fig. 11.2 Estimated nonlinear (logit) effects of age and Body Mass Index (BMI) on hypertension in South Africa. Shown are the posterior logit within the 95 % and 80 % credible intervals (DHS 1998)

crude prevalence in Table 11.2 indicating slightly higher magnitudes provincial point estimates. The highest prevalence was still observed in North West, Free State, and Northern Cape provinces, followed by Gauteng, Western Cape, Kwazulu Natal and Eastern Cape provinces, with the lowest prevalence in Northern province and Mpumalanga provinces (see Table 11.2). Kwazulu Natal and Gauteng provinces were among the highest prevalence rates provinces compared to the national average but surprisingly, have now moved down the rank in the adjusted POR model (Table 11.3).

In general, for both the observed prevalence and adjusted marginal ORs, Northern Province and Mpumalanga provinces were associated with the lowest prevalence.

The estimates of the spatial effects of hypertension were also mapped (Figs. 11.3 and 11.4). Before adjustment for the geographic location, which acts as a surrogate for cultural, ethnic and environmental differences, a higher prevalence of hypertension was concentrated in the central provinces and the southern west provinces (Tables 11.1 and 11.2). However, after multiple adjustments, the effect normalised in South West provinces but became more pronounced in Free State and North West provinces (Fig. 11.3). In Fig. 11.4, the left-hand maps show estimated posterior Odd Ratio (OR) of total residual spatial province effects (i.e. adjusted odds ratios after multiple adjustment of the geographical location, taking into account the autocorrelation structure in the data and other risk factors) for hypertension in each province, with the dark colour indicating the maximum posterior OR recorded (1.33) while grey denotes a lower prevalence (OR: 0.68).

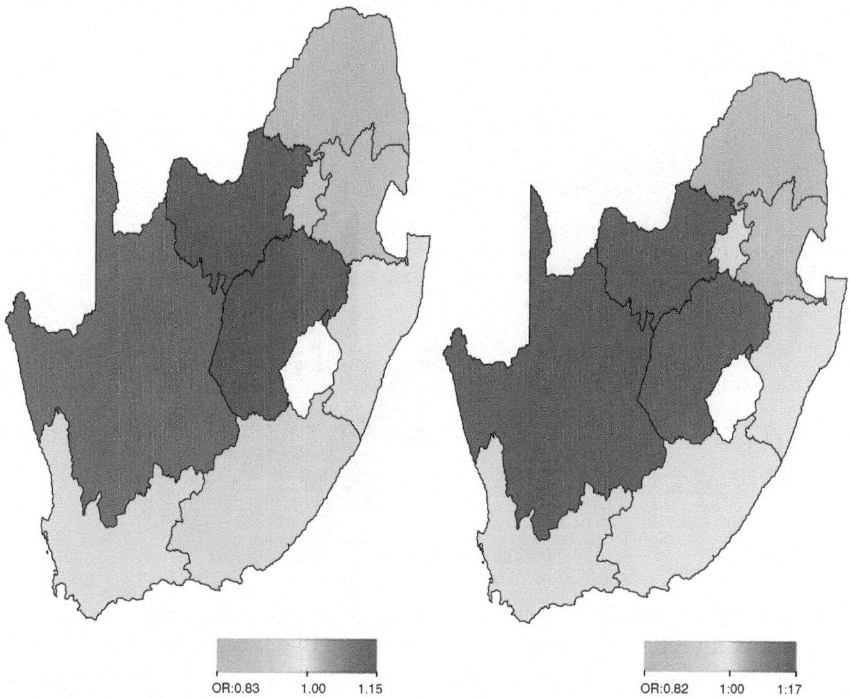

Dark coloured – high risk
Grey coloured – low risk

Fig. 11.3 Unstructured (*left*) and structured (*right*) residual spatial provincial effects of the risk of hypertension in South Africa (DHS 1998) (*Dark* coloured – high risk, *Grey* coloured – low risk)

A high prevalence of hypertension was concentrated in North West, Free State and Northern Cape provinces. The right-hand maps (Fig. 11.4) show the 95 % posterior probability maps of hypertension. White colour indicates a negative spatial effect (associated with reduced risk of hypertension), black colour a positive effect (an increased risk).

The pattern of the prevalence of hypertension by province differed markedly between the estimated models, though there was consistently higher prevalence in North West, Free State and Northern Cape and lower prevalence in Northern Province and Mpumalanga (Table 11.3). The marginal odds ratios of hypertension prevalence at the provincial level shown in Table 11.3 left column indicate that the two provinces in which hypertension prevalence is lowest and below the national prevalence are Northern Province and Mpumalanga provinces.

Table 11.3 (2nd column) contains the fixed effects from the multivariable Bayesian geo-additive regression analyses, and the non-linear effects of respondent's age and BMI are shown in Fig. 11.2. In the left-hand map of Fig. 11.4 we show the posterior OR by province predicted by considering the socioeconomic

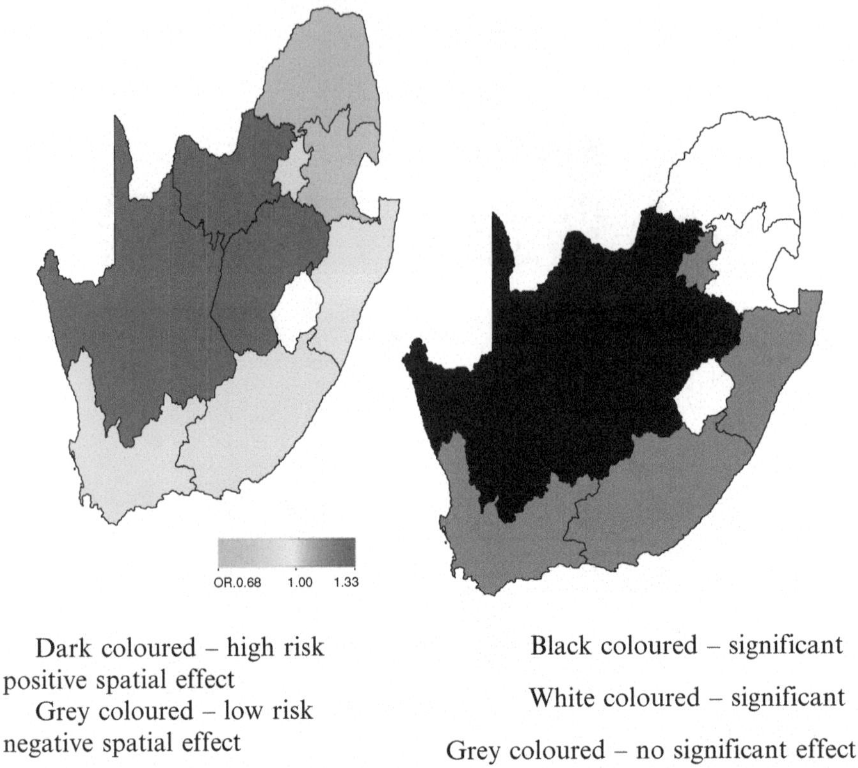

Fig. 11.4 Total residual spatial provincial effects (*left*) and 95 % posterior probability map (*right*) of the risk of hypertension in South Africa (DHS 1998) (*Dark* coloured – high risk, *Black* coloured – significant positive spatial effect, *Grey* coloured – low risk, *White* coloured – significant negative spatial effect, *Grey* coloured – no significant effect)

covariates and many other risk factors consisting of the residual spatial effects by province that are not explained by the socioeconomic and other variables in our data. These residual spatial effects are then allocated to structured and unstructured effects (Fig. 11.3). The posterior OR estimate of the structured spatial effects f_{str} is shown in the maps of Fig. 11.3a. Figure 11.3b shows the unstructured spatial effects. The total residual spatial effects (i.e. the sum of the unstructured and structured spatial effects) are shown in Fig. 11.4a. In addition, posterior probability maps (Fig. 11.4b) indicate significance of the spatial effects (white = significantly negative effect (lower risk); black = significantly positive (higher risk), grey = not significant). Note that the spatial effects are centred on zero, i.e. the average over all provinces is zero, while the overall level is estimated through the intercept term. Before commenting on the substantive results, it is important to point out that the spatial model has the best fit after evaluation of the fit criteria using Deviance Information Criteria (DIC).

The results for the fixed effects from the multivariable Bayesian geo-additive regression analyses in Table 11.3 (2nd column) suggest that, current smokers [OR & 95 % Credible Region (CR): 1.14 (1.03, 1.26)], current drinkers [OR & 95 % CR: 1.17 (1.05, 1.29)], sleep problems [OR & 95 % CR: 1.16 (1.02, 1.31)] and diabetes [OR & 95 % CR: 2.49 (1.92, 3.13)], heart attack [OR & 95 % CR: 2.41(2.01, 2.86)], and stroke [OR & 95 % CR: 2.11(1.36, 3.16)], were consistently associated with higher prevalence of hypertension.

It is observed that after controlling for socio-economic life-style variables there still remains a substantial residual spatial effect that begs for an explanation (Figs. 11.3 and 11.4), and the province of residence remained a significant risk factor for hypertension. Overall, results of the 1998 SADHS (Fig. 11.4) show that provinces with the highest prevalence of hypertension included only North West, Free State and Northern Cape after accounting for spatial auto-correlation in the data, while Eastern Cape, Gauteng and Kwazulu Natal no longer ranked among the highest prevalence provinces as suggested by the marginal OR (Table 11.3).

Figure 11.2 shows the non-linear relationship (as a continuous variable), and between the risk of hypertension and age and BMI of the respondent at the time of the survey for the whole national sample. Shown are estimated posterior logits of the effects of the respondent's age and BMI within the 80 % and 90 % credible intervals. There is a clear linear association between respondent's age and BMI. Age and BMI of the respondent appear to be almost linearly positively related to the prevalence of hypertension. As expected, as age and BMI increase, the likelihood of respondent's hypertension status per age also significantly increases.

11.9 Discussion

Our novel and most important findings are illustrated in the contrast between 1st, 2nd column of Table 11.3 (marginal ORs obtained using the traditional logistic regression model and the posterior ORs using the Bayesian model). We observed a pronounced change in the odd ratios in the provincial effects for Western and Eastern Cape, Kwazulu Natal and Gauteng following adjustment of the geographical location (spatial auto-correlation) arising from environmental factors and age structure of the population.

Figures 11.3 and 11.4 (left) shows that the socioeconomic effects are able to explain a fair amount of the spatial variation of hypertension in South Africa. We calculate that the average residual spatial effect in the left-hand panel of Fig. 11.4 is about 22 % lower than the observed prevalence and marginal OR in Table 11.2, showing that the socioeconomic and other risk factors explain some but not all of the spatial variation.

However, the spatial residuals in the left-hand side of Fig. 11.4 show that much of the variation in hypertension remains unexplained. These spatial effects are then allocated by the model into structured effects, which are shown in Fig. 11.3 left, and unstructured residual effects in Fig. 11.3 right and the total effects in Fig. 11.4.

Several important findings emerged. First, the structured spatial effects point to some spatial variation in the risk of hypertension although they are not significant as indicated by the probability map (not shown here).

Thus we clearly have a pattern of higher hypertension in the western provinces: North West, Free State, and Northern Cape.

Conversely, ORs are significantly lower in Northern Province and Mpumalanga. Second, while these structured effects suggest hypertension is higher in the southern provinces in a belt ranging from Gauteng to Western Cape, it is interesting to note that the province of Gauteng is not a significant component in that belt. Thus while some spatial residuals do spill significantly across borders, e.g. between Northern Cape and North West and Free State, some borders do seem to matter in the sense that spatial residuals remain noticeably distinct in the analysis on the two sides of the border.

Third, the unstructured spatial effects shown in Fig. 11.3 left, while being much smaller and not significant, also displayed an interesting pattern. While the Western Cape and Eastern Cape have significantly higher observed prevalence of hypertension this was not the case in the structured map in Fig. 11.3 right and Fig. 11.4 left where these provinces actually have lower prevalence, though not statistically significant. This may be related to the effect of life style factors specific to certain provinces as the unstructured spatial effects convey a localised effect.

The clear structured pattern begs for an explanation. None of the socioeconomic variables we tried in addition to the ones mentioned are able to completely explain these pronounced spatial effects. One common factor to most of the areas that are negatively affected is that these areas are comparatively at the centre of the country and are mostly poor provinces. This distinction is most noticeable and clear in the South–north divide observed in the structured and total spatial effects. The difference could well be due to differences in life style, level of urbanisation, share of poverty, access to medical facilities, and other diseases that thrive in these provinces. Indeed, looking at the ranking of hypertension by provinces, there is a positive correlation between provinces with higher poverty and provinces with high hypertension. Free State is a typical example of this association between hypertension and poverty. There might well be some other factors such as climate and associated environmental factors (Dennison et al. 2007; Seedat 1999, Cappuccio et al. 2008; Thorogood et al. 2007a, b).

Moreover, the higher prevalence in Northern Cape, Free State and North West could additionally be related to the poor access to health facilities and the general remoteness of these areas, which are poorly served with health facilities. These issues deserve closer attention and this procedure is merely able to highlight the important spatial patterns of hypertension without being able to fully explain them.

Quite clearly, the methods used here are able to identify more subtle life style, socioeconomic and spatial influences on hypertension than reliance on linear models with regional dummy variables. As such, they are useful for diagnostic purposes to identify the need to find additional variables that can account for this spatial structure. Moreover, even if the causes of spatial structure are not fully explained, one can use this spatial information for chronic diseases mapping for planning purposes and educational programmes on life-style, which is gaining increasing importance in policy circles that attempt to focus the allocation of public resources to the most affected areas of the population.

Another important fact to highlight is co-morbidity associated with vascular conditions such as hypertension, heart attacks or angina, stroke and high blood cholesterol in Sub-Saharan Africa (Dennison et al. 2007). Little is known about environmental and geographic overlaps in these illnesses. The epidemiology and aetiology of the diseases may be improved by joint spatial modelling for management, planning and cost-effective control. In this chapter a univariate spatial model was applied to a single disease hypertension, in which provincial specific geographic variation of high blood pressure in South Africa was fitted. In Chap. 14, however, a multivariate spatial model is applied to analyse more than one vascular disease (hypertension, heart attacks or angina, stroke and high blood cholesterol) simultaneously which enable to quantify the correlation between relative risks for each disease as well as enable disease-specific residuals to be mapped, while at the same time, examining the influence of covariates on each disease.

There are some limitations in the present study that deserve attention. First, the cross-sectional nature of the present study does not allow establishing temporality and thus causality of the observed associations. Given the self-reporting of lifestyle factors, we cannot disregard the likelihood that health outcomes such as hypertension may influence reports of habitual smoking, drinking habits, and sleep problems and not vice versa. Second, the analysis was based on data collected in 1998, which is likely to underestimate the current prevalence of hypertension in South Africa, as reported by several recent reports (10–13). However, since 1998 there are no recent nationally representative reliable data from SA with information on hypertension. Thus, this limits our ability to apply our approach to more recent data. In addition, there was limited or lack of information for variables such as dietary habits, physical activity, and biomarker data, which are relevant to hypertension aetiology. Nevertheless, our findings corroborate the notion that high blood pressure is an increasing public health issue in these settings, with evidence of considerable spatial variation in hypertension prevalence across different provinces in South Africa.

Another important issue in the use of this data is the issue of data quality because of the fact that national surveys in developing countries are prone to incomplete or partial reporting of responses. Moreover, the use of complex questionnaires inevitably allows scope for inconsistent responses to be recorded for different questions resulting in a further complication in the assessment of health outcomes. Luckily, the MEASURE DHS program primary goals are to produce high-quality data and make it available for analysis in a coherent and consistent form. Therefore, the DHS program has a strict primary data quality policies by adopting a policy of editing and imputation which results in a data file that accurately reflects the population studied and may be readily used for analysis which ultimately reduce bias in the reporting of health outcomes including hypertension.

11.10 Conclusion

In this chapter we re-analysed the 1998 Demographic and Health surveys of South Africa to model the socioeconomic and spatial determinants of hypertension. We find strong association between poverty and the prevalence of hypertension by using a flexible approach to modelling hypertension that clearly has spatial structure. The spatial analysis shows distinct patterns that point to the influence of omitted variables with strong spatial structure or possibly life-style, health accessibility, environment and epidemiological processes that account for this spatial structure.

By re-examining the data, we are able to establish that the prevalence of chronic diseases in Sub-Saharan Africa is even higher than reported and for the case of South Africa, the prevalence of hypertension was under-estimated. With the novel approach, we are able to depict the higher hypertension in Free State and North West, which begs for an explanation.

The maps generated are novel tools to help policy-makers re-evaluate the lack of focus on non-communicable diseases (chronic diseases) in Sub-Saharan Africa and focus on integrated diseases management approach, which we believe will accelerate the achievement of the Millennium Development Goals (MDGs) for maternal and child health in the region.

References

Addo, J., Smeeth, L., & Leon, D. A. (2007). Hypertension in Sub-Saharan Africa: A systematic review. *Hypertension, 50*, 1012–1018.

Cappuccio, F. P. (2004). Epidemiologic transition, migration and cardiovascular disease. *International Journal of Epidemiology, 33*, 387–388.

Cappuccio, F. P., Kerry, S. M., Adeyemo, A., Luke, A., Amoah, A. G., Bovet, P., Connor, M. D., Forrester, T., Gervasoni, J. P., Kaki, G. K., Plange-Rhule, J., Thorogood, M., & Cooper, R. S. (2008). Body size and blood pressure: An analysis of Africans and the African diaspora. *Epidemiology, 19*(1), 38–46.

Craig Schwabe. (2004). *Fact sheet: Poverty in South Africa*. Human Sciences Research Council. http://www.sarpn.org.za/documents/d0000990/

Dennison, C. R., Peer, N., Lombard, C. J., Kepe, L., Levitt, N. S., Steyn, K., & Hill, M. N. (2007). Cardiovascular risk and comorbid conditions among Black South Africans with hypertension in public and private primary care settings: The HiHi study. *Ethnicity & Disease, 17*(3), 477–483.

Department of Health. (2002). *South Africa demographic and health survey (SADHS) 1998. Full report*. Pretoria: Department of Health.

DHS. (1998). *South Africa demographic and health survey (SADHS) 1998. Full report*. Pretoria: Department of Health.

Eilers, P. H. C., & Marx, B. D. (1996). Flexible smoothing with B-splines and penalties (with discussion). *Statistical Science, 89*, 89–121.

Everatt, D. (2005). The Politics of poverty. *Bangladesh e-Journal of Sociology*. Vol 2:1. Access: www.bangladeshsociology.org/BEJS%20-%202.1.2%20-%20Everatt.pdf. Accessed 9 April 2006. pp. 78–80.

Fahrmeir, L., & Lang, S. (2001). Bayesian inference for generalized additive mixed models based on Markov random field priors. *Applied Statistics (JRSS C), 50*, 201–220.

Gelb, S. (2003). *Inequality in South Africa: Nature, Causes and Responses*. The EDGE Institute, Johannesburg. www.tips.org.za/events/forum2004/Papers/Gelb_Inequality_in_SouthAfrica.pdf. Accessed July 10–25 2011. pp. 1–21.

Kandala, N.-B., Brodish, P., Buckner, B., Foster, S., & Madise, N. (2011). Millennium development goals (MDG 6) and HIV infection in Zambia: What can we learn from successive household surveys? *AIDS, 25*(1), 95–106.

Kandala, N.-B., & Ghilagaber, G. (2006). A Geo-additive Bayesian discrete-time survival model and its application to spatial analysis of childhood mortality in Malawi. *Quality and Quantity, 40*(6), 935–957.

Kammann, E. E., & Wand, M. P. (2003). Geoadditive models. *Journal of the Royal Statistical Society C, 52*, 1–18.

Landman, J. P. (2003). Breaking the grip of poverty and inequality in South Africa 2004–2014 Current trends, issues and future policy options. Ecumenical Foundation of South Africa (EFSA). Stellenbosch.

May, J. (1998). *Poverty and inequality in South Africa*. http://www.polity.org.za/html/govdocs/reports/poverty.html?rebookmark=1. Accessed 25 July 2011.

Medical Research Council (MRC). (2006). *Chronic diseases of lifestyle in South Africa: 1995–2005*. Medical Research Council.

Seedat, Y. K. (1999). Hypertension in black South Africans. *Journal of Human Hypertension, 13*, 97–103.

Spiegelhalter, D., Best, N., Carlin, B., & Van der Line, A. (2002). Bayesian measures of models complexity and fit. *Journal of the Royal Statistical Society B, 64*, 1–34.

Statistics South Africa. (2010). *Mid-year population estimates 2011*. July 2010. www.statssa.gov.za.

Steyn, K., Gaziano, T. A., Bradshaw, D., Laubscher, R., Fourie, J., & South African Demographic and Health Coordinating Team. (2001). Hypertension in South African adults: Results from the demographic and health survey, 1998. *Journal of Hypertension, 10*, 1717–1725.

Thorogood, M., Connor, M. D., Hundt, G. L., & Tollman, S. M. (2007a). Understanding and managing hypertension in an African sub-district: A multidisciplinary approach. *Scandinavian Journal of Public Health, 69*(Supplement), 52–59.

Thorogood, M., Connor, M., Tollman, S., Hundt, G. L., Fowkes, G., & Marsh, J. A. (2007b). Cross-sectional study of vascular risk factors in a rural South African population: Data from the Southern African Stroke Prevention Initiative (SASPI). *BMC Public Health, 7*, 326.

UNDP. (2009). Human Development Report 2009. *Economy and Inequality*. http://hdrstats.undp.org/en/indicators

World Bank. (2008). *World development indicators database 2008*.

Woolard, I. (2002). *A comparison of wage levels and wage inequality in the public and private sectors, 1995 and 2000*. Working Papers 9660, University of Cape Town: Development Policy Research Unit.

Chapter 12
A Semiparametric Stratified Survival Model for Timing of First Birth in South Africa

Samuel O.M. Manda, Renate Meyer, and Bo Cai

12.1 Introduction

In many parts of the world, pregnancy in adolescence has been found to be associated with adverse reproductive and maternal health, economic, educational and social consequences. In particular, as a result of biological immaturity and social disadvantage, teenage pregnancy is linked to high risk of low birth weight, premature birth, unsafe abortion and miscarriage that may result in high child and maternal mortality and morbidity (Acsadi and Johnson-Acsadi 1990; Sharma et al. 2003; Gupta and Mahy 2003; Magadi 2004). These adverse effects are compounded in populations where maternal health care among teenage mothers is very poor (Borja and Adair 2003). A reduction in education and employment opportunities hinders women from contributing effectively to social and economic development of a country (Siu-Man and Boachang 1995). As a consequence of limited life opportunities, young mothers face gender inequalities, which subject them to subordinate positions in a society (Jewkes et al. 2009). Improvement in maternal health is one of the eight Millennium Development Goals (MDGs) (United Nations 2012). It is now widely accepted that high rates of teenage pregnancy contribute to the cycle of maternal mortality and indicate poorer reproductive health.

S.O.M. Manda (✉)
Biostatistics Unit, South African Medical Research Council, Pretoria, South Africa
e-mail: Samuel.Manda@mrc.ac.za

R. Meyer
Department of Statistics, University of Auckland, Auckland, New Zealand

B. Cai
Department of Epidemiology and Biostatistics, University of South Carolina, Columbia, SC 29208, U.S.A

N.-B. Kandala and G. Ghilagaber (eds.), *Advanced Techniques for Modelling Maternal and Child Health in Africa*, The Springer Series on Demographic Methods and Population Analysis 34, DOI 10.1007/978-94-007-6778-2_12,

Rates of teenage pregnancy have been declining across the world, albeit with differing success. For instance, in South Africa, there were 124 births per 1,000 women, aged between 15 and 19 years, in the period 1987–1989; the rate was 81 and 54 by 1998 and 2003, respectively (Department of Health 2002, 2007). Even though this shows a substantial decline, the rates are high compared to the developed countries where there are only 24 births per 1,000 women in the same age group. In particular, rates of teenage pregnancy in South Africa are more than twice those of the United Kingdom, which itself has the highest rates in Western Europe (Jewkes et al. 2009). The declining rates in South Africa may be explained by the country having high use of modern methods of contraception and legalized termination of pregnancy up to 20 weeks. However, lack of information about the abortion services and inadequate access create uncertainty of termination rates (Jewkes et al. 2009). Thus, teenage pregnancy rates might be higher than estimated. A distinct feature of South Africa compared to most sub-Saharan countries is that Black African women tend to marry late at around 28 years, if at all (Kalule-Sabiti et al. 2007). Thus, a high proportion of teenage pregnancies are pre-marital leading to high pre-marital teenage fertility rate. In this scenario, timing of first birth may be a more important predictor of fertility in South Africa. In other sub-Saharan Africa countries, early age at marriage in the absence of contraceptives has been shown to be associated with high rates of fertility (Manda and Meyer 2005).

Despite the high risks associated with pregnancy in adolescence in the sub-Saharan region, there is a scarcity of research studies in this area. The sociocultural and economic determinants favouring early pregnancy are analysed so that suitable preventive measures can be taken up. There are many sociocultural and economic factors that have consistently been found to be associated with early pregnancy in the developing countries (U.S. Bureau of the Census 1996; Singh 1998; Maitra 2004; Uwaezuoke et al. 2004; Manda and Meyer 2005). Through its influence on poverty and modernisation, the level of education is the overwhelming determinant of adolescent pregnancy (Were 2007). However, its relationship with early childbearing is compromised by prevailing sociocultural and economic factors that may favour early marriage and pregnancy (Sharma et al. 2003; Were 2007). In many instances, after dropping out of school, young girls grow up in residential areas where poverty is entrenched. In these conditions, they have poor access to healthcare services, experience gender power imbalances, low socio-economic status and poor life opportunities to further education or to establish livelihoods. The overall consequences are that young women struggle to meet immediate material needs and have very few opportunities to negotiate safe sex, thus increasing the risk of pregnancy (Jewkes et al. 2009; Human Sciences Research Council [HSRC] 2009). In societies where there is a great stigma attached to adolescent sexuality, there are few opportunities for open communication about sex with parents and partners. These barriers constrain young girls from accessing maternal health services, resulting in gaps in knowledge on how to access contraception.

The foundations of the paper are methodologically and empirically driven to investigate socio-economical and geographical determinants that are independently predictive of early pregnancy in South Africa. In particular, the paper investigates a number of substantive themes including quantifying provincial, racial, urban–rural, birth cohort, poverty and educational differential effects on teenage pregnancy rates. The available data on time to first child birth was obtained using stratified sampling.

A standard analysis for survival data collected over many strata is fitting a stratified proportional hazards model. This, however, fails to borrow strength by implicitly assuming that the strata are completely unrelated. An unstratified analysis, on the other hand, is risky when the strata have different underlying baseline hazards. Thus, a better approach models each stratum-specific baseline hazard function as an overall hazard function multiplied by a frailty, where a collection of strata units are regarded as frailties. The frailties are defined as independent and identically distributed random variables. This frailty model is regarded as a compromise between fully stratified and unstratified analyses. However, attempting to describe the variability of a whole function by a single random variable will obviously be insufficient in most situations. Therefore, in this paper we use a modelling approach where instead of including frailties we consider treating the entire stratum-specific baseline hazard function as a random effect using a Bayesian nonparametric approach. Each stratum-specific baseline hazard function is thus treated as a random draw from a population of hazard functions and the data will provide information about the variability of the hazard functions between units. If the baseline hazard functions are highly variable between strata, the analysis moves towards a stratified analysis whereas if they are similar to each other, it moves towards an unstratified analysis. In general, it will provide results that can be regarded as a compromise between the two extreme situations. We employ simultaneous estimation of the unknown baseline hazard functions using a nonparametric approach based on mixtures of triangular distributions and the covariate effects using a parametric approach based on the Cox proportional hazard regression model. The estimation procedure is Bayesian in formulation using a Markov chain Monte Carlo algorithm for posterior computation. The results are compared to those of fitting a fully parametric Weibull proportional hazards model.

The rest of the paper is organized as follows. Section 12.2 briefly describes the study data, with some preliminary results. In Sect. 12.3, we present the parametric Weibull and the semiparametric Cox proportional hazards model based on mixtures of triangular distributions together with issues of posterior computation. The models are fitted to the example data and results presented in Sect. 12.4. Section 12.5 concludes with a discussion of the models and results.

12.2 The Study Data

The data available for this study were collected from 7,041 women aged 15–49 years who were interviewed in the 2003 South Africa Demographic and Health Survey (2003 SADHS) (Department of Health 2007). The 2003 SADHS selected a nationally representative probability sample of nearly 10,000 households using a two-stage stratified cluster sampling technique. The country was primarily stratified into the nine provinces, and each province was further stratified into urban and rural areas. The first stage selected a proportional sample of 630 primary sampling units (enumerate areas (EA)) and the second stage sampled a total of just over 10,000 households from each selected EA with systematic sampling. All women aged between 15 and 49 years in the selected households were eligible for the interviews, resulting in just over 7,000 interviews. In order to obtain sufficient numbers from the minority Indian population, there was an oversample of EAs with a large Indian ethnicity. This resulted in differing sample proportions; thus, the sample is not self-weighting at the national level and appropriate weighting needs to be considered when deriving national indicators. We do not pursue these issues in this paper. For purposes of this study, we restrict the analyses to those 5,591 women aged 20 or more years as these women were exposed to teenage pregnancy for the full teenage period, below 20 years.

We consider a number of explanatory variables for inclusion in the analyses: *province of residence*, whose boundaries largely define social and cultural norms, is used to investigate sociocultural differentials; *urban or rural residence* captures effects of urbanisation and modernisation; *birth cohort* is used to capture effects of time period on early childbearing; education level of woman is used to capture effects of social status and modernisation of women. The inclusion of woman's education in the hazard regression equation for age at first child birth may result in the endogeneity of education. A teenage woman may leave school after getting pregnant, resulting in reverse causality. In order to minimise the possibility of endogeneity of education, we follow Manda and Meyer (2005) by including categories of no and little education. The reasoning is that not many young women in the first few years of schooling would be forced to leave school due to being mothers. However, formally, a two-stage modelling process could be used, with the first stage being a regression model on education using covariates such as women birth cohort, province of residence and rural–urban residence. Then its predicted value could be used as an explanatory variable in a model for age at first child birth, an approach adopted by Maitra (2004) but not here.

Some of the above explanatory variables act as proxies for socio-demographic status and traditional beliefs, which may influence family planning decisions and female independence. Inclusion of province and ethnicity may capture differentials in general levels of education, beliefs and sanctions against premarital childbirth, culturally approved motherhood ages and religious beliefs that would have the effect of increasing or decreasing the timing of childbearing (Gupta and Mahy 2003; Maitra 2004).

It is conventionally accepted that income and expenditure measurements adequately describe poverty at a household level. However, in many developing countries, especially in rural areas, measuring income may be problematic since many people work in agriculture and informal sectors. Even though, Demographic and Health Surveys do not collect adequate data on household income and expenditure, they nonetheless provide information on household assets. This has prompted many researchers to use the information on household assets to calculate a composite measurement of household-level poverty (Booysen 2001). In particular, a DHS data set provides a wealth index, which indirectly measures long-term economic status of

Table 12.1 Distributions of characteristics for women aged 20–49 years, SADHS 2003

Characteristic	Frequency	Percent
1979–1983	1,227	21.95
1974–1978	1,019	18.23
1969–1973	901	16.12
1964–1968	972	17.39
1969–1963	782	13.99
1954–1958	690	12.24
Place of residence		
Urban	3,348	59.88
Rural	2,946	40.12
Province of residence		
Western Cape	596	10.48
Eastern Cape	382	6.83
Northern Cape	610	10.91
Free State	624	11.16
Kwazulu-Natal	995	17.80
North West	613	10.96
Gauteng	615	11.00
Mpumalanga	613	10.96
Limpopo	553	9.89
Ethnicity of woman		
Black African	4,097	73.33
Coloured	749	13.41
White	237	4.29
Asian/Indian	504	9.02
Total	5,591	100.00
Education level of woman		
No education	331	5.92
Grade 1–7	1,103	19.73
Grade 8–11	2,200	39.36
Grade 12	1,396	39.36
Higher	560	10.02
Wealth index quintile		
I (Least wealth)	1,026	18.37
II	1,159	20.75
III	1,159	20.75
IV	1,052	18.84
V (Most wealth)	1,189	21.29

a household. It is the first principal component from a principal component analysis (PCA) on the measured household assets (Rutstein and Johnson 2004).

The distributions of the explanatory variables are shown in Table 12.1. We also used the Kaplan-Meier product limit method to calculate fractions of women that were mothers at each teenage age across the different 5-year birth-cohorts (Fig. 12.1). There appears to be an overall increase in age at motherhood as the birth cohort gets younger. For instance, about 5 % of women born in 1978 or earlier

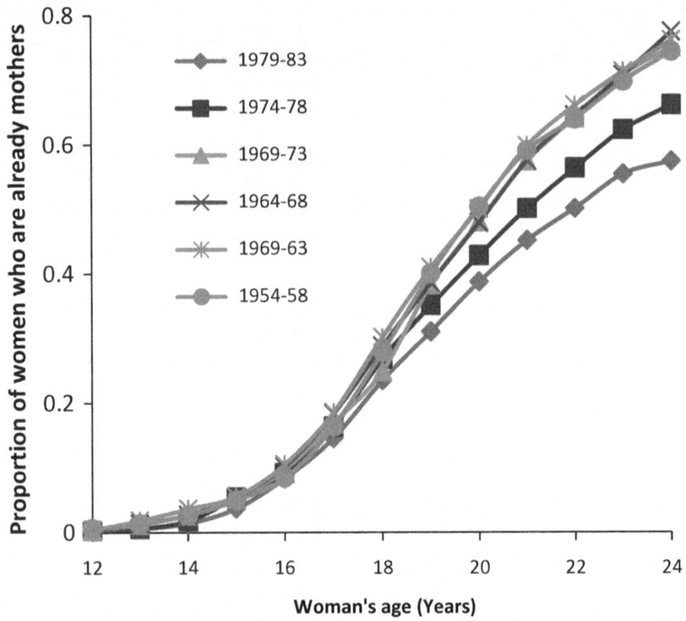

Fig. 12.1 Fraction of birth cohorts that are mothers by various teenage ages

would have been mothers by age 15 years as opposed to only 3 % of women born between 1978 and 1983. By 20 years, nearly half of the women born in 1973 or earlier would have had a child, but only 40 % and 43 % of the women born in 1979–1983 and 1974–1978 birth cohorts, respectively would have had a child, . There have been concerns that women respondent in the 2003 SADHS underreported their birth histories, which may have impacted negatively on the estimated national fertility declines and teenage motherhood rates (Department of Health 2007). However, the data are of reasonable quality such that under-reporting and mis-reporting errors would not have a major impact on the results arising from this study.

12.3 Statistical Methods

To set notation, let n_l denote the number of women in the lth stratum, $l = 1, \ldots, n$, t_{lj} denote the age (or censoring time) of the jth woman in stratum l, $j = 1, \ldots, n_i$ and let δ_{lj} be a censoring indicator variable (1 if first child born, 0 if not). In a proportional hazards model, the hazard function in stratum l for a woman with explanatory variables vector z_{lj} is given by

$$h(t;\, z_{lj}) = h_{0l}(t)\, \exp(\beta z_{lj}) = h_{0l}(t)\, \exp(\beta_1 z_{lj1} + \ldots\, \beta_p z_{ljp}), \qquad (12.1)$$

where $h_{0l}(t)$ denotes the baseline hazard in stratum l.

In our first model, we use a parametric assumption for the baseline hazards in each stratum and assume that these follow the Weibull distribution with stratum-specific hazard function

$$h_{0l}(t) = \rho_l t^{\rho_l - 1} \exp(\beta_{0l}\rho_l), \tag{12.2}$$

where β_{0l} is a stratum-specific time-scale accelerator, and the parameters ρ_l are stratum-specific shape parameters. If ρ_l is positive or negative, we obtain an increasing or decreasing baseline hazard function, respectively. The ρ_l are given a Gamma (α, α^{-1}) prior distribution, where a Gamma (a, b) distribution has mean ab and variance ab^2. Thus, the prior specification for ρ_l reflects a prior expectation of a constant baseline hazard as the prior mean of ρ_l is 1; its prior variance of $1/\alpha$ implies that smaller values of α correspond to a wide distribution around 1. The stratum-specific time-scale accelerator β_{0l} is given a Normal prior, i.e. $\beta_{0l} \sim N(\mu_0, \sigma_0^2)$. The hierarchical model specification is completed by adding a flat normal prior on parameter μ_0 and Gamma (c_1, d_1) and Gamma (c_2, d_2) priors on $\tau_0 = 1/\sigma_0^2$ and α, respectively. Furthermore, flat normal priors are used for the regression parameters $\beta_1, \ldots, \beta_p$. This parametric model can be implemented using the Bayesian software package WinBUGS (Spiegelhalter et al. 2004) that implements the Gibbs sampler for sampling from the joint posterior distribution of all model parameters.

By making rigid parametric assumptions, parametric models like the Weibull model for the stratum-specific baseline hazards have restricted flexibility compared to nonparametric approaches that allow a fully data-driven specification of the functional form of the baseline hazard. The main advantages of nonparametric models are that they have the potential to detect local trends; they can provide additional information and thus prevent model misspecification. And they can, of course, verify the validity of simpler parametric models as well.

In our second model, we follow the nonparametric approach by Carlin and Hodges (1999), which models a suitable transformation of the integrated baseline hazard $H_{0l}(t) = \int_0^t h_{0l}(s)\,ds$ as a mixture of beta distributions. We first note that modeling the integrated baseline hazard function $H_{0l}(t)$ is equivalent to modeling a stratum-specific cumulative distribution function (cdf) F_{0l}. This is because any integrated hazard $H(t)$ is a nondecreasing function on the positive real line; thus, there exists a cdf F on [0,1] such that $H(t) = J^{-1}(F(J(t)))$ where $J(t) = \frac{at}{at+b}$ for some $a, b > 0$. But instead of using a mixture of beta distributions as in Carlin and Hodges (1999), we use a mixture of triangular distributions that allows a closer approximation (Perron and Mengersen 2001; Cai and Meyer 2011).

Let $J_{0l} : \mathcal{R}^+ \to [0, 1]$ with $J_{0l}(t) = J(H_{0l}(t)) = \frac{aH_{0l}(t)}{aH_{0l}(t)+b}$ where a and b are global pre-specified positive constants. Each J_{0l} can be represented by a cdf F_l on [0, 1], i.e. $J(H_{0l}(t))$ and these are modelled as a mixture of triangular cumulative distributions with stratum-specific knots $x_l = (x_{0l}, x_{1l}, \ldots, x_{kl})$ as follows:

$$J_{0l}(t) = \sum_{i=-1}^{k-1} w_{il} IT(J(t); x_{i,l}, x_{i+1,l}, x_{i+2,l})\ for\ l = 1, \ldots, n, \tag{12.3}$$

where $IT(t, x_i, x_{i+1}, x_{i+2})$ denotes the cumulative distribution function of the triangular distribution based on the knots x_i, x_{i+1}, x_{i+2} with mode at x_{i+1} and the weights $w_{0l} = w_{1l} = \ldots = w_{k-1,l} = \frac{1}{k}$ and $w_{-1,l} = w_{k-1,l} = \frac{1}{2k}$ are fixed. A candidate integrated baseline hazard function $\tilde{H}_0$, such as $\tilde{H}_0(t) = t$ of the exponential distribution, is chosen at which we nonparametrically center each of the stratum-specific baseline hazards via the transformation J_{0l}.

Denoting the collection of knot vectors by $\mathbf{x} = (\mathbf{x_1}, \ldots, \mathbf{x_n})$ the likelihood is given by

$$L(\beta|x, y, z, \delta) = \prod_{l=1}^{n}\prod_{j=1}^{n_l} \{h_{0l}(t_{lj}) \exp(\beta z_{lj})\}^{\delta_{lj}} \times \exp\left[-H_{0l}(t_{lj}) \exp(\beta z_{lj})\right]$$

To evaluate the likelihood function, we need expressions for $H_{0l}(t)$ in terms of $J_{0l}(t)$ and thereby $\mathbf{x}$ or $\mathbf{w}$, respectively. The former is

$$\begin{aligned} H_{0l}(t) &= \frac{b J_{0l}(t)}{a\left[1 - J_{0l}(t)\right]} \\ &= \frac{b \sum_{i=-r}^{k-1} w_{il} b_i^{(r)}\left(J(t); x_{il}, \ldots, x_{i+r+1,l}\right)}{b\left[1 - \sum_{i=-r}^{k-1} w_{il} b_i^{(r)}\left(J(t); x_{i+r+1,l}\right)\right]} \end{aligned}$$

while the latter is obtained by differentiating the integrated hazard above and using the quotient and chain rules. The joint posterior density (up to normalization constant) is then obtained by multiplying the likelihood by the prior density of the parameters. We choose a Dirichlet prior for the knot spacings, i.e. $(x_{1l} - x_{0l}, \ldots, x_{k-1,l}) \sim$ Dirichlet $(\phi_0, \ldots, \phi_{k-1})$ with hyperparameter $(\phi = \phi_0 = \ldots = \phi_{k-1})$. The hierarchical models are completed by a prior distribution for the hyperparameters $\phi \sim$ Gamma(a, b) with $a = 0.5$ and $b = 2$. We used $k = 10$ knots and set the global transformation constants to be $a_0 = 1$ and $b_0 = 20$ to cover the largest range of [0,1]. We ran multiple MCMC chains from highly dispersed starting values for 30,000 iterations after discarding a burn-in of 10,000. We performed the Gelman and Rubin (1992) convergence diagnosis, and it confirmed adequate convergence by iteration 1,000. We also conducted the sensitivity analysis for the triangular mixture model with different choices of hyperparameters, which provide a robust result. We also calculated the deviance information criterion (DIC) (Spiegelhalter et al. 2002) for the model based on triangular mixtures. The DIC is 29220.22. The posterior mean and the 95 % credible interval for ϕ is 0.5 (0.411, 0.603). The proposed semiparametric model can be conceptually implemented by using either WinBUGS or R. However, due to the large sample size, we experienced an intensive computation. Instead, a C program was written for implementing the approach.

12.4 Results

We fitted the stratified proportional hazards model to the age at first birth dataset using both the Weibull and the triangular mixture distributions for stratum-specific baseline hazards. The stratum-specific time-scale accelerator hyper-parameter μ_0 and fixed-effect parameters $\beta_1, \ldots, \beta_p$ were assigned exchangeable flat normal priors with mean zero and variance 1,000. The hyperparameter $\tau_0 = \sigma_0^{-2}$ of the stratum-specific time-scale accelerator was assigned a Gamma (3, 0.5) prior and, as in Carlin and Hodges (1999), we used a low-information Gamma (3,10) prior for α. Three multiple chains were run from different starting values for 10,000 iterations after discarding the first 1,000 as being in the *burn-in* period. Trace plots and Gelman-Rubin convergence diagnostic statistic (Brooks and Gelman 1998) all confirmed adequate convergence.

Plots of the stratum baseline hazards using the Weibull and triangular mixtures models are shown in Figs. 12.2 and 12.3, respectively. Both plots show substantive provincial variations in baseline risk on the timing of first child birth. The stratum-specific baseline risks from fitting the parametric Weibull model are shown in Fig. 12.2. Both urban and rural areas of the Eastern Cape, North West, Mpumalanga and Limpopo provinces show early motherhood rates; likewise for Gauteng province. Higher rates of delayed motherhood are seen in Northern Cape and Free State. Kwazulu-Natal is seen as having low rates of teenage child birth, but this should be treated with great caution as the reproductive health data from this province was found to be inconsistent (Department of Health 2007). The problem with the Weibull model is the per se increasing hazard rate, which is not realistic

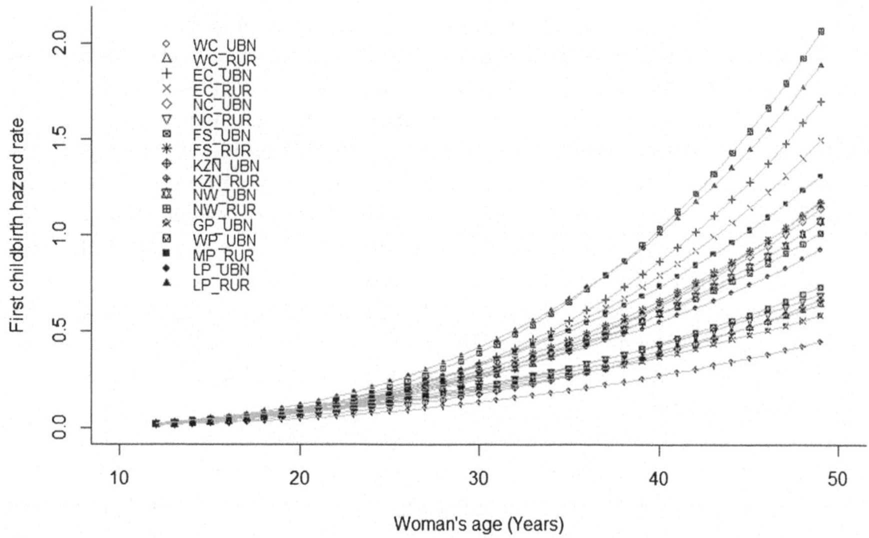

Fig. 12.2 Stratum-specific timing of first child baseline hazards using the Weibull model

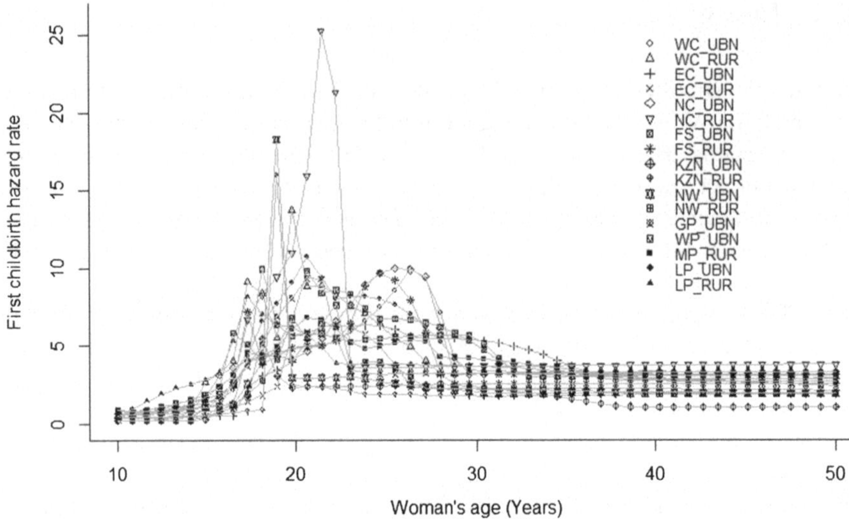

Fig. 12.3 Stratum-specific timing of first child baseline hazards using the triangular mixture model

in the context of South Africa and the Sub-Saharan African region (Kalule-Sabiti et al. 2007; HSRC 2009). The differences in baseline hazards between provinces only show which ones increase more quickly.

The restrictions inherent in Weibull models are removed when we use mixtures of triangular distributions, where we can detect peaks, periods of increase and decrease or even multi-modal function of hazards. From Fig. 12.3, the baseline risk of timing of first child birth shows general bi-modal peak hazards around 20 and 30 years of age. In particular, rural areas of the Northern Cape and Free State have baseline risk with a bi-modal distribution. It also shows that early adolescent child birth is highest in the North West province and in the urban parts of the Gauteng province.

Table 12.2 presents posterior medians and 95 % credible intervals of fixed effect hazard ratios using the Weibull parametric and triangular mixture distribution models. Also, shown are results from an unstratified analysis, where stratum factor was included as a fixed effect and results from an analysis where the strata were treated as random effects using a frailty model. A frailty model is seen as a compromise between a fully stratified and unstratified Cox regression model. We assumed that the stratum-specific random effects follow an exchangeable normal distribution with mean zero and a precision parameter drawn from a Gamma (0.01, 100) distribution.

The fixed effects results from both the frailty and Weibull models confirm the findings of the unstratified model. The triangular mixture approach is consistent with the other three models, but there are a few exceptions. The more realistic triangular mixture model has significantly higher hazard ratios for older birth cohorts 1954–1958 and 1959–1963 than the 1979–1983 cohort, not smaller as the other models seem to suggest. The Triangular mixture model even shows a more consistent and

Table 12.2 Median (95 % CI) hazards ratios estimates of fixed effects parameters

Parameter	Unstratified model	Frailty model	Weibull model	Triangular mixture model
Birth cohort				
1979–1983	1 (–, –)	1 (–, –)	1 (–, –)	1 (–, –)
1974–1978	1.12 (1.01, 1.25)	1.11 (1.00, 1.25)	1.11 (0.99, 1.23)	1.25 (1.12, 1.38)
1969–1973	1.17 (1.06, 1.31)	1.16 (1.05, 1.30)	1.16 (1.04, 1.29)	1.45 (1.30, 1.60)
1964–1968	1.18 (1.06, 1.32)	1.17 (1.04, 1.30)	1.16 (1.05, 1.30)	1.55 (1.40, 1.71)
1959–1963	0.93 (0.82, 1.04)	0.91 (0.81, 1.03)	0.93 (0.83, 1.04)	1.46 (1.31, 1.62)
1954–1958	0.83 (0.74, 0.94)	0.82 (0.73, 0.93)	0.84 (0.74, 0.94)	1.39 (1.24, 1.56)
Education				
None	1 (–, –)	1 (–, –)	1 (–, –)	1 (–, –)
Grade 1–7	1.14 (0.98, 1.31)	1.12 (0.99, 1.31)	1.15 (1.01, 1.31)	1.08 (0.96, 1.24)
Grade 8–11	1.19 (1.04, 1.37)	1.17 (1.04, 1.37)	1.20 (1.06, 1.37)	1.07 (0.95, 1.22)
Grade 12	0.97 (0.75, 1.01)	0.86 (90.75, 1.02)	0.87 (0.76, 1.01)	0.78 (0.68, 0.91)
Higher	0.69 (0.59, 0.83)	0.70 (0.57, 0.84)	0.69 (0.59, 0.82)	0.63 (0.53, 0.74)
Ethnicity				
Black/African	1 (–, –)	1 (–, –)	1 (–, –)	1 (–, –)
Coloured	0.97 (0.85, 1.09)	0.96 (0.86, −1.09)	0.96 (0.85, 0.1.09)	0.94 (0.87, 1.04)
White	0.75 (0.62, 0.89)	0.75 (0.63, 0.89)	0.74 (0.62, 0.89)	0.84 (0.71, 0.99)
Indian/Asian	1.14 (0.98, 1.32)	1.13 (0.97, 1.30)	1.15 (0.99, 1.35)	1.19 (1.05, 1.35)
Wealth				
I	1 (–, –)	1 (–, –)	1 (–, –)	1 (–, –)
II	1.00 (0.91, 1.11)	1.01 (0.91, 1.11)	1.01 (0.91, 1.11)	1.01 (0.92, 1.11)
III	0.95 (0.85, 1.05)	0.95 (0.85, 1.05)	0.94 (0.86, 1.06)	0.93 (0.85, 1.03)
IV	1.03 (0.93, 1.16)	1.03 (0.92, 1.15)	1.05 (0.94, 1.17)	0.94 (0.84, 1.04)
V	0.89 (0.78, 1.02)	0.89 (0.78, 1.02)	0.91 (0.80, 1.04)	0.85 (0.85, 0.96)

significant reduction in the hazard ratio for women with higher education than the other models. The same picture emerges with women in the higher wealth groups. Thus, using the results from the mixture model, rates of early childbearing are higher among older birth cohorts, low educated women, Black/African or Indian/Asian women and women with low economic status.

12.5 Discussion and Conclusion

This paper introduces novel Bayesian nonparametric approaches to model baseline hazards in a stratified proportional hazards regression model using data on timing of first birth in South Africa. The computations of the model parameters are embedded within a Bayesian hierarchical model framework. This is an important application as teenage pregnancies are associated with adverse health and socioeconomical consequences, particularly in the developing countries. Thus, this paper adds valuable insights into the social and public health knowledge base on maternal health. We have modelled the influence of a number of important explanatory variables. Important features of our modelling and estimation approaches are the avoidance of parametric assumptions for the stratum-specific hazard functions and flexible modelling using a nonparametric mixture of triangular distributions. This innovative feature relaxes the typical parametric assumptions for the baseline hazard yielding a more realistic analysis. The commonly used Weibull model, for instance, has per se either increasing or decreasing hazard rates, whereas a mixture of triangular distributions has the ability to detect peaks, periods of increase and decrease and multi-modality in the baseline hazards.

The results show that teenage pregnancy was significantly associated with low education, rural residence and being of Black African, Indian/Asian, or Coloured ethnicity. Teenage pregnancy also depended on birth cohorts where rates were higher among the women born between the 1960s and 1970s than among women born in the 1980s. The rates also varied according to the province of residence, with higher rates in Eastern Cape, North West, Mpumalanga, Limpopo and Gauteng provinces. These findings point to an association between socio-cultural and economic determinants and pregnancy in adolescence, which is consistent with results obtained in previous studies (Singh 1998; Sharma et al. 2003; Gupta and Mahy 2003). These findings should be treated with caution as there have been grave concerns about the accuracy of reproductive history data (Department of Health 2007). The observed differentials in education operate through other elements of socioeconomic development that are associated with education. Educated women are an urbanised and modernized subgroup with better socio-economic status conducive towards delayed childbearing (Maitra 2004). Moreover, they are more likely to use modern contraceptives in order to develop careers (US Bureau of the Census 1996). Although improvements have been achieved, levels of women's education in the rural areas of the sub-Sahara region remain low (Kirk and Pillet 1998). Thus, the status of education among rural women in the region indicates that the environment is not conducive to any significant increase in age at first child birth.

The government of South Africa has acknowledged the importance of improving maternal health and has put in place policies that focus on empowering teenagers to prevent pregnancy. In this respect contraception is freely and widely available from clinics, which are easily accessible (Jewkes et al. 2009). It can be argued that the declines in rates of teenage pregnancy are more attributable to increasing use of contraception by teenagers. However, quantifying the net gains in teenage pregnancies is complicated as there are legal provisions for termination of pregnancy up to 20 weeks gestation. This policy is so liberal that teenagers do not need parental consent to terminate a pregnancy. A proper empirical study is needed to examine important factors contributing to reduction of rates of early pregnancy. As a complement to helping young women to avoid conception, the government has put in place policies devised to mitigate the adverse consequences for the young mother and baby. These policies have made it possible for girls to remain in school until the end of their pregnancy and return at an appropriate stage after the birth. This has had some success but many African girls still have their education interrupted by pregnancy. As most teenage pregnancies happen to the more economically deprived teenagers, the government has also introduced policies to prevent extreme child poverty. A monthly child support grant is disbursed to the primary care giver of a child up to 14 years of age. Even though this is well intended, a greater number of beneficiaries are, for various reasons, not able to access it (Jewkes et al. 2009).

In conclusion, South Africa has made positive steps in improving maternal health among teenagers and in combating the adverse effects of early childbearing on both the mother and child. It is apparent that through its influence on poverty and modernisation, the level of education is the overwhelming direct and indirect determinant of adolescent pregnancy. Women with higher education levels possess better socio-economic status that is conducive to delayed childbearing in that they are more likely to use contraceptives in order to develop careers (US Bureau of the Census 1996; Maitra 2004). Although improvements have been achieved, levels of African/Black women's education in the country are comparatively low (Kirk and Pillet 1998). The government has acknowledged the importance of improving women's education as a way of curbing the negative social and economic consequences of teenage pregnancy. Programs that strengthen education, employment and family planning have been embarked on. An improvement in accessibility to information on reproductive health services for young people will enhance maternal health among adolescents. However, there is a need for better understanding of factors, including cultural practices, contributing to unusually high incidence of teenage pregnancies in South Africa to enable formulation of most effective programmes for prevention of teenage pregnancy. The programmes should comprehensively empower teenagers with relevant information and skills to negotiate safe sex and motherhood. However, any such programs need strong and sustained commitment by the government, a task made even harder by the adverse economic conditions and resources (Caldwell and Caldwell 2002).

References

Acsadi, G. T. F., & Johnson-Acsadi, G. (1990). *Effects of timing of marriage on reproductive health*. A World Bank Symposium, Washington, DC.

Booysen, F. (2001). The Measurement of poverty. In D. Bradshaw & K. Steyn (Eds.), *Poverty and chronic disease in South Africa, Technical Report* (pp. 15–38). Cape Town: Medical Research Council.

Borja, J. B., & Adair, L. S. (2003). Assessing the net effect of young maternal age on birthweight. *American Journal of Human Biology, 15*, 735–740.

Brooks, S. P., & Gelman, A. (1998). Alternative methods for monitoring convergence of iterative simulations. *Journal of Computational and Graphical Statistics, 7*, 434–455.

Cai, B., & Meyer, R. (2011). Bayesian semiparametric modeling of survival data based on mixtures of B-spline distributions. *Computational Statistics and Data Analysis, 55*, 1260–1272.

Caldwell, J., Caldwell, P. (2002). *The fertility transition in sub-Saharan Africa*. A paper presented at the conference: Fertility and the Current South African Issues of Poverty, HIV/AIDS and Youth, Pretoria.

Carlin, B. P., & Hodges, J. S. (1999). Hierarchical proportional hazards regression models for highly stratified data. *Biometrics, 55*, 1162–1170.

Department of Health, Medical Research Council, Measure DHS+. (2002). *South Africa demographic and health survey 1998*. Pretoria: Department of Health.

Department of Health, Medical Research Council, OrcMacro. (2007). *South African demographic and health survey 2003*. Pretoria: Department of Health.

Gelman, A., & Rubin, D. B. (1992). Inference from iterative simulation using multiple sequences. *Statistical Science, 7*, 457–472.

Gupta, N., & Mahy, M. (2003). Adolescent childbearing in sub-Saharan Africa: Can increased schooling alone raise ages at first birth? *Demographic Research, 8*, 93–106.

Human Sciences Research Council. (2009). *Teenage pregancy in South Africa-with specific focus on school-going children. Full Report*. Pretoria: Human Sciences Research Council.

Jewkes, R., Morrell, R., & Christofides, N. (2009). Empowering teenages to prevent pregnancy: Lessons from South Africa. *Culture, Health and Sexuality, 11*, 675–688.

Kalule-Sabiti, I., Palamuleni, M., Makiwane, M., & Amoateng, A. Y. (2007). Family formation and dissolution patterns. In A. Y. Amoateng & T. B. Heaton (Eds.), *Families and households in post-apartheid South Africa: Socio-demographic perspectives* (pp. 89–112). Cape Town: HSRC Press.

Kirk, D., & Pillet, B. (1998). Fertility levels, trends and differentials in sub-Saharan African in the 1980s and the 1990s. *Studies in Family Planning, 29*, 1–22.

Magadi, M. (2004). *Poor pregnancy outcomes among adolescents in South Nyansa Region of Kenya* (Working Paper: A04/04). Southampton: Statistical Sciences Research Institute, University of Southampton.

Maitra, P. (2004). Effect of socioeconomic characteristics on age at marriage and total fertility in Nepal. *Journal of Health, Population, and Nutrition, 22*, 84–96.

Manda, S. O. M., & Meyer, R. (2005). Age at first marriage in Malawi: A Bayesian multilevel analysis using a discrete time-to-event model. *Journal of the Royal Statistical Society A, 168*, 439–455.

Perron, F., & Mengersen, K. (2001). Bayesian nonparametric modelling using mixtures of triangular distributions. *Biometrics, 57*, 518–528.

Rutstein, S. O., & Johnson, K. (2004). *The DHS wealth index* (DHS Comparative Reports No. 6). Calverton: ORC Macro.

Sharma, A. K., Verma, K., Khatri, S., & Kanan, A. T. (2003). Determinants of pregnancy in adolescents in Nepal. *Indian Journal of Pediatrics, 69*, 19–22.

Singh, S. (1998). Adolescent childbearing in developing countries: A global review. *Studies in Family Planning, 29*, 117–136.

Siu-Man, N. G., & Boachang, G. U. (1995, April 6–8). *Dimensions of fertilitytransition in the Third World: Level, timing and equality*. Paper presented at the 1995 Population Association of America Annual Meeting, San Francisco.

Spiegelhalter, D. J., Best, N. G., Carlin, B. P., & Linde, A. V. D. (2002). Bayesian measures of model complexity and fit. *Journal of Royal Statistical Society B, 64*, 1–34.

Spiegelhalter, D. J., Thomas, A., Best, N. G., & Lunn, D. (2004). *BUGS: Bayesian inference Using Gibbs Sampling, version 1.4.1*. Medical Research Council Biostatistics Unit, Cambridge University.

U.S. Bureau of the Census. (1996). *Trends in adolescent fertility and contraceptive use in the developing World* (Report IPC/95-1). Washington, DC: U.S. Government Printing Office.

United Nations. (2012). *The millennium development goals report 2012*. New York: United Nations.

Uwaezuoke, A. I. O., Uzochukwu, B. S. C., Nwagbo, D. F. E., & Onwujekwe, O. E. (2004). Determinants of teenage pregnancy in rural communities of Abia State, South East Nigeria. *Journal of College of Medicine, 9*, 28–33.

Were, M. (2007). Determinants of teenage pregnancies: The case of Busia District in Kenya. *Economics and Human Biology, 5*, 322–339.

Chapter 13
Stepwise Geoadditive Regression Modelling of Levels and Trends of Fertility in Nigeria: Guiding Tools Towards Attaining MDGs

Samson Babatunde Adebayo and Ezra Gayawan

13.1 Introduction

African countries are beginning to experience fertility transition like other parts of the world. This belated transition is, however, slow and as a result, fertility rates are still at very high levels in majority of the countries going by the standard of the rest of the world. Whereas only a few countries in the continent e.g. South Africa, Ghana, Lesotho, Namibia, and Swaziland, are now maintaining a total fertility rates (TFR) of about 4.0 births per woman or less, others, Nigeria inclusive, are still having a rate above 5.0.

Relative to other countries in the continent, the transition from high to low fertility in Nigeria appears to be one of the least and slowing. In 1981–1982, report of the National Fertility Survey (NFS) put the TFR of the country at 6.3 births per woman. This dropped to 6.0 in 1990 in the 1990 Nigeria Demographic and Health Survey (NDHS) and then slightly to 5.9 in 1991 (Population Census). The rate further reduced to 5.7 in 2003 (NPC [Nigeria] and ORC Macro 2004); a rate that is still being maintained as at 2008 NDHS (NPC [Nigeria] & ICF Macro). However, Cohen (1998) and Kirk and Pillet (1997) have observed a comparable small and slow decline in countries like Burkina Faso, Burundi, Liberia, Mali, Niger and Uganda.

In response to the pattern and trend of population growth and its adverse effects on national development, the Federal Government of Nigeria in 1988

S.B. Adebayo (✉)
Planning, Research and Statistics, National Agency for Food and Drug Administration and Control (NAFDAC), Plot 2032 Olusegun Obasanjo Way, Wuse Zone 7, PMB 5116, Abuja, Nigeria
e-mail: adebayo_sba@yahoo.com

E. Gayawan
Department of Mathematical Sciences, Redeemer's University, Redemption City, Nigeria
e-mail: gayawane@run.edu.ng

N.-B. Kandala and G. Ghilagaber (eds.), *Advanced Techniques for Modelling Maternal and Child Health in Africa*, The Springer Series on Demographic Methods and Population Analysis 34, DOI 10.1007/978-94-007-6778-2_13,

set up the National Policy on Population for Development. As other emerging issues such as HIV/AIDS, poverty, gender inequality, among others, gained wider recognition, the 1988 Policy was reviewed giving way to the National Policy on Population for Sustainable Development in 2005. The policy recognizes that population factors, environmental issues and social and economic developments are irrevocably interconnected and are critical to the achievement of sustainable development in Nigeria which in turn can lead to the country's attainment of the Millennium Development Goals (MDGs). One of the set targets as a consequence of the 2005 policy is the reduction of the TFR by at least 0.6 children every 5 years by encouraging child spacing through the use of family planning.

Studies on the major determinants of fertility in Nigeria have therefore become inevitable. Several authors (Bongaarts and Potter 1983; Foote et al. 1993; Cleland et al. 1994; Cohen 1998) have shown interest in studying the proximate determinants of fertility in the African region as these determinants are considered important developmental problems that are related to economic growth and poverty as well as maternal and child health (Shen and Willianson 1999). Using Bongaart's framework (Bongaarts 1982), Jolly and Gribble (1993) and Adlakha et al. (1991) found that fertility inhibiting effect of age at marriage is significant in African countries. Makinde-Adebusoye and Ebigbola (1992); Makinde-Adebusoye (2001) and Norville et al. (2003) identified some social-economic and socio-cultural factors to include couple's relative income, kinship and community institutions, as well as lineage and decent; and explained how they determine fertility level especially in African countries. According to Bongaarts's (1982) framework, all the important variation in fertility is captured by variation in the proximate determinants of fertility. Therefore if we have quality and enough individual-level data on contraceptive use, breastfeeding and post-partum amenorrhoea and the other proximate determinants, we should be able to capture all variation in individual-level fertility. Baschieri and Hinde (2007) also opined that changes in fertility are the direct result of changes in the proximate determinants, which thus mediate the effect of changes in social, economic and cultural factors. Looking at these determinates from modelling point of view, Kazembe (2009) asserted that modelling determinants of fertility may assist in designing effective interventions that can lead to improved child and maternal well-being as well as economic growth.

In a typical regression situation where the dependence of an outcome variable of interest is to be modelled on several independent variables, a better way to achieve a more parsimonious model is to consider screening of the variables. In this Chapter, we adopted a modelling technique that permits screening and selection of variables (i.e. the determinants of fertility) using stepwise geoadditive regression model as proposed in Belitz and Lang (2008).

Although many studies on determinates of fertility have been carried out especially in sub-Saharan African countries, see Kazembe (2009); Baschieri and Hinde (2007), not much work has been done with the Nigerian data especially considering joint estimation of trend, nonlinear effects of continuous covariates, spatial effect and possible random effect to account for unobserved heterogeneity that may be present in the data. Often, effects of continuous covariates are modelled by assuming a linear dependence of the outcome variable on the predictor. It has become evident that assumption of linear dependence is often too rigid in many realistically complex situations. Therefore, classical parametric regression models for analysing fertility data have severe problems with estimating small area effects and simultaneously adjusting for other covariates, in particular when the effects of some covariates are non-linear or time-varying. Usually a very high number of parameters will be needed for the modelling purposes, which may result in unstable estimates with high variance. Therefore, flexible geoadditive approaches are needed which allow one to incorporate small area spatial effects, non-linear or time-varying effects of covariates and usual linear effects in a joint model.

In this Chapter, we explore level and trend of total fertility in Nigeria using the total number of children ever born per woman. As highlighted by Kazembe (2009), total number of children ever born per woman measures lifetime fertility for women of reproductive age. Similarly, Becker and Lewis (1973); Famoye and Wang (1997); and Olfa and El Lahga (2002) used children ever born per woman as a better approximate measure of fertility rate. In this case, children ever born per woman results in a count variable. Therefore, we adopted a Poisson stepwise geoadditive regression approach through a Bayesian perspective for screening of the variables.

13.2 The Data

The most common set of data used to study fertility differentials in developing countries are the Demographic and Health Surveys (DHS). These are large, nationally representative sample surveys collected for many countries around the world, which provide information about fertility and family planning, including knowledge and current use of contraceptive methods, and detailed fertility histories with records of children's birth and death dates.

Several scholars have examined the quality of DHS data. Studies by, Arnold (1990), Blanc and Rutenberg (1990), Arnold and Blanc (1990) and Makinde-Adebusoye and Feyisetan (1994) have noted the limitations of the data with respect to the estimations of levels and trend in fertility. Inaccuracies result from age misreporting, under-reporting of births, inaccurate reporting of births and its consequent intentional or unintentional displacements of birth and age heaping. However, in order to avoid these problems and to ensure the data properly reflect the situations they intend to describe, the DHS programme developed standard procedures, methodologies and manuals to guide the survey process. Also, appropriate policies guiding the editing and imputation of data are put in place. The standard methodologies permit comparison of indicators across all countries where these surveys are being conducted. Hence, many researchers who have carried out demographic studies preferred DHS data.

Therefore, we used three waves of datasets from 1999, 2003 and 2008 Nigeria Demographic and Health Surveys (NDHS). This avails us opportunity to explore trend in fertility between 1999 and 2008 in Nigeria NPC ([Nigeria] (2000), NPC [Nigeria] and ORC Macro (2004), NPC [Nigeria] and ICF Macro (2009)). The 2008 survey was a significant improvement on the 1999 and 2003 surveys in scope and content. Whereas a nationally representative sample of 34,070 households were successfully interviewed in the 2008 survey, 7,647 and 7,225 households were interviewed in the 1999 and 2003 surveys respectively. Of these, the response rates for the eligible women in the households were 92 %, 95 % and 97 %, for the 1999, 2003 and 2008 surveys respectively.

The NDHS was designed to provide estimates for demographic and health indicators at the national, zonal and states levels as well as for rural and urban areas. The sampling frame used for the survey was the Population and Housing Census of the Federal Republic of Nigeria conducted in 1991 and 2006. The primary sampling unit (PSU), referred to as a cluster for the survey was defined on the basis of enumeration areas (EAs) from the census frames. The NDHS sample was selected using a stratified two-stage cluster design. Due to the hierarchical nature of which the data were collected, conventional regression approach that assumes independent observations may not be suitable. Therefore, a modelling technique that accounts for possible within cluster correlation is required. Our modelling technique permits incorporation of random effect and spatially correlated observations which may assist in explaining some unobserved heterogeneity that may be present in the data.

One of the eligibility criteria for women component of the survey is that female respondents must be in the age range 15–49 years. As mentioned earlier, the data include the total number of children per woman. Of the independent variables considered in the analyses, age at marriage is an important proximate determinate of fertility and is therefore included in this study. It is evident in developing countries that marriage affects fertility via frequent and regular exposure to sexual relations. Given the fact that fertility often takes place within marriage, there is an inverse relationship between age at first marriage and fertility (Blanc and Poukouta 1997). This is because age at first marriage determines the length of exposure to the risk of becoming pregnant and the actual commencement of the process of child bearing (Islam 2009). Previous studies have also shown that the level of women's education and fertility are inversely related. It affects the woman's knowledge and awareness of modern contraceptive methods and usage; delays entry into marriage which reduces the exposure time to risk of child bearing thus, more educated women are known to have fewer children than the less educated ones. Other studies have investigated possible association between respondent's working status and fertility level. However, this was not the case in this study. Among other covariates suspected to be related to fertility and considered in this study are: *type of place of residence* given as *urban* or *rural* (reference category), partner's education, respondent's age, marital status, time the respondent wanted the last child, respondent's and partner's desire for children, parity, use of modern contraceptive, desire for last child, age at first sex, use of a modern family planning method before birth, and geopolitical zones. Finally, the state of residence is an important factor as it captures the large-scale socio-economic difference that exits in Nigeria. In all, there are 37 states (36 states and the Federal Capital Territory, Abuja). All categorical covariates are dummy coded. We present the variables included in the analyses in Table 13.1.

Table 13.1 Description of variables included in the analysis

Variables	Description of variables
totchid	Total number of children ever given birth to (count and outcome variable)
yearstud	Year of study: 1999, 2003 and 2008 (2 dummies $time_2$ – 2003 and $time_3$ – 2008 were created; 1999 as reference)
agecont	A continuous variable of age in years
maryyr	Duration of marriage measured in years
agesex1	Age at first sexual intercourse measured in years (continuous)
agemar	Age at marriage (continuous)
wantedlc	Desire for last child
usingcon	Current use of modern Family Planning
Useb4b	Whether respondent used modern FP before birth
Educ	Educational attainment (no formal education – *ref category*)
idealchd	Ideal number of children grp (7 and above – ref category)
whendes	Respondents desire for more children (wants no more, infecund & sterilised – ref category)
husbdes	Husband's desire for children (Others – ref category)
married	Marital status (formerly or never married – ref category)
zones	Geopolitical zones (North Central – ref category)
p_educ	Partner's educational attainment (No formal education – ref category)
urban	Place of residence (rural – ref category)

13.3 Stepwise Geoadditive Regression Model for Count Outcomes

13.3.1 Bayesian Stepwise Regression

Stepwise regression technique is a model building approach that permits choice of predictive variables in a model according to a specific criterion (Hocking 1976). This can be achieved through either a forward selection or backward selection procedure by using partial correlations of the explanatory variables. Usually in many practical situations, one is faced with a large number of potential explanatory variables, and no underlying theory on which to base the model selection (as in this case study). The procedure is used primarily in regression analysis, though the basic approach is applicable in many forms of model selection. This is a variation on forward selection. At each stage in the process, after a new variable is added into the model, a test is made to check if some variables can be deleted without appreciably increasing the residual sum of squares. The procedure terminates when the measure is (locally) maximized, or when the available improvement falls below some critical value. The basic idea is to find a best model from a number of possible models. This technique has been well discussed in literature. For details about stepwise regression, see Draper and Smith (1981), Chaterjee and Price (1991), Neter et al. (1996) among others.

Variable selection for complex regression models has been an area of research that recently attracts attention. In realistically complex models, the decision as to which variables (covariates) to be included in a model, the inclusion of continuous covariates whether as linear or nonlinear, etc., is difficult to make. In some situations when the methodology exists, user-friendly methods of implementing such can as well be challenging. Also in a number of applications, one is confronted with large datasets with many potential covariates of different types and a lack of theory guiding the analysts as to the specification promising models. Moreover, the existence or non existence of complex interactions between covariates is often difficult and challenging. In their efforts to contribute to this area, Belitz and Lang (2008) proposed a *stepwise* regression approach for regression models with structure additive predictors. Within a structured additive regression procedure (Fahrmeir et al. 2004; Kneib and Fahrmeir 2006, 2007), stepwise regression simultaneously performs model selection and estimation with inferences based on penalised likelihood. Markov chain Monte Carlo (MCMC) techniques are partly used for computing interval estimates. This was first proposed by Belitz (2007) and incorporated into BayesX – software for Bayesian inference in Structured Additive Regression Models by Belitz and Lang (2008). In this case, model choice and estimation of the parameters is done simultaneously. The algorithm for Bayesian variable selection technique determines whether a particular covariate enters the model; determines whether a continuous covariate enters the model linearly or nonlinearly; determines whether a spatial effect enters the model, determines whether a unit or cluster specific heterogeneity effects enter the model, selects complex interaction effects, determine the degree of smoothness of nonlinear covariates, spatial or cluster specific heterogeneity effects.

Inference is based on penalized likelihood in combination with fast algorithms for selecting relevant covariates and model terms. Different models are compared via various goodness-of-fit criteria, e.g. Akaike's Information Criterion (AIC), Bayesian Information Criterion (BIC), Generalized Cross Validation (GCV) and 5 or 10 fold cross validation (Belitz and Lang (2008)). Stepwise regression analysis is estimated with object '*stepwisereg*' in BayesX. For more details, see the software manuals (http://www.stat.uni-muenchen.de/~bayesx/manual/tutorials_manual.pdf).

13.3.2 Bayesian Inference

Suppose that observations (y_i, x_i, s_i, v_i), $i = 1, \ldots, n$, where y_i is a Poisson response variable, a vector $x = (x_{i1}, \ldots, x_{ip})'$ of metrical covariate, $s_i = (1, \ldots, S)$ the state (district) where respondent i lived during the survey and a further vector $v = (v_{i1}, \ldots, v_{iq})'$ of categorical covariates. Usually one intends to jointly model the dependence of y_i on metrical, spatial and categorical covariates within the context of generalized additive model (Hastie and Tibshirani 1990). The predictor η_i for the Structured Additive Regression (STAR) model can be defined as

$$\eta_i = time_2 + time_3 + \sum_{j=1}^{p} f_j(x_{ij}) + \sum_{k=1}^{K} g_k(x_{ik}, x_{ik'}) + f_{spat}(s_i) + v_i' \beta \quad (13.1)$$

where $f_1, \ldots, fp$ are nonlinear (unknown) smooth functions of the metrical covariates, $g_1, \ldots, g_k$ are the interaction[1] effects of continuous variables x_{ik} and x_{ik}', f_{spat} is the nonlinear effect of spatial covariates and $\beta_i = (\beta_1, \ldots, \beta_L)'$ is a vector of fixed effect parameters for the categorical covariates, $time_2$ and $time_3$ are the second and third rounds of the NDHS data: 2003 and 2008 (i.e. year of study with 1999 as the reference category). One may further split up spatial effects f_{spat} into spatially correlated (structured) and uncorrelated (unstructured) effects as

$$f_{spat}(s_i) = f_{str}(s_i) + f_{unstr}(s_i).$$

A rationale behind this is that a spatial effect is a surrogate of many unobserved influential factors, some of which may be a strong spatial structure and others may only be present locally.

Within a Bayesian context, all parameters and functions are usually considered as random variables upon which appropriate priors are assumed. Independent diffuse priors are assumed on the parameters of fixed effects. For the non-linear effects, a Bayesian P-splines prior based on Lang and Brezger (2004); and Brezger and Lang (2006) was assumed. Omitting indices, each function f is represented or approximated through a linear combination

$$p(z) = \sum_{j=1}^{J} \beta_j B_j(z)$$

of B-spline basis functions. Smoothness of function f is achieved by penalizing differences of coefficients of adjacent B-splines (Eilers and Marx 1996) or, in our Bayesian approach, by assuming first or second order Gaussian random walk smoothness priors

$$\beta_1 = \beta_{j-1} + u_1 \qquad \beta_1 = 2\beta_{j-1} - \beta_{j-2} + u_1,$$

with *i.i.d.* errors $u_l \sim N(0, \tau^2)$. The variance τ^2 controls the smoothness of f. Assigning a weakly informative inverse Gamma prior $\tau^2 \sim IG(\varepsilon, \varepsilon)$, ε small, it is estimated jointly with the basis function coefficients.

[1]This can also be a varying coefficient effect.

For the geographical effects $f_{spat}(s)$, $s = 1, \ldots, S$, we assume a Gaussian Markov random field prior. Basically, this is an extension of first order random walk priors to two-dimensional spatial arrays, see Rue and Held (2005) for general information.

For the structured spatial effects $f_{str}(s)$ we chose a Gaussian Markov random field prior (13.2) which is common in spatial statistics, see Besag et al. (1991). Unstructured spatial effects are *i.i.d.* random effects.

$$(f_{str}(s)|f_{str}(t); t \neq s, \tau^2) \sim N\left(\sum_{t \in \partial_s} f_{str}(t)/N_s, \tau^2/N_s\right) \tag{13.2}$$

In order to be able to estimate the smoothing parameters for non-linear and spatial effects simultaneously, highly dispersed but proper hyper-priors are assigned to them. Hence for all variance components, an inverse gamma distribution with hyperparameters a and b is chosen, e.g. τ^2 IG(a,b). Standard choices of hyperparameters are $a = 1$ and $b = 0.005$ or $a = b = 0.001$.

Basis of inference in this study is a penalized least squares with pointwise confidence intervals for non-linear effects. The variable selection procedure aims at minimising a goodness-of-fit criterion.

13.4 Bayesian Stepwise Regression Analysis of Fertility Data

Modelling count data has received considerable attention in the recent time, see Cameron and Trivedi (1998), Chib et al. (1998), Winkelmann (2000), Chib and Winkelmann (2001), and Fahrmeir and Osuna (2006), also Kazembe (2009) for modelling fertility which is more related to this work. In our application in this study, fertility is known to depend on a number of factors such as age at marriage, age at first sex, respondent's and partner's educational attainment, desire and preference for children, and district (state) of residence. The decision as to which of these covariates should be included in an attempt to model the dependence of total number of children ever given birth to per woman, how the continuous covariates should enter the model (whether linear or nonlinear) and possible interactions of the covariates is often too difficult to make a priori.

In this case study, we adopted a structured additive regression predictor for count data as proposed by Fahrmeir and Osuna (2006). The approach provides flexible modelling that can deal with most problems inherent in traditional Poisson regression such as overdispersion, zero inflated outcomes, estimation of temporal or spatial correlation, and possibly nonlinear effects of metrical covariates available in that data. The models are fully Bayesian and inference is carried out through computationally efficient MCMC techniques. To incorporate variable selection and estimation of the smoothing parameters simultaneously, the object name *stewisereg* in BayesX was used for all analyses. Through this, we are able to adequately address the issues of variable selection and model building. These consist of including continuous covariates, spatial correlation, interaction of continuous covariates, and exclusion of heterogeneity among respondents through the approach.

In this case study, we fitted the model (as the primary model) that includes all the possible covariates as

totchid=time$_2$ + *time*$_3$ + f_{spat}*(state)* + f_1*(agecont)* + f_2*(agesex1)* + f_3*(agemar)* + f_4*(maryyr)* + *g(agecont*maryyr)* + *state(random)* + *cluster(random)* + *zones(factor)* + *urban* + *married* + *educ(factor)* + *part_educ(factor)* + *chd_0* + *chd_13* + *chd_45* + *chd_6* + *withn2* + *later2* + *unsuretm* + *undecided* + *wantsame* + *husbmore* + *husbfew* + *usedb4b* + *usingcon* + *wantedlc,*

In BayesX, categorical variable can be specified with *factor*. This permits estimation of categorical variable without user necessarily creating the dummies for such categorical variables.

13.5 Results

13.5.1 Applications to Fertility Data

The final model was achieved at the 10th step with AIC −177589.19. This is extracted from the output and displayed below:

Final model totchid = const + year03 + year08 + northe + northw + southe + southw + married + primary + secondry + higher + chd_0 + chd_13 + chd_45 + chd_6 + withn2 + later2 + unsuretm + usingcon + wantedlc + usedb4b + agesex1(psplinerw2,df=8.03645,(lambda=418.645)) + undecide + wantsame + *husbfew* + husbmore + agemar(psplinerw2,df=4.95213,(lambda=6578.29)) + agecont(psplinerw2,df=3.96368,(lambda=37166.4)) + maryyr(psplinerw2, df=15.037,(lambda=32.768)) + sstate(spatial,df=26.9899,(lambda=255.59)) + maryyr_c*agecont_c(psplineinteract,df=6.56474,(lambda=5302.73))

Also automatically estimated and included as part of the fitted model are the degrees of freedom and smoothing parameters. This model is more parsimonious than the full model. For instance, partner's educational attainment, unstructured spatial effects and cluster specific random effects were excluded from the model. Moreover, the selected model still contains the interaction between respondent's age and duration of marriage. The final model was later fitted with object 'bayesreg' in BayesX. Therefore, we based the discussion of our results (fixed, spatial and nonlinear effects) on the '*bayesreg*' output and not on the *stepwisereg* output. As mentioned earlier, the variable selection approach applied prior to the main estimation of the fitted model has availed us opportunity to reasonably determine which covariates and form (linear or nonlinear for continuous variables) should be included in the model, inclusion of complex interaction effect. In the same manner, variable selection made it clear that inclusion of cluster and unstructured spatial effect will not lead to a better fit, hence, the need to drop them from the analysis. This would not have been possible without a scientific means of determining which variables should be explored.

13.5.2 Results

Trend and Linear Effects

Table 13.2 presents the results of fixed effects. A possible significant trend was evident based on total number of children given birth to per woman. Comparing 2003 with 1999 and 2008 with 1999, the total number of children given birth to has not substantially decreased. Respondent's educational attainment was significantly related to fertility with respondents with secondary education or higher having fewer number of children compared with those that do not have any formal education. On ideal number of children the respondents desire, those who desire at most 5 children are likely to have given birth to fewer children than those who desire 7 children and more; and in other words, contribute less to the overall total fertility level of the country. The surveys elicited information about husband's desire for children. The respondents who said that their husband's desire more children are more likely to give birth to more children and this is positively significant.

Contraceptive use has been shown in some studies to be significantly related to fertility. In this study, effect of current use of a modern contraceptive and use before the last birth on fertility was explored. As shown in Table 13.2, contraceptive use (either currently or before the last birth) does not show any reduction effect on the number of children given birth to per woman. However, those who are currently using are more likely to have fewer number of children compared with those who used before last birth. Respondents who claimed to have wanted last child are associated with fewer number of children.

Nonlinear Effects

Now turning attention to the nonlinear effect of the continuous variables, see Fig. 13.1 a–d. While effect of age at first sex and effect of respondent's current age are approximately linearly related to number of children given birth to, the stepwise regression approach reveals that estimating these nonparametrically fits better than assuming a parametric model. Moreover, the DIC of models with linear dependence of these effects are better off. Therefore, we still maintained the model with non parametric effect of age at first sex and current age of the respondents. With age at first sex, an obvious reduction in number of children given birth to was apparent among respondents who had their first sexual experience at an older age. On the other hand, an obvious increase in number of children given birth to was evident among older respondents. Respondents who married at an early age: say 10–25 years are more likely to have given birth to more children compared with their counterparts who married at older age (25 years and above). Year or duration of marriage is positively associated with fertility with number of children increasing as duration of marriage increases. A sharp increase was noticed, however, between 0 and 10 years.

Table 13.2 Estimates of posterior means with 95 % credible interval for the Poisson regression model of fertility rate

			95 % Credible interval (CI)	
Variable	Post mean	Std. Dev.	Lower	Upper
Constant	1.380	0.088	1.203	1.549
Year of study				
Year 1999 (ref)	ref			
Year 2003	0.058	0.012	0.035	0.080
Year 2008	0.044	0.010	0.026	0.065
Geopolitical zones				
North Central (ref)	ref			
North East	0.050	0.030	−0.013	0.105
North West	0.029	0.028	−0.027	0.087
South East	0.047	0.023	8.23e-05	0.090
South West	−0.045	0.025	−0.093	0.004
Married	0.113	0.017	0.080	0.146
Respondent's education				
None (ref)	ref			
Primary	0.016	0.008	0.002	0.032
Secondary	−0.029	0.009	−0.047	−0.012
Higher	−0.133	0.017	−0.165	−0.099
Ideal number of children				
7 and above (ref)	ref			
None	−0.046	0.024	−0.094	0.006
1–3	−0.186	0.019	−0.223	−0.149
4–5	−0.144	0.010	−0.164	−0.123
6	−0.027	0.008	−0.044	−0.011
Desire for more children				
Wanted no more/sterilised/infecund	ref			
Within 2 years	−0.174	0.009	−0.190	−0.156
Later than 2 years	−0.105	0.008	−0.121	−0.090
Unsure of time	−0.126	0.013	−0.149	−0.100
Undecided	−0.063	0.010	−0.082	−0.042
Husband's desire for children				
Others (ref)	ref			
Want same	0.004	0.007	−0.010	0.017
Husband wants more	0.016	0.006	0.004	0.028
Husband wants few	−0.004	0.018	−0.0412	0.031
Currently using FP method	0.019	0.009	0.001	0.038
Wanted last child	−0.051	0.008	−0.067	−0.034
Used FP before last birth	0.027	0.009	0.009	0.046

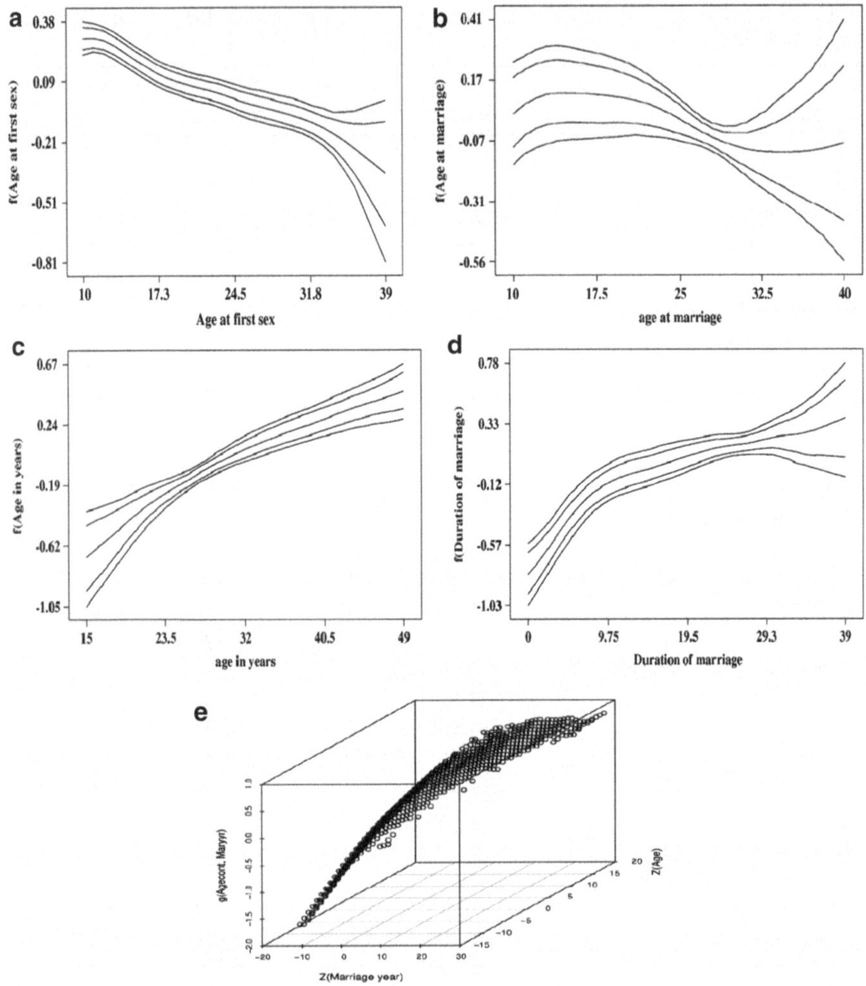

Fig. 13.1 Nonlinear effects of (**a**) age at first sex, (**b**) age at marriage, (**c**) respondent's age, (**d**) duration of marriage with their corresponding 95 % and 80 % credible intervals. Also included is the surface plot of interaction effect of duration of marriage and respondent's age

Interaction Effect

Figure 13.1e displays the interaction effect of duration of marriage and respondent's age. It was evident that as the duration of marriage and age of the respondent also increase, they both have positive impact on increase number of children given birth to per woman. This 3 dimensional plot was obtained with '*plotsurf*' command in R. It can also be obtained using the same function in Splus. BayesX automatically generates the graph command for plotting the interaction effect of any two variables. Model with interaction effect of duration of marriage and respondent's age was found to be more parsimonious based on the stepwise regression procedure in BayesX.

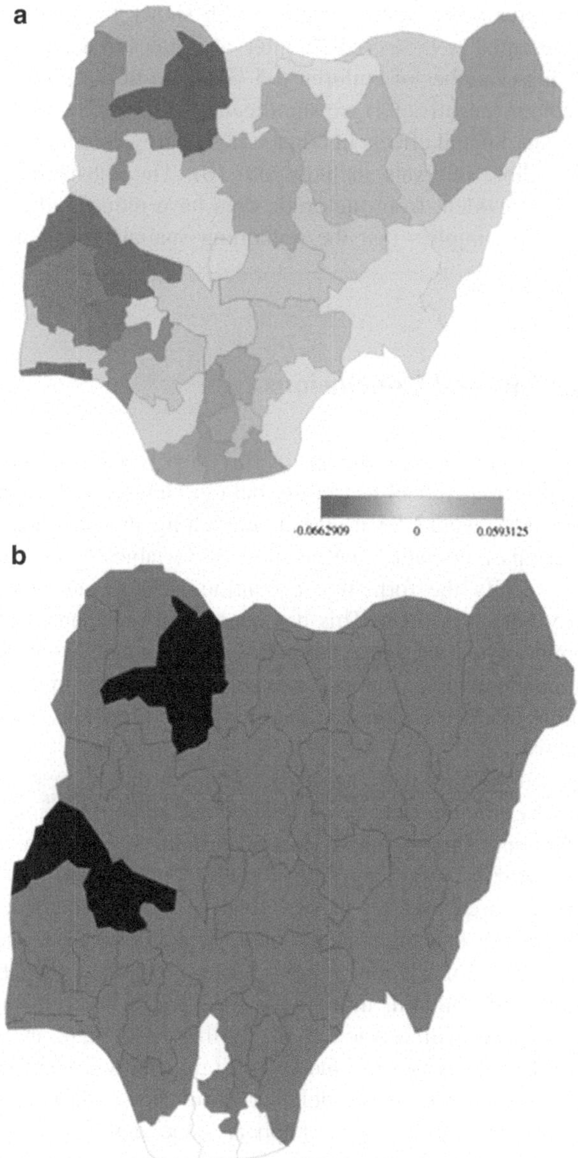

Fig. 13.2 Map of Nigeria showing spatial effect (**a**) and significance of spatial effect (**b**)

Spatial Effects

Figure 13.2a, b shows the results of spatial effect in the fitted model. In Fig. 13.2a, an interesting West–east spatial pattern was noticed. Respondents in the Western zones are associated with fewer number of children. However, this spatial pattern is only significant for a few states. Figure 13.2b shows the map of significance with estimates presented at 95 % credible intervals. States in white are significantly associated with high number of children (95 % CI lie in the positive side) while states in black colour (negative CI) are significantly associated with low number of children per woman. Spatial effects in other states in grey colour are not significant i.e. the 95 % credible intervals include zero (0). The substantial geographical variations that were evident from the crude data have reduced after adjusting for some covariates. This implies that the remaining spatial effects are the residual spatial effects.

13.6 Discussions and Conclusions

In this Chapter, we demonstrated the use of Bayesian variable selection procedure for fitting a parsimonious model to fertility data in Nigeria. Rather than assuming all available variables would be useful in modelling the phenomenon at hand, the approach permits automatic identification of variables to be included in the model and also specify the form that a continuous covariate enters the model (whether linearly or nonlinearly). This has been a very challenging task in many realistically complex situation where modelling involves many components such as trend, spatial, random, nonlinear, interaction and spatial effects. In this application, a more parsimonious model was achieved and model interpretations could be assumed to be more objective.

In the analysis of fertility data, it became apparent that highest level of educational attainment by women could be considered as a major proximate determinant of fertility in Nigeria. This is similar to other findings. For such, see Bhargava (2007); and Kazembe (2009). Therefore, for the country to achieve the planned reduction of 0.6 children every 5 years, effective intervention that will address and encourage women's education should be designed. Whereas those respondents that acquired at most primary education are found to be significantly associated with more number of children, those with secondary education and above are significantly associated with reduction of fertility. Although, in other studies, respondents in urban areas were found to be significantly associated with fewer number of children, however, this variable was eliminated in the course the variable selection procedure. Therefore, it did not appear in the final model.

Inter-spousal communication on contraceptive use has been found to play major role in uptake of a family method. For instance, Ujuju et al. (2010) found male involvement to be a useful approach towards acceptability of a family planning method. The link between use of family method and fertility is inter-twined. In this study, however, respondents who claimed that their husbands desire fewer children are more likely to have contributed towards reduction of fertility. Although this was not significant, the result suggests a possible and important implication of findings. Similarly, those respondents who claimed that their husbands want more children than them are significantly likely to adversely affect the reduction of fertility. One important programmatic implication of this is that, policy makers should intensify behavioural change in communications that will be targeted at men which will encourage couples discussion to deciding on the benefits of reduced fertility to the family and not only to the mother alone.

Although contraceptive use was found to be significantly associated with fertility, however, there was no evidence to show that its use could result in reduction of fertility in Nigeria. Other studies have found similar result as regards contraceptive use in sub Saharan Africa. Notable among them are Agyei-Mensah (2007) and Kazembe (2009) among others. Nigeria is one of the countries in sub Saharan African with low contraceptive prevalence. One implication of this finding is that, possibly there could be an unmet need for family planning method. On the other hand, it may be an evidence of contraceptive failure. However, the cause of this cannot be established in this study. A point for follow-up research here may be to conduct qualitative studies which may assist in unravelling this difficult knot. On ideal number of children a respondent would like to have, respondents who desired at most six children are significantly associated with reduction in fertility compared with their counterparts who desired at least seven children.

A steady decline in fertility with increase in age at first sex is biologically not unusual. Firstly, it is expected that those that had the first sex at an older age have reduced intervals between onset of sexual initiation and age of menopause. In other words, the older a respondent is before initiation of sex, the fewer the number of children that person can give birth to. This same explanation goes for age at marriage. On respondent's current age and duration of marriage, almost similar pattern are evident here. Under a normal circumstance and all things being equal, older respondents, who were married at a reasonably normal time (say 25 years); and who did not experience death of children are very likely to have more children compared with their counterparts who experienced delay in getting married, delay in conception and possibly death of children. Early marriage and the onset of childbearing at young ages are strongly associated with high fertility (Foote et al. 1993),

The significant spatial effect that was evident in this study could be as a result of some unexplained factors that may be associated with number of children given birth to per woman. For instance, Nigeria has a diverse cultural and ethnic structure. This, sometimes, is difficult to separate from religion. After adjusting for possible determinants of fertility, Akwa Ibom, Anambra, Bayelsa, and Rivers states are significantly associated with high fertility; while Kwara and Zamfara states are significantly associated with low fertility. This method of analysis has permitted opportunity that will assist policy makers in prudently making use of the scarce resources which is the situation in developing countries (including Nigeria).

Of the seven components of the Millennium Development Goals (MDGs), fertility is directly or indirectly linked with four of them, these are MDG 1 (eradicating extreme poverty), MDG 2 (achieve universal education), MDG 4 (reduce child mortality) and MDG 5 (improve maternal health). Therefore, if findings from this study are judiciously used, it will assist policy makers in designing strategies that will contribute towards attaining the goals.

Appendix

Example of output from fitting 'Stepwise' regression in BayesX
> stepwisereg s
> s.outfile= C:\Collaborations\Yahya\Fertility\m12
> s.regress totchid = sstate(spatial,map=m,lambda=0.1) + agecont(psplinerw2) + agesex1(psplinerw2) + agemar(psplinerw2) + maryyr(psplinerw2) + agecont*maryyr(psplineinteract) + agecont*agesex1(psplineinteract) + agesex1*agemar(psplineinteract) + sstate(random) + Hholdno(random) + year03 + year08 + northe + northw + southe + southw + souths + urban + married + primary + secondry + higher + chd_0 + chd_13 + chd_45 + chd_6 + withn2 + later2 + unsuretm + undecide + wantsame + husbmore + husbfew + usedb4b + usingcon + wantedlc, CI=MCMCselect step=10 iterations=10000 family=poisson predict using d

STEPWISE OBJECT s: stepwise procedure
GENERAL OPTIONS:

Performance criterion: AIC_imp
Maximum number of iterations: 100

RESPONSE DISTRIBUTION:

Family: Poisson
Number of observations: 33482

OPTIONS FOR STEPWISE PROCEDURE:

OPTIONS FOR LINEAR EFFECTS TERM: year03

Startvalue of the 1. startmodel is "effect excluded"

OPTIONS FOR LINEAR EFFECTS TERM: year08

Startvalue of the 1. startmodel is "effect excluded"

OPTIONS FOR LINEAR EFFECTS TERM: northe

Startvalue of the 1. startmodel is "effect excluded"

OPTIONS FOR LINEAR EFFECTS TERM: northw

Startvalue of the 1. startmodel is "effect excluded"

OPTIONS FOR LINEAR EFFECTS TERM: southe

Startvalue of the 1. startmodel is "effect excluded"

OPTIONS FOR LINEAR EFFECTS TERM: southw

Startvalue of the 1. startmodel is "effect excluded"

OPTIONS FOR LINEAR EFFECTS TERM: souths

Startvalue of the 1. startmodel is "effect excluded"

OPTIONS FOR LINEAR EFFECTS TERM: urban

Startvalue of the 1. startmodel is "effect excluded"

OPTIONS FOR LINEAR EFFECTS TERM: married

Startvalue of the 1. startmodel is "effect excluded"

OPTIONS FOR LINEAR EFFECTS TERM: primary

Startvalue of the 1. startmodel is "effect excluded"

OPTIONS FOR LINEAR EFFECTS TERM: secondry

Startvalue of the 1. startmodel is "effect excluded"

OPTIONS FOR LINEAR EFFECTS TERM: higher

Startvalue of the 1. startmodel is "effect excluded"

OPTIONS FOR LINEAR EFFECTS TERM: chd_0

Startvalue of the 1. startmodel is "effect excluded"

OPTIONS FOR LINEAR EFFECTS TERM: chd_13

Startvalue of the 1. startmodel is "effect excluded"

OPTIONS FOR LINEAR EFFECTS TERM: chd_45

Startvalue of the 1. startmodel is "effect excluded"

OPTIONS FOR LINEAR EFFECTS TERM: chd_6

Startvalue of the 1. startmodel is "effect excluded"

OPTIONS FOR LINEAR EFFECTS TERM: withn2

Startvalue of the 1. startmodel is "effect excluded"

OPTIONS FOR LINEAR EFFECTS TERM: later2

Startvalue of the 1. startmodel is "effect excluded"

OPTIONS FOR LINEAR EFFECTS TERM: unsuretm

Startvalue of the 1. startmodel is "effect excluded"

OPTIONS FOR LINEAR EFFECTS TERM: undecide

Startvalue of the 1. startmodel is "effect excluded"

OPTIONS FOR LINEAR EFFECTS TERM: wantsame

Startvalue of the 1. startmodel is "effect excluded"

OPTIONS FOR LINEAR EFFECTS TERM: husbmore

Startvalue of the 1. startmodel is "effect excluded"

OPTIONS FOR LINEAR EFFECTS TERM: husbfew

Startvalue of the 1. startmodel is "effect excluded"

OPTIONS FOR LINEAR EFFECTS TERM: usedb4b

Startvalue of the 1. startmodel is "effect excluded"

OPTIONS FOR LINEAR EFFECTS TERM: usingcon

Startvalue of the 1. startmodel is "effect excluded"

OPTIONS FOR LINEAR EFFECTS TERM: wantedlc

Startvalue of the 1. startmodel is "effect excluded"

OPTIONS FOR NONPARAMETRIC TERM: agecont

Minimum value for the smoothing parameter: 42.59841875
This is equivalent to degrees of freedom: approximately 15, exact 15.0445
Maximum value for the smoothing parameter: 561250
This is equivalent to degrees of freedom: approximately 2, exact 1.9873
Number of different smoothing parameters with equidistant degrees of freedom: 20
Startvalue of the 1. startmodel is "effect excluded"

OPTIONS FOR NONPARAMETRIC TERM: agesex1

Minimum value for the smoothing parameter: 4.300834375
This is equivalent to degrees of freedom: approximately 15, exact 15.0073
Maximum value for the smoothing parameter: 122500
This is equivalent to degrees of freedom: approximately 2, exact 2.03467
Number of different smoothing parameters with equidistant degrees of freedom: 20
Startvalue of the 1. startmodel is "effect excluded"

OPTIONS FOR NONPARAMETRIC TERM: agemar

Minimum value for the smoothing parameter: 11.4688125
This is equivalent to degrees of freedom: approximately 15, exact 14.9876
Maximum value for the smoothing parameter: 203750
This is equivalent to degrees of freedom: approximately 2, exact 2.02288
Number of different smoothing parameters with equidistant degrees of freedom: 20
Startvalue of the 1. startmodel is "effect excluded"

OPTIONS FOR NONPARAMETRIC TERM: maryyr

Minimum value for the smoothing parameter: 32.7680375
This is equivalent to degrees of freedom: approximately 15, exact 15.0367
Maximum value for the smoothing parameter: 403750
This is equivalent to degrees of freedom: approximately 2, exact 2.02664
Number of different smoothing parameters with equidistant degrees of freedom: 20
Startvalue of the 1. startmodel is "effect excluded"

OPTIONS FOR NONPARAMETRIC TERM: sstate

Minimum value for the smoothing parameter: 7.5776421875
This is equivalent to degrees of freedom: approximately 27, exact 35.5912
Maximum value for the smoothing parameter: 1470.23
This is equivalent to degrees of freedom: approximately 1, exact 14.519
Number of different smoothing parameters with equidistant degrees of freedom: 20
Startvalue of the 1. startmodel is "effect excluded"

OPTIONS FOR NONPARAMETRIC TERM: sstate

Minimum value for the smoothing parameter: 1074.7904359375
This is equivalent to degrees of freedom: approximately 27, exact 27.0357
Maximum value for the smoothing parameter: 141250
This is equivalent to degrees of freedom: approximately 1, exact 0.963917
Number of different smoothing parameters with equidistant degrees of freedom: 20
Startvalue of the 1. startmodel is "effect excluded"

OPTIONS FOR NONPARAMETRIC TERM: Hholdno

Minimum value for the smoothing parameter: 6.5536
This is equivalent to degrees of freedom: approximately 220, exact 220.004
Maximum value for the smoothing parameter: 12968.8
This is equivalent to degrees of freedom: approximately 10, exact 10.0044
Number of different smoothing parameters with equidistant degrees of freedom: 20
Startvalue of the 1. startmodel is "effect excluded"

OPTIONS FOR NONPARAMETRIC TERM: agecont_c*maryyr_c

Minimum value for the smoothing parameter: 6.71875e-07
This is equivalent to degrees of freedom: approximately 310, exact 310.032
Maximum value for the smoothing parameter: 5302.73
This is equivalent to degrees of freedom: approximately 50, exact 49.9928
Number of different smoothing parameters with equidistant degrees of freedom: 20
Startvalue of the 1. startmodel is "effect excluded"

OPTIONS FOR NONPARAMETRIC TERM: agecont_c*agesex1_c

Minimum value for the smoothing parameter: 1.97362723338301e-08
This is equivalent to degrees of freedom: approximately 330, exact 329.971
Maximum value for the smoothing parameter: 9375
This is equivalent to degrees of freedom: approximately 50, exact 50.0202
Number of different smoothing parameters with equidistant degrees of freedom: 20
Startvalue of the 1. startmodel is "effect excluded"

OPTIONS FOR NONPARAMETRIC TERM: agesex1_c*agemar_c

Minimum value for the smoothing parameter: 1.5e-06
This is equivalent to degrees of freedom: approximately 260, exact 259.988
Maximum value for the smoothing parameter: 1639.47
This is equivalent to degrees of freedom: approximately 50, exact 50.0083

Number of different smoothing parameters with equidistant degrees of freedom: 20
Startvalue of the 1. startmodel is "effect excluded"

STEPWISE PROCEDURE STARTED

Startmodel:

totchid = const

AIC_imp = -137982.08

Startmodel:

totchid = const + year03 + year08 + northe + northw + southe + southw + souths + urban + married + primary + secondry + higher + chd_13 + chd_45 + withn2 + later2 + unsuretm + undecide + wantsame + husbmore + husbfew + usedb4b + usingcon + wantedlc + agesex1_c*agemar_c + agecont(psplinerw2,df=8.38737,(lambda=1671.22)) + agesex1(psplinerw2,df=5.15948,(lambda=3879.49)) + agemar(psplinerw2,df= 4.16032,(lambda=16239.4)) + sstate(spatial,df=28.2258,(lambda=168.912)) + sstate(random,df=2.16761,(lambda=9511.92))
AIC_imp = -170003.9

Startmodel:

totchid = const + year03 + year08 + northe + northw + southe + southw + souths + urban + married + secondry + higher + chd_13 + chd_45 + withn2 + later2 + unsuretm + undecide + husbmore + usedb4b + usingcon + wantedlc + agecont(psplinerw2,df=9.02973,(lambda=967.445)) + agesex1(psplinerw2,df=10.0038,(lambda=125.019)) + agemar(psplinerw2,df= 4.99049,(lambda=6578.29)) + maryyr(psplinerw2,df=15.1087,(lambda=32.768)) + sstate(spatial,df=22.1851,(lambda=168.912)) + sstate(random,df=9.12529, (lambda=1651.18)) + agecont_c*maryyr_c(psplineinteract,df=8.34503,(lambda= 5302.73)) + agecont_c*agesex1_c(psplineinteract,df=8.47754,(lambda=9375)) + agesex1_c*agemar_c(psplineinteract,df=7.37864,(lambda=1639.47))
AIC_imp = -177017.85

Startmodel:

totchid = const + year03 + year08 + northe + northw + southe + southw + souths + married + primary + secondry + higher + chd_13 + chd_45 + chd_6 + withn2 + later2 + unsuretm + undecide + husbmore + usedb4b + usingcon + wantedlc + agecont(psplinerw2,df=6.04443,(lambda=6172.44)) + agesex1(psplinerw2,df=4.99068,(lambda=3879.49)) + agemar(psplinerw2,df= 4.9667,(lambda=6578.29)) + maryyr(psplinerw2,df=15.0388,(lambda=32.768)) + sstate(spatial,df=26.5994,(lambda=66.5082)) + sstate(random,df=6.98566, (lambda=1074.79)) + agecont_c*maryyr_c(psplineinteract,df=7.73487,(lambda =5302.73)) + agecont_c*agesex1_c(psplineinteract,df=13.4769,(lambda= 2043.22)) + agesex1_c*agemar_c(psplineinteract,df=12.2985,(lambda=1.5e-06))
AIC_imp = -177541.1

Startmodel:

totchid = const + year03 + year08 + northe + northw + southe + southw + souths + married + secondry + higher + chd_13 + chd_45 + chd_6 + withn2 + later2 + unsuretm + undecide + husbmore + usedb4b + usingcon + wantedlc + agecont(psplinerw2,df=4.96975,(lambda=14419.5)) + agesex1(psplinerw2,df=4.00305,(lambda=9619.72)) + agemar(psplinerw2,df=6.02728,(lambda=2859.82)) + maryyr(psplinerw2,df=15.0327,(lambda=32.768)) + sstate(spatial,df=25.5783,(lambda=77.6428)) + sstate(random,df=7.74974,(lambda=1074.79)) + agecont_c*maryyr_c(psplineinteract,df=7.26835,(lambda=5302.73)) + agecont_c*agesex1_c(psplineinteract,df=15.9844,(lambda=1.97363e-08)) + agesex1_c*agemar_c(psplineinteract,df=11.9434,(lambda=1.5e-06))
AIC_imp = -177633.66

Startmodel:

totchid = const + year03 + year08 + northe + northw + southe + southw + souths + married + secondry + higher + chd_0 + chd_13 + chd_45 + chd_6 + withn2 + later2 + unsuretm + undecide + husbmore + usedb4b + usingcon + wantedlc + agecont(psplinerw2,df=3.96519,(lambda=37166.4)) + agesex1(psplinerw2,df=2.95082,(lambda=31303.9)) + agemar(psplinerw2,df=6.02686,(lambda=2859.82)) + maryyr(psplinerw2,df=15.0375,(lambda=32.768)) + sstate(spatial,df=26.6013,(lambda=66.5082)) + sstate(random,df=6.98631,(lambda=1074.79)) + agecont_c*maryyr_c(psplineinteract,df=6.58284,(lambda=5302.73)) + agecont_c*agesex1_c(psplineinteract,df=9.86227,(lambda=1.97363e-08)) + agesex1_c*agemar_c(psplineinteract,df=9.08355,(lambda=1.5e-06))
AIC_imp = -177651.74

Startmodel:

totchid = const + year03 + year08 + northe + northw + southe + southw + souths + married + primary + secondry + higher + chd_0 + chd_13 + chd_45 + chd_6 + withn2 + later2 + unsuretm + undecide + husbmore + usedb4b + usingcon + wantedlc + agecont(psplinerw2,df=3.96485,(lambda=37166.4)) + agesex1(psplinerw2,df=2.95079,(lambda=31303.9)) + agemar(psplinerw2,df=6.02644,(lambda=2859.82)) + maryyr(psplinerw2,df=15.0365,(lambda=32.768)) + sstate(spatial,df=25.5786,(lambda=77.6428)) + sstate(random,df=7.74987,(lambda=1074.79)) + agecont_c*maryyr_c(psplineinteract,df=6.58136,(lambda=5302.73)) + agecont_c*agesex1_c(psplineinteract,df=9.86105,(lambda=1.97363e-08)) + agesex1_c*agemar_c(psplineinteract,df=9.08291,(lambda=1.5e-06))
AIC_imp = -177659.5

Startmodel:

totchid = const + year03 + year08 + northe + northw + southe + southw + souths + married + primary + secondry + higher + chd_0 + chd_13 + chd_45 + chd_6 + withn2 + later2 + unsuretm + undecide + husbmore + usedb4b

+ usingcon + wantedlc + agecont(psplinerw2,df=3.9648,(lambda=37166.4)) + agesex1(psplinerw2,df=2.95078,(lambda=31303.9)) + agemar(psplinerw2, df=6.02628,(lambda=2859.82)) + maryyr(psplinerw2,df=15.0365,(lambda= 32.768)) + sstate(spatial,df=25.5783,(lambda=77.6428)) + sstate(random,df= 7.74977,(lambda=1074.79)) + agecont_c*maryyr_c(psplineinteract,df=6.58102, (lambda=5302.73)) + agecont_c*agesex1_c(psplineinteract,df=9.86082,(lambda =1.97363e-08)) + agesex1_c*agemar_c(psplineinteract,df=9.08301,(lambda= 1.5e-06))
AIC_imp = -177662.58

Startmodel:

totchid = const + year03 + year08 + northe + northw + southe + southw + souths + married + primary + secondry + higher + chd_0 + chd_13 + chd_45 + chd_6 + withn2 + later2 + unsuretm + undecide + husbmore + usedb4b + usingcon + wantedlc + agecont(psplinerw2,df=3.96479,(lambda=37166.4)) + agesex1(psplinerw2,df=2.95079,(lambda=31303.9)) + agemar(psplinerw2,df =6.0262,(lambda=2859.82)) + maryyr(psplinerw2,df=15.0366,(lambda=32.768)) + sstate(spatial,df=24.3966,(lambda=91.9764)) + sstate(random,df=8.63275, (lambda=1074.79)) + agecont_c*maryyr_c(psplineinteract,df=6.58091,(lambda= 5302.73)) + agecont_c*agesex1_c(psplineinteract,df=9.86074,(lambda=1.97363e-08)) + agesex1_c*agemar_c(psplineinteract,df=9.08311,(lambda=1.5e-06))
AIC_imp = -177664.52

Startmodel:

totchid = const + year03 + year08 + northe + northw + southe + southw + souths + married + primary + secondry + higher + chd_0 + chd_13 + chd_45 + chd_6 + withn2 + later2 + unsuretm + undecide + husbmore + usedb4b + usingcon + wantedlc + agecont(psplinerw2,df=3.96479,(lambda=37166.4)) + agesex1(psplinerw2,df=2.95079,(lambda=31303.9)) + agemar(psplinerw2,df= 6.02614,(lambda=2859.82)) + maryyr(psplinerw2,df=15.0366,(lambda=32.768)) + sstate(spatial,df=24.3965,(lambda=91.9764)) + sstate(random,df=8.63272, (lambda=1074.79)) + agecont_c*maryyr_c(psplineinteract,df=6.58088,(lambda= 5302.73)) + agecont_c*agesex1_c(psplineinteract,df=9.8607,(lambda=1.97363e-08)) + agesex1_c*agemar_c(psplineinteract,df=9.0832,(lambda=1.5e-06))
AIC_imp = -177665.39

Startmodel:

totchid = const + year03 + year08 + northe + northw + southe + southw + souths + married + primary + secondry + higher + chd_0 + chd_13 + chd_45 + chd_6 + withn2 + later2 + unsuretm + undecide + husbmore + usedb4b + usingcon + wantedlc + agecont(psplinerw2,df=3.9648,(lambda=37166.4)) + agesex1(psplinerw2,df=2.9508,(lambda=31303.9)) + agemar(psplinerw2,df= 6.02609,(lambda=2859.82)) + maryyr(psplinerw2,df=15.0366,(lambda=32.768)) + sstate(spatial,df=24.3964,(lambda=91.9764)) + sstate(random,df=8.6327,

(lambda=1074.79)) + agecont_c*maryyr_c(psplineinteract,df=6.5809,(lambda=5302.73)) + agecont_c*agesex1_c(psplineinteract,df=9.86069,(lambda=1.97363e-08)) + agesex1_c*agemar_c(psplineinteract,df=9.08325,(lambda=1.5e-06))
AIC_imp = -177666.11

Final Model:

totchid = const + year03 + year08 + northe + northw + southe + southw + souths + married + primary + secondry + higher + chd_0 + chd_13 + chd_45 + chd_6 + withn2 + later2 + unsuretm + undecide + husbmore + usedb4b + usingcon + wantedlc + agecont(psplinerw2,df=3.9648,(lambda=37166.4)) + agesex1(psplinerw2,df=2.9508,(lambda=31303.9)) + agemar(psplinerw2,df=6.02609,(lambda=2859.82)) + maryyr(psplinerw2,df=15.0366,(lambda=32.768)) + sstate(spatial,df=24.3964,(lambda=91.9764)) + sstate(random,df=8.6327,(lambda=1074.79)) + agecont_c*maryyr_c(psplineinteract,df=6.5809,(lambda=5302.73)) + agecont_c*agesex1_c(psplineinteract,df=9.86069,(lambda=1.97363e-08)) + agesex1_c*agemar_c(psplineinteract,df=9.08325,(lambda=1.5e-06))
AIC_imp = -177666.76

Used number of iterations: 11

Final Model:
totchid = const + year03 + year08 + northe + northw + southe + southw + souths + married + primary + secondry + higher + chd_0 + chd_13 + chd_45 + chd_6 + withn2 + later2 + unsuretm + undecide + husbmore + usedb4b + usingcon + wantedlc + agecont(psplinerw2,df=3.9648,(lambda=37166.4)) + agesex1(psplinerw2,df=2.9508,(lambda=31303.9)) + agemar(psplinerw2,df=6.02609,(lambda=2859.82)) + maryyr(psplinerw2,df=15.0366,(lambda=32.768)) + sstate(spatial,df=24.3964,(lambda=91.9764)) + sstate(random,df=8.6327,(lambda=1074.79)) + agecont_c*maryyr_c(psplineinteract,df=6.5809,(lambda=5302.73)) + agecont_c*agesex1_c(psplineinteract,df=9.86069,(lambda=1.97363e-08)) + agesex1_c*agemar_c(psplineinteract,df=9.08325,(lambda=1.5e-06))
AIC_imp = -177687.06

References

Adlakha, A., Ayad, M., & Kumar, S. (1991). The role of nuptiality in fertility decline: A comparative analysis. In *Proceedings of the demographic and health surveys world conference*, Washington, DC. 1991, vol. 2. Columbia, Maryland: IRD/Macro International Inc., Demographic and Health Surveys, 947–964.

Agyei-Mensah S. (2007, December). *New times, new families: The stall in Ghanaian fertility*. Paper presented at the African Population Conference. Arusha, Tanzania.

Arnold, F. (1990). Assessment of quality of birth history data in the Demographic and Health Surveys. Assesment of DHS-1 Data Quality, Institute for Resource Development (IRD). DHS methodological reports, no. 1, IRD, Columbia.

Arnold, F., & Blanc, A. K. (1990). *Fertility levels and trend* (DHS comparative studies, Vol. 2). Columbia: IRD/Macro Systems Inc.
Baschieri, A., & Hinde, A. (2007). The proximate determinants of fertility and birth intervals in Egypt: An application of calendar data. *Demographic Research, 16*(3), 59–96.
Becker, G. S., & Lewis, H. G. (1973). On the interaction between quantity and quality of children. *Journal of Political Economy, 81*, 279–299.
Belitz, C. (2007). Model selection in generalized structured additive regression models. Ph.D. thesis, University of Munich
Belitz, C., & Lang, S. (2008). Simultaneous selection of variables and smoothing parameters in structured additive regression models. *Computational Statistics and Data Analysis, 53*, 61–81.
Besag, J., York, Y., & Mollie, A. (1991). Bayesian image restoration with two applications in spatial statistics (with discussion). *Annals of the Institute of Statistical Mathematics, 43*, 1–59.
Bhargava, A. (2007). Desired family size, family planning and fertility in Ethiopia. *Journal of Biosocial Science, 39*, 367–381.
Blanc, A., & Poukouta, P. (1997). *Components of unexpected fertility decline in sub-Saharan Africa*. Demographic and health surveys analytical reports No. 5, Calverton: Macro International Inc.
Blanc, A. K., & Rutenberg (1990). Assessment of quality of data at first sex, age at first marriage and age at first birth in Demographic and Health Surveys. Assessment of DHS-1 Data Qulaity, Institute for Resource Development (IRD). DHS methodological reports, no. 1, IRD, Columbia.
Bongaarts, J. (1982). The fertility-inhibiting effects of the intermediate fertility variables. *Studies in Family Planning, 13*, 178–189.
Bongaarts, J., & Potter, R. G. (1983). *Fertility biology and behavior: An analysis of the proximate determinants*. New York: Academic.
Brezger, A., & Lang, S. (2006). Generalized structured additive regression based on Bayesian P splines. *Computational Statistics and Data Analysis, 50*, 967–991.
Cameron, A., & Trivedi, P. (1998). *Regression analysis of count data*. New York: Cambridge University Press.
Chatterjee, S., & Price, B. (1991). *Regression analysis by example*. New York: Wiley.
Chib, S., & Winkelmann, R. (2001). Markov chain Monte Carlo analysis of correlated count data. *Journal of Business and Economic Statistics, 19*, 428–435.
Chib, S., Greenberg, E., & Winkelmann, R. (1998). Posterior simulation and Bayes factors in panel count data models. *Journal of Econometrics, 86*, 33–54.
Cleland, J., Onuoha, N., & Timaeus, I. (1994). Fertility change in sub-Saharan Africa: A review of evidence. In T. Locoh & V. Hertrich (Eds.), *The onset of fertility transition in Sub-Saharan Africa* (pp. 1–20). Liège: Ordinal editions.
Cohen, B. (1998). The emerging fertility transition in sub-Saharan Africa. *World Development, 26*, 1431–1461.
Draper, N., & Smith, H. (1981). *Applied regression analysis* (2nd ed.). New York: Wiley.
Eilers, P. H. C., & Marx, D. B. (1996). Flexible smoothing with B-splines and penalties. *Statistical Science, 11*(2), 89–121.
Fahrmeir, L., & Osuna, L. (2006). Structured additive regression for overdispersed and zero-inflated count data. *Applied Stochastic Models in Business and Industry, 22*, 351–369.
Fahrmeir, L., Kneib, T., & Lang, S. (2004). Penalized structured additive regression for space-time data: A Bayesian perspective. *Statistica Sinica, 14*, 715–745.
Famoye, F., & Wang, W. (1997). Modeling household fertility decisions with generalised poisson regression. *Journal of Population Economics, 10*, 273–283.
Foote, K. A., Hill, K. H., & Martin, L. G. (Eds.). (1993). *Demographic change in sub-Saharan Africa population dynamics of sub-Saharan Africa*. Washington, DC: National Academy Press.
Hastie, T., & Tibshirani, R. (1990). *Generalized additive models*. London: Chapman and Hall.
Hocking, R. R. (1976). The analysis and selection of variables in linear regression. *Biometrics, 32*(1), 1–49.
Islam, S. (2009). Differential determinants of birth spacing since marriage to first live birth in rural Bangladesh. *Pertanika Journal of Social Science and Humanities, 17*(1), 1–6.

Jolly, C. L., & Gribble, J. N. (1993). The proximate determinants of fertility. In K. A. Foot, K. H. Hill, & L. G. Martin (Eds.), *Demographic change in sub-Saharan Africa*. Washington, DC: National Academy Press.

Kazembe, L. N. (2009). Modelling individual fertility levels in Malawian women: A spatial semiparametric regression model. *Statistical Methods and Applications, 18*(2), 237–255.

Kirk, D., & Pillet, B. (1997). Fertility levels, trends, and differentials in sub-Saharan Africa in the 1980s and 1990s. *Studies in Family Planning, 29*, 1–22.

Kneib, T., & Fahrmeir, L. (2006). Structured additive regression for categorical space-time data: A mixed model approach. *Biometrics, 62*, 109–118.

Kneib, T., & Fahrmeir, L. (2007). A mixed model approach to structured hazard regression. *Scandinavian Journal of Statistics, 34*, 207–228.

Lang, S., & Brezger, A. (2004). Bayesian P-splines. *Journal of Computational and Graphical Statistics, 13*, 183–212.

Makinde-Adebusoye, P. (2001, July 9–11). *Social-cultural factors affecting fertilityin Sub Saharan Africa*. Paper presented at the Workshop on Prospects for Fertility Decline in High Fertility Countries, Population Division, Department of Economic and Social Affairs, UN Secretariat, New York.

Makinde-Adebusoye, P., & Ebigbola J. (1992). *Socio-cultural factors affecting fertilityand family planning in Nigeria. Federal Republic of Nigeria: Implementing the National Policy on Population*. Sectoral reprot. Vol. II Annexes, World Bank, West Department, Population and Human Resources Operations Division. Annex B. pp. 1–33.

Makinde-Adebusoye, P., & Feyisetan, B. J. (1994). The quantum and tempo of fertility in Nigeria. In *Fertility trends and determinants in six African countries*. DHS regional analysis. Workshop for anglophone Africa, Macro International Inc., pp. 41–86.

National Population Commission [Nigeria]. (2000). *Nigeria demographic and health survey 1999*. Calverton: National Population Commission and ORC Macro.

National Population Commission [Nigeria] and ICF Macro. (2009). *Nigeria demographic and health survey 2008*. Abuja: National Population Commission and ICF Macro.

National Population Commission [Nigeria] & ORC Macro. (2004). *Nigeria demographic and health survey 2003*. Calverton: National Population Commission and ORC Macro.

Neter, J., Kutner, M., Nachtsheim, C., & Wasserman, W. (1996). *Applied linear statistical models* (4th ed.). Chicago: McGraw-Hill/Irwin.

Norville, C., Gomez, R., & Brown, R. L. (2003). *Some causes of fertilityrates movements* (Research Report 03–02). University of Waterloo, Institute of Insurance and Pension Research.

Olfa, F., & El-Lahga, A. R. (2002). A socioeconomic analysis of fertility determinants with a count data model: the case of Tunisia. In Proceedings of the 9th annual conference of the economic research forum for the Arab countries, Sharjah, United Arab Emirates, 26–28th Oct 2002.

Rue, H., & Held, L. (2005). *Gaussian Markov random fields: Theory and applications*. Boca Raton/London/NewYork/Singapore: Chapman & Hall/CRC.

Shen, C., & Williamson, J. B. (1999). Maternal mortality, women's status, and economic dependency in less developed countries: A cross national analysis. *Social Science & Medicine, 49*, 197–214.

Ujuju, C., Anyanti, J., Adebayo, S. B., Muhammad, F., Oluigbo, O., & Gofwan, A. (2010). Religion, culture and male involvement in the use of family planning: Evidence from Enugu and Katsina States of Nigeria. *International Nursing Review* (Published online on 6th Sept 2010). doi: 10.1111/j.1466-7657.2010.00820.x.

Winkelmann, R. (2000). Seemingly unrelated negative binomial regression. *Oxford Bulletin of Economics and Statistics, 62*, 553–560.

Chapter 14
A Spatial Analysis of Age at Sexual Initiation Among Nigerian Youth as a Tool for HIV Prevention: A Bayesian Approach

Alfred A. Abiodun, Samson Babatunde Adebayo, Benjamin A. Oyejola, Jennifer Anyanti, and Olaronke Ladipo†

14.1 Introduction

Age at first sex has been associated with increased risk of unplanned pregnancy and sexually transmitted infections, including HIV and human papilloma-virus (HPV) (Cooper et al. 2007). Studies have examined early sexual activity largely as a potential risk factor for adverse outcomes rather than identifying the correlates of the timing of sexual debut (Pettifor et al. 2005; Harrison et al. 2005).

There have been changes in the age at which young males and females initiate sex in Nigeria over years. The median age at sexual initiation has been steadily lower for females aged 15–24 than for males in the same age group. This was evident from the findings from the 2003 and 2005 National HIV/AIDS and Reproductive Health Survey. In 2003, the median age at sexual initiation (MASI) for youth aged 15–24 years was 19.8 and 16.9 for male and female respectively. These values increased to 20.1 and17.4 for male and female respectively in 2005. The national average (males

† deceased

A.A. Abiodun (✉) • B.A. Oyejola
Department of Statistics, University of Ilorin, Ilorin PMB 1515, Nigeria
e-mail: manfredwole@yahoo.com; boyejola2003@yahoo.com

S.B. Adebayo
Planning, Research and Statistics, National Agency for Food and Drug Administration and Control (NAFDAC), Plot 2032 Olusegun Obasanjo Way, Wuse Zone 7, PMB 5116, Abuja, Nigeria
e-mail: adebayo_sba@yahoo.com

J. Anyanti
Technical Services Directorate, Society for Family Health, Wuse, Abuja PMB 5116, Nigeria
e-mail: janyanti@sfhnigeria.org

N.-B. Kandala and G. Ghilagaber (eds.), *Advanced Techniques for Modelling Maternal and Child Health in Africa*, The Springer Series on Demographic Methods and Population Analysis 34, DOI 10.1007/978-94-007-6778-2_14,

and females combined) are 18.4, 18.8 and 16.5 in 2003 and 2005 respectively. There has been a steady decline in the average age at sexual initiation in the urban areas of the country over this period (2003 = 19.3 and 2005 = 18.7), while a slight delay in sexual debut was noticeable in the rural areas (2003 = 18.1 and 2005 = 18.7). In Nigeria, majority of male youth experience first sexual intercourse at older age than their female counterparts.

The median age at sexual initiation is consistently higher over the period 2003–2005 for males in the Northern part of the country than in the Southern part. This is, however, consistently lower in the North than South for females. For 2003 survey, median age at sexual initiation (MASI) for males in the North was 20.2 compared with 18.7 in the South, and 17.5 in the North compared with 18.5 in the South. From 2005, MASI is 21.8 in the North compared with 18.7 in the South while for females it is 16.9 in the North compared with 18.9 in the South.

Findings from Demographic and Health Surveys (DHS) conducted in six African countries (Ghana, Kenya, Tanzania, Uganda, Zambia and Zimbabwe) between 1988 and 2000 show that the median age at sexual initiation is generally lower for females youth (age 15–24 years) than their male counterparts (see Zaba et al. 2004), a finding which is similar to Nigeria's experience.

One major focus of the Millennium Development Goals (MDGs) is combating the spread of HIV and AIDS, malaria and other infectious diseases by 2015. Recent studies indicate that about one half of all new HIV infections in sub-Saharan Africa occur among youth aged 15–24 years (Garcia-Calleja et al. 2006; Mishra et al. 2006). Studies show that globally, an estimated 12 million people age 15–24 were living with HIV/AIDS in 2002 and three-quarters of these lived in sub-Saharan African countries. Since most HIV infections are through heterosexual activity, the vulnerability of young people is strongly influenced by sexual behaviour and their ability to protect themselves.

Situation analysis on HIV and AIDS in Nigeria revealed that the HIV prevalence rate has reduced from 5.8 % in 2001 (the peak) to 4.4 % in 2005 (FMOH 2006). However, substantial state level variation exists as prevalence ranges between 1.6 % and 10 % throughout the country. Early intercourse exposes one to increased risk of sexually transmitted diseases and unwanted pregnancies; which may result in long term health and social disadvantages (Dickson et al. 1998). Studies from the U.S. have suggested that adolescents who have fewer interpersonal and community resources to draw upon are likely to initiate their sexual activity earlier (Coleman 1988; Brewster 1994).

Sexual behaviour among Nigerian youth age 15–24 is not only influenced by socio-economic, demographic and health factors, but it also varies considerably across regions, districts and ethnic groups. Most studies in sub-Saharan Africa have focused on the social, demographic and familial factors associated with sexual initiation and reasons adolescents begin having consensual intercourse (Andersson-Ellstrom et al. 1996; Kinsman et al. 1998; Rink et al. 2007). Such studies have only reported geographical variations at a highly aggregated regional level and trends for data collected from similar multi-round surveys (see for instance, Agha et al. 2006; Chiao and Mishra 2007). Very little is known about the geographical factors and some unobserved heterogeneity at high level of aggregation, which expectedly may help identify the extent of regional, state and ethnic disparities in age at first sex.

A major challenge with this is that information is concealed within regions and has an adverse influence on policy formulation. First, policy is not usually formulated at a zonal level since five to seven states may constitute a zone. Second, in multi-ethnic country such as Nigeria, designing interventions at a zonal level seems impracticable and not suitable for the political and administrative convenience of the country.

Various indicators have been used to measure age at first sex from cross-sectional data in various surveys and to assess changes over time from data in multiple surveys. Also studies have been carried out on the individual and contextual factors influencing age at first sex. For example, Agha et al. (2006) examined individual and community-level determinants of early sexual initiation among males and females aged 15–24, using multilevel analysis. In their study, censored observations were ignored in which case binary variable was created for response, where value 1 was assigned if a respondent reported that he/she initiated sex before age 15 and 0 assigned if otherwise. Little had been done on timing of sexual initiation among Nigerians aged 15–24 by accounting for those who had not initiated sex by the survey time. This approach is limited by the fact that information is grossly lost from the ignored censored observations. To fill the gaps highlighted above, this study examines individual bio-demographic and knowledge covariates influencing early sexual initiation. It also examines spatial effects as well as adjusting for frailty components by controlling for clustering effects under the same model framework. Demographic covariates include age, sex, level of education and other covariates that describe the background characteristics of the survey population. Covariates on knowledge provide information about awareness of HIV, knowledge about how it can be transmitted.

14.2 Model Specification

Time-to-event principle that is commonly encountered in survival analysis often occurs in many practical situations and has a wide coverage with industrial, economic, demographic and medical applications. Age at initiation of sexual intercourse can also be viewed within this principle. In demographic studies, proportional hazards model, a popular methodology in survival analysis is used widely to model event history data such as age at marriage, age at first pregnancy and age at sexual initiation. Further, Cox proportional hazards model, which leaves the baseline distribution arbitrary has been used in modelling data on age at sexual initiation (see Fatusi and Blum 2008).

Often, time-to-event studies involve hierarchical data with structured and unstructured geographical information grouped into identified clusters such as clinical sites, states, geographic regions, census block or location of residence. In such settings, subjects residing within the same cluster are often exposed to similar unmeasured physical and social environments, which may be different from subjects residing in adjacent clusters. Therefore, there is need to take into account such unmeasured or unobserved heterogeneity during analysis. One way of analyzing such data is to include in the model cluster specific random effects (frailties) to account for the unexplained heterogeneity that cannot be included as fixed effects. In its simplest form, a frailty is an unobserved random proportionality factor that modifies the hazard function of an individual, or of related individuals (Wienke 2003). The concept of frailty dates back to the work of Greenwood and Yule (1920) on accident proneness and the term itself was introduced by Vaupel et al. (1979). An analysis that ignores frailty if present in data and assumes independence of observations across clusters may result in an underestimation of variances thereby leading to an inflation of the significance of the effects (Goldstein 1991).

Until recently, previous studies involving frailties have focused mainly on models with one level of frailty (Sastry 1997; Sargent 1998). Often, the study data may be composed of more than one level of random effects in which case we have one level nested within the other. A three-level hierarchical Cox model with nested random effects structure was presented by Sastry (1997) with an application to the study of child survival in northeast Brazil, where the children were clustered at both community and family levels.

It is observed that a flexible exploratory analysis that considers spatial variability at a highly disaggregated level of states as considered in this application is lacking in literature especially for Nigeria. Rather, analyses that consider spatial variation at highly aggregated regional (or zonal) level, which conceals local and district specific information are common in literature.

The main focus of this Chapter, therefore, is to examine the demographic factors as well as knowledge about modes of transmission and prevention of HIV/AIDS that may be associated with age at sexual initiation among Nigerian youths (males and females aged 15–24 years). It also aims at investigating the influence of geographical heterogeneity on sexual initiation, taking advantage of structured spatial information at highly disaggregated level of states as well as frailty information due to census blocks and ethnic groups.

The justification for the study is that it will help in identifying geographical areas of increased or decreased risks of early sexual initiation as well as studying the variability in age at first sex among youths aged 15–24 years which are attributable to measured covariates and unobservable heterogeneity.

14.3 Data

The data used for this Chapter was obtained from the 2005 National HIV/AIDS and Reproductive Health Survey (NARHS). It is a nationally representative survey in Nigeria conducted to provide information on the reproductive and sexual health in Nigeria and the factors that influence them. Eligible respondents for the survey were females aged 15–49 years and males aged 15–64 years. One specific objective of NARHS, 2005 is to collect quantitative data on key sexual behaviours and reproductive health indicators among these age groups in Nigeria, and also provide information that will be used to monitor behavioural patterns that may influence HIV/AIDS as well as the impact of reproductive health interventions.

Selection of sample in the survey involved a three-level multistage sampling procedure, employing a probability sampling technique. The first stage involved selection of rural and urban localities from the sampling frame of all the rural and urban localities maintained by the Nigeria National Population Commission. At the second stage, enumeration areas were randomly selected within each locality; and at the third stage, individual respondents were selected within each enumeration area.

The development and management of survey protocol was handled by the technical committee and survey management committee. Ethical approval was granted by the appropriate institutional review board. Consents, both written for the literate respondents and verbal with thumb printing for non-literate respondents were sought from the eligible respondents. As contained in the survey protocol, confidentiality of information provided by the respondents was emphasized and ensured. For detailed description of the survey protocol, see FMOH [Nigeria] (2006).

The survey was undertaken by the Federal Ministry of Health (FMOH) with the Society for Family Health providing technical support in planning, implementation, data processing, analysis and report writing of the survey. The British Department for International Development (DFID) and the United States Agency for International Development (USAID) provided the financial support to undertake this project while the National Population Commission provided assistance in the design of the sampling methodology for the survey.

In the survey questionnaire, question on whether or not the respondents ever had sexual intercourse was asked. The respondent was also asked to give the age at which he/she first had sexual intercourse and this was recorded to the nearest whole year. A respondent who had not initiated sex at the time of survey was right censored at current (survey) age.

For the purpose of the study in this Chapter, data for young respondents, males and females, aged 15–24 years were retrieved from the entire survey data. 4,301 respondents in this age range participated in the survey. These consisted of 2,162 (52.27 %) males and 2,139 (49.73 %) females. Of these, 2,050 (47.75 %) reported ever had sex. 798 (37.0 %) of male respondents ever had sex while 1252 (58.61 %) of the females did. The number of respondents that ever had sex varied across the geopolitical zones. It was highest in the South, where of 940 respondents, 431(45.9 %) have engaged in sexual activities whereas South East recorded the least where only 34 % (183of 528) of the respondents ever had sex. Of 1,512 respondents aged 15–24 years who were urban dwellers, 661 (43.7 %) had initiated sex while 1,389 (49. 0 %) of the 2,781 residing in the rural locations had ever engaged in sex.

14.4 Survival Model with Nested Frailties

One popular model for analyzing continuous survival data is the Cox proportional hazards model (Cox 1972). The hazard function for a given individual describes the instantaneous risk of experiencing an event of interest within an infinitesimally small interval of time, given that the individual has not experienced that event prior to the beginning of the interval. The interesting feature about Cox proportional hazard model is that it does not make any assumption about the shape of the underlying hazards, but rather keeps the baseline hazard as an arbitrary, nonnegative function of time.

We consider that data collected on n respondents are denoted by (t_i, δ_i, Z_i), $i = 1,. . .n$, where t_i is the age at which the ith respondent had sexual initiation, δ_i is the censoring indicator such that $\delta_i = 1$ if the respondent was observed to have initiated sex at time (age) t_i and $\delta_i = 0$ if the respondent has not yet initiated sexual intercourse as at the time of the survey and hence right censored at the current (survey) age. We suppose that Z_i is a vector of covariates (including metrical and categorical) collected on the ith respondent.

For the data used in this study, respondents were sampled from 344 clusters across the country and such cluster information is necessary to assist in capturing heterogeneity in the attitude towards sexual behaviour of Nigerian youth. This is often introduced into the model as a random effect (frailty) ω_g, shared by all members of the cluster g, $g = 1,. . .,344$. Thus in the frailty setting, the classical Cox (1972) proportional hazard model assumes that the hazard function for the ith subject with covariate value Z_i has the form

$$\lambda(t_{ig}\,|Z_{ig}\,,\omega_g) = \omega_g \lambda_o(t)\exp(Z_{ig}^{/}\gamma), \tag{14.1}$$

where $\lambda_o(t)$ is an unspecified baseline hazard function and γ is the vector of regression coefficients.

Suppose the study is composed of G independent clusters indexed by g, and within each cluster g, there are Jg sub-clusters indexed by j, if we consider Cox model with two-level random effects structure as in this study, then conditional on the frailties (random effects) w_{jg} and v_g for sub-cluster j and cluster g respectively, the model of ith individual ($i = 1,\ldots,G_{ij}$), with covariate vector Z_{ijg} in the sub-cluster j ($j = 1,\ldots, J_g$), nested within cluster g ($g = 1,\ldots,G$) can be given by

$$\lambda(t_{ijg}\,|Z_{ijg}\,, w_{jg}, v_g) = w_{jg}v_g\lambda_o(t_{ijg})\exp(Z_{ijg}^{/}\gamma), \tag{14.2}$$

Model in (14.2) is based on assumption that the cluster level frailties v_g are assumed to be independent and identically distributed with $v_g \sim (0,\sigma^2)$ and also that given the cluster level frailties v_g, the sub-cluster random effects w_{jg} are conditionally independent with $w_{jg}|v_g \sim (0,{\sigma_g}^2)$.

For the data used in this chapter, respondents were sampled from 344 clusters based on the urban-rural localities in Nigeria, which is distributed over more than 250 ethnic groups. It is conjectured that analysis of data on the age at sexual initiation of respondents based on independent and identically distributed assumption may be grossly inadequate. In a nested sample, respondents within the same census block or the same ethnic group are more likely to have similar sexual behaviours such that their responses can no longer be treated as independent. Grouping data at the levels of the census blocks (sub-clusters) within ethnic group (cluster) can therefore be described by two- level hierarchical nested random effects (frailties) structure. In the setting, w_{jg} represent the frailties for the census blocks and v_g are for the ethnic groups. Studies of this kind on age at sexual initiation, that incorporate frailties at more than one level is not common in survival analysis literature.

Model (14.2) assumes that effects of covariates (metrical and categorical) are linear on the log hazard and are often modelled parametrically as fixed effects. However, in this study continuous covariate (current age of respondents at survey) is supposed to have a nonlinear effect. Also, classical parametric regression models for analysing data containing geographical information may become unrealistic in estimating small area effects and simultaneously adjusting for other covariates, especially when the effects of some covariates are non-linear or time-varying. In such a situation, a very high number of parameters may be required for modelling purposes; which may result in unstable estimates with high variance (Adebayo and Fahrmeir 2005). For example, the dataset used in this chapter contains 36 states and the Federal Capital Territory (FCT, Abuja) of Nigeria. Therefore model (14.2) was extended to a geo-additive regression model by including the state as a structured spatial covariate so as to adequately explore geographical effects. Geo-additive model allows one to simultaneously incorporate small area spatial effects, non-linear effects of continuous variables as well as the usual linear fixed effects for categorical variables in a unifying model framework. Such models have been used in some studies. For example, Adebayo and Fahrmeir (2005) analyzed data on child mortality in Nigeria using geo-additive discrete-time survival model. In this Chapter, a flexible geo-additive regression model, similar to Kammann and Wand (2003), and developed in Fahrmeir and Lang (2001a), which is an extension of Hastie and Tibshirani (1990) was used under Cox proportional hazards model framework.

Model (14.2), on re-parameterization with inclusion of spatial effects, extending Hennerfeind et al. (2006), may be written as

$$\lambda_i(t) = \exp(\eta_i(t)),$$

with

$$\eta_i(t) = f_o(t) + \sum_{j=1}^{p} f_j(x_{ij}) + f_{spat}(s_i) + Z_i^{/}\gamma + b_{jg} + b_g, \tag{14.3}$$

where $f_o(t) = \log \lambda_o(t_{ijg})$, suppressing the index (ijg), is the log-baseline effect, f_j is the nonlinear function of a continuous covariate x_j, γ is the vector of the usual linear fixed effects, $f_{spat}(s_i)$ is a structured spatial effect of area or state, such as the 36 states of Nigeria plus the Federal Capital Territory where s, $s = 1, \ldots, 37$ is a spatial index, with $s_i = s$ if respondent i is from state s, $b_{jg} = \exp(w_{jg})$ are the sub-cluster specific unstructured random effects (frailties) such as the census block in our data and $b_g = \exp(w_g)$ are the cluster specific frailties such as ethnic group in Nigeria.

The log frailties b_{jg} and b_g are typically assumed to be independent and identically distributed variables from normal distributions (Biggeri et al. 2001).

One practical obstacle to the application of (14.3) has been the lack of available software. However, the Cox survival model with normal frailty can now be fitted in BayesX (Belitz et al. 2009). It is a software for Bayesian Inference in structured Additive Regression Models.

To estimate smooth effect functions and model parameters in (14.3), a fully Bayesian approach, extended from Lang and Brezger (2004) and Brezger and Lang (2006) was used. In Bayesian analysis, the proposed model of the observed data is combined with the prior distributions of all the unknown model parameters and functions. Therefore in (14.3), a diffuse prior $p(\gamma_j) \propto const$ was assigned for fixed effect parameters γ. For the function f_j of continuous covariate x_j, a Bayesian P-splines prior based on Lang and Brezger (2004) which is an extension of Eilers and Marx (1996) was assigned. A spline of degree l can be written in terms of a linear combination of $m = s + l$ B-spline basis functions B_t in which each function f can be approximated through a linear combination

$$f(x) = \sum_{t=1}^{m} \beta_t B_t(x) \tag{14.4}$$

where $\beta = (\beta_{1,}, \ldots \beta_m)$ corresponds to the vector of unknown regression coefficients. Smoothness of function f can be achieved within the Bayesian context by a first or a second order random walk model

$$\beta_t = \beta_{t-1} + u_t,\ \beta_t = 2\beta_{t-1} - \beta_{t-2} + u_t \tag{14.5}$$

for the regression coefficients, with identically distributed Gaussian errors $u_t \sim N(0, \tau^2)$ (see Fahrmeir and Lang 2001b). A first order random walk penalizes abrupt jumps $\beta_t - \beta_{t-1}$ between successive states and a second order random walk penalizes deviations from the linear trend $2\beta_{t-1} - \beta_{t-2}$. The variance τ^2 controls the amount of smoothness of f.

For the structured spatial effects $f_{str}(s)$, the Gaussian Markov random field prior (GMRF), which is common in spatial statistics was chosen, see Besag et al. (1991). This is given as

$$\{f_{str}(s) | f_{str}(t); t \neq s, \tau^2\} \sim N\left(\sum_{t \in \partial_s} \frac{f_{str}(t)}{N_s}, \frac{\tau^2}{N_s}\right), \tag{14.6}$$

where N_s is the number of adjacent sites and $t \in \partial_s$ denotes that site t is a neighbour of site s. Thus the (conditional) mean of $f_{str}(s)$ is an average of function evaluations $f_{str}(t)$ of neighbouring sites t. Again τ^2 controls the amount of spatial smoothness.

A highly dispersed but proper hyper-prior was assigned to the smoothing parameter τ^2 to allows its estimation and for all variance components, an inverse gamma distribution with hyper-parameters a and b was chosen, e.g. $\tau^2 \sim IG(a, b)$. For this study, inverse gamma priors for the variance components with hyperparameters $a = b = 0.001$ were used.

For the unstructured random effects b_{jg} due to the census blocks, independent and identically distributed Gaussian prior, $b_{jg} \sim N(0, \tau_b^2)$ was assigned and $b_g \sim N(0, \tau_e^2)$ assigned for the ethnic group random effects b_g.

Fully Bayesian inference was based on the posterior distribution of the model parameters. Because posterior distribution is numerically intractable in some practical situations involving structured additive regression models, Markov chain Monte Carlo (MCMC) method has been widely used in Bayesian Statistics as a simulation method that allows one to draw random samples from the posterior and approximates joint distributions involving difficult integrals (Manda and Meyer 2005). The algorithm requires that sampling be done from all full conditional posterior distributions of the parameters. Each of the full conditional posterior distributions involves only those terms from the joint posterior distribution that are relevant to the parameter under consideration. In this study therefore, MCMC sampling from full conditionals for nonlinear effects, spatial effects, fixed effects, and smoothing parameters was used for posterior analysis utilizing, the sampling scheme based on iteratively weighted least squares (IWLS) proposals. This is generally designed for responses from an exponential family within which the data used in this chapter fall.

14.5 Data Analysis and Results

14.5.1 Data Analysis

Using the 2005 National HIV/AIDS and Reproductive Health Survey (NARHS), the impacts of some demographic covariates and covariates about the knowledge about HIV/AIDS on age at sexual initiation of Nigerian youths aged 15–24 years were explored. As a result of missing observations in some of the covariates, 4,194 observations were included in the final analysis.

Due to the hierarchical nature of the data, frailty terms were included at two levels (census blocks nested within ethnic groups) to investigate the impact of unmeasured covariates and unobserved heterogeneity on the sexual behaviours of the Nigerian youths.

Analyses were based on the following variables: Outcome variable: Age at sexual initiation (measured in years). The only continuous independent variable included in the analysis is the respondent's age (measured in years) as at the last birthday prior to the survey. All categorical variables were dummy-coded.

Several models, with and without spatial effects were investigated at the exploratory data analysis stage, utilizing various explanatory variables which were thought to be associated with sexual initiation.

Model fit and complexity were compared by examining the distribution of the posterior deviance using Deviance Information criterion (DIC) (Spiegelhalter et al. 2002). The smaller the value of DIC the better the model.

All analyses were carried out using BayesX. To ensure identifiability, BayesX automatically imposes sum-to-zero constraints on the parameters representing the smooth functions f_j's and includes an additional intercept term. This is implemented during the MCMC by subtracting the mean from the current estimate at each iteration (Crook et al. 2003).

Models were run by including demographic independent variables, knowledge variables and combined variables in different analyses. Current age of respondent was dichotomized as "age (15–19)" (reference category) or "age (20–24)". Best model based on DIC was selected for further analyses.

Model Building

M_1: Baseline with fixed effects of the six geopolitical zones with no further covariates

$$\eta = f_o(t) + NE^{/}\gamma_1 + NW^{/}\gamma_2 + SE^{/}\gamma_3 + SW^{/}\gamma_4 + SS^{/}\gamma_5$$

M_2: Baseline, state-specific structured spatial effects with GMRF priors with no further covariates.

$$\eta = f_o(t) + f_{spat}(s)$$

M_3: Baseline, fixed effects of geopolitical zones and fixed effects of combined demographic and knowledge covariates (U)

$$\eta = f_o(t) + NE^{/}\gamma_1 + NW^{/}\gamma_2 + SE^{/}\gamma_3 + SW^{/}\gamma_4 + SS^{/}\gamma_5 + U_i^{/}\gamma$$

M_4: Baseline, state-specific structured spatial effects with GMRF priors and both demographic and knowledge covariates

$$\eta = f_o(t) + f_{spat}(s) + U_i^{/}\gamma$$

M_5: Baseline, state-specific structured spatial effects with GMRF priors and reduced set of bio-demographic and knowledge covariates (V)

$$\eta = f_o(t) + f_{spat}(s) + V_i^{/}\gamma$$

M_6: Same as **M_5** but also with nonlinear effect of age

$$\eta = f_o(t) + f_{spat}(s) + f(age) + V_i^{/}\gamma$$

$\mathbf{M_7}$: Same as $\mathbf{M_6}$ but with census blocks frailties

$$\eta = f_o(t) + f_{spat}(s) + f(age) + V_i^{/}\gamma + b_{jg}$$

$\mathbf{M_8}$: Same as $\mathbf{M_6}$ but with ethnic groups frailties

$$\eta = f_o(t) + f_{spat}(s) + f(age) + V_i^{/}\gamma + b_g$$

$\mathbf{M_9}$: Same as $\mathbf{M_6}$ but with census blocks frailties nested within ethnic groups frailties.

$$\eta = f_o(t) + f_{spat}(s) + f(age) + V_i^{/}\gamma + b_{jg} + b_g$$

where $f_o(t)$ is the log-baseline effect in all the models, γ's are the effects of the usual linear fixed effects of the geopolitical zones, demographic and knowledge covariates; $f_{spat}(s)$ is a structured spatial effect of the 36 states and Federal capital territory with Gaussian Markov Random Field (GMRF) prior.

At the second stage of the analyses, models were first fitted with inclusion of the geographical information as fixed effects of geopolitical zones (M_1) and also as structured spatial effects of states (M_2), both without any further covariate included. More complex models were fitted thereafter by progressively adding covariates. Analyses at the second stage allowed us to closely examine the possible information loss due to concealment of geographic information within the highly aggregated level of geopolitical zone when compared to the less aggregated level of states.

Tables 14.1 and 14.2 present some descriptive information about the covariates included in the analysis and the median age at sexual initiation among males and females aged 15–24 years.

14.5.2 Results

Table 14.3 presents the results of DIC of the selected models from the second stage analyses. It is observed that models without covariates (Models M_1 and M_2) were generally worst in performances with DIC values of 12955.8 and 12911.6 respectively. However, Model M_1 where geographical information were condensed into six geopolitical zone at high level of aggregation performed worse than M_2 which incorporated geographical information as spatial effect of states at less level of aggregation.

Clear improvements were seen when covariates were included. Models M_3 and M_4 were obtained from M_1 and M_2 respectively by including demographic and knowledge covariates. Better performances were observed when M_3 and M_4 were compared with M_1 and M_2, The DIC were M_3 (11856.7) and M_4 (11810.5) respectively.

Table 14.1 Descriptive information about some selected covariates included in the analysis

Indicators/variables	Male (%)	Female (%)	Total (%)
Locality			
Urban	35.9	34.4	35.2
Rural	64.1	65.6	64.8
Education			
Qur'anic	9.6	11.8	10.6
Primary	19.7	20.3	20.0
Secondary	63.2	60.1	61.8
Higher	7.5	7.8	7.6
Region			
North-Central	17.4	17.8	17.6
North-East	16.3	15.3	15.8
North-West	21.0	23.1	22.0
South-West	17.9	16..8	17.4
South-East	11.6	13.0	12.3
South-South	15.8	14.0	14.9
Religion			
Islam	46.6	48.8	47.7
Protestant	37.5	36.0	36.7
Catholic	15.0	14.7	14.8
Traditional	0.9	0.5	0.8
Knowledge about male condom			
Ever heard	80.2	55.0	65.3
Never heard	19.7	44.7	34.3
Age of Respondents			
15–19	41.6	45.5	43.6
20–24	58.4	54.5	56.4
Mean Age (st.dev)	18.7 (2.84)	18.9 (2.87)	18.8 (2.86)
Knowledge of HIV			
Yes	94.8	90.0	92.4
No	5.2	10.0	7.6
Knowledge that a healthy looking person can be HIV positive			
Yes	72.4	67.2	59.6
No	27.6	32.8	40.4
Knowledge of cure for AIDS			
Yes	86.7	83.3	85.0
No	13.3	16.7	15.0
Total	50.3	49.7	100.0

During the second stage analyses some of the demographic and knowledge covariates were found not to be significant and were removed from further analyses and this resulted in the reduced model M_5. Model M_6 was obtained from M_5 by the inclusion of nonlinear effect of age. This was aimed at exploring whether

Table 14.2 Median age at first sex among youth 15–24 years

	Male (%)	Female (%)
Locality		
Rural	20.3	17.1
Urban	19.8	17.8
Region		
North-Central	19.0	17.6
North-East	22.7	17.6
North-West	23.8	15.5
South-East	19.6	20.2
South-South	19.3	17.8
South-West	19.2	17.8
Total	**20.1**	**17.4**

Source: FMOH [Nigeria] (2006, p. 22)

Table 14.3 Model comparison based on the deviance information criterion (DIC)

Model	Model description	pD	DIC
M1	$\eta = f_o(t) + NE^{/}\gamma_1 + NW^{/}\gamma_2 + SE^{/}\gamma_3 + SW^{/}\gamma_4 + SS^{/}\gamma_5$	15.2	12955.8
M2	$\eta = f_o(t) + f_{spat}(s)$	38.1	12911.6
M3	$\eta = f_o(t) + NE^{/}\gamma_1 + NW^{/}\gamma_2 + SE^{/}\gamma_3 + SW^{/}\gamma_4 + SS^{/}\gamma_5 + W_i^{/}\gamma$	49.9	11856.7
M4	$\eta = f_o(t) + f_{spat}(s) + W_i^{/}\gamma$	47.4	11810.5
M5	$\eta = f_o(t) + f_{spat}(s) + V_i^{/}\gamma$	46.5	11804.7
M6	$\eta = f_o(t) + f_{spat}(s) + f(age) + V_i^{/}\gamma$	49.4	11758.3
M7	$\eta = f_o(t) + f_{spat}(s) + b_g$	140.8	11743.3
M8	$\eta = f_o(t) + f_{spat}(s) + f(age) + V_i^{/}\gamma + b_g$	104.6	11757.9
M9	$\eta = f_o(t) + f_{spat}(s) + f(age) + V_i^{/}\gamma + b_{jg} + b_g$	103.5	11723.5

considering nonlinear effect of age will result in a more appropriate model. Models M_7 and M_8 included frailty components of census blocks and ethnic groups respectively in separate analyses and Model M_9 included census blocks frailty nested within that of ethnic group. It was observed that model M_9 performed best of all the models considered in this study. Therefore, discussion of results for all components of the model is based on model M_9.

Results of Fixed Effects

Table 14.4 presents the posterior estimates (means) of the fixed effect parameters in model M_9 along with the standard errors, hazard ratios and 95 % credible intervals. The results show significant gender differentials of age at sexual initiation. Females were more likely to initiate sexual activities earlier than their male counterparts, (hazards ratio of male to that of female is 0.690). As observed, respondents in the

Table 14.4 Posterior estimates of the fixed effects of Bio-demographic covariates Model M9

Variable	Coefficient	Std. error	2.5 %	97.5 %	Hazard ratio	2.5 %	97.5 %
Male	−0.373	0.051	−0.474	−0.269	0.689	0.623	0.764
Age (20–24)	−0.228	0.137	−0.514	−0.198	0.793	0.598	0.820
Primary	−0.525	0.080	−0.686	−0.369	0.592	0.504	0.691
Secondary	−0.432	0.075	−0.576	−0.274	0.649	0.562	0.760
Higher edu.	−0.542	0.106	−0.743	−0.332	0.582	0.476	0.717
Urban	−0.207	0.063	−0.334	−0.081	0.813	0.716	0.922
Singles	−1.187	0.058	−1.303	−1.077	0.305	0.272	0.341
Ever heard of AIDS	0.012	0.112	−0.207	0.251	1.012	0.813	1.285
Knew one who died of AIDS	0.049	0.087	−0.125	0.214	1.050	0.882	1.239
Knew correct of modes of HIV transmission	−0.144	0.057	−0.248	−0.032	0.866	0.780	0.969
Healthy looking person can be HIV positive	0.143	0.058	0.029	0.253	1.154	1.029	1.288
Variance of random effects							
Model M7	0.058	0.020					
Model M8	0.014	0.015					
Model M9 (census blocks)	0.044	0.018					
Model (Ethnic group)	0.014	0.016					

cohort of age group 15–19 years initiated sexual activity earlier than those in age group 20–24 years. On level of educational attainment, respondents with higher education were less likely to initiate sexual activities at younger age than their counterparts with no formal education. Muslims, Protestant and Catholic youth were more likely to delay sexual debut than those belonging to other or no religions. Results also show that respondents living in urban areas were likely to initiate sexual activities later than those living in the rural areas. Ever heard of diseases that can be transmitted through sexual intercourse (STIs) lowered the risk of early sexual initiation than those who never heard of it. Also, respondents who never heard of AIDS were likely to initiate sex earlier than those who have heard of it. Respondents with correct knowledge of mode of HIV transmission were likely to delay sexual initiation compared with those with incorrect knowledge.

Results of Spatial Effects

Map of Nigeria showing the 36 states and the Federal Capital Territory is shown in Fig. 14.1. Results of spatial effects for models M_2 and M_9 are presented in Fig. 14.2. Shown are the posterior means (a) and (c) with the 95 % posterior probabilities

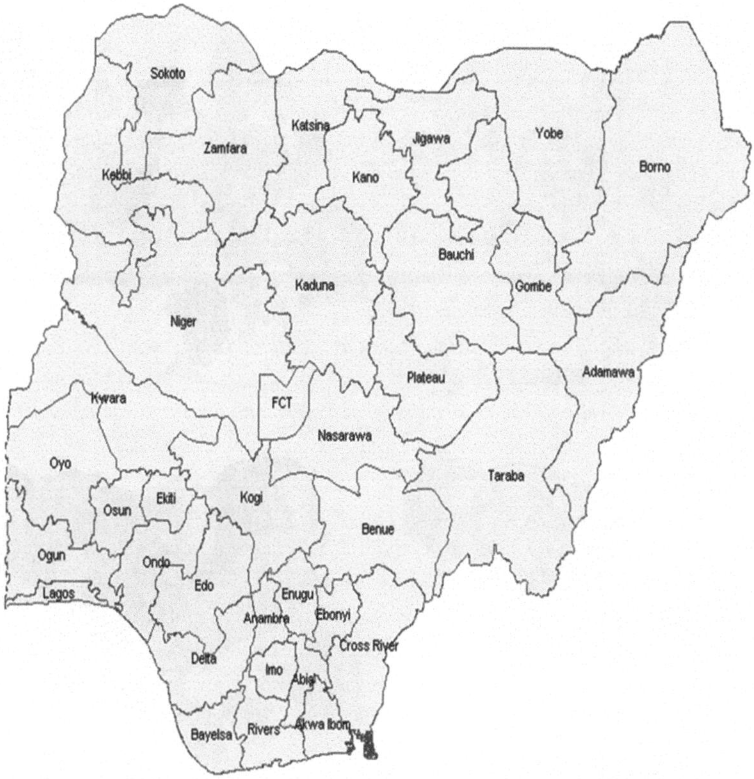

Fig. 14.1 Map of Nigeria showing 36 states and the Federal Capital Territory

of spatial effects (b) and (d). It is evident that there exist geographical variations at state level on age at sexual initiation in Nigeria. From the maps of posterior probabilities (b) and (d), states with black colours are associated with negatively significant spatial effects implying that early sexual initiation was experienced in those states. States with white colours were associated with positively significant spatial effects implying that respondents in those states are likely to delay sexual initiation. However, the spatial effects in states with grey colour are not significant, implying that the credible intervals include zero (0).

Regarding the impact of relevant covariates in this model, it is clearly observed that when no other covariates were controlled for (model M_2), as presented in the upper panel (b), early sexual initiation was prominent in Abia, Anambra, Borno, Ebonyi, Enugu, Imo, Kano and Plateau states. On the other hand, states associated with significant delayed sexual debut include Bayelsa, Cross-River, Delta, Jigawa, Katsina, Kebbi, Kwara, Ondo and Rivers. Model M_9 explored net-effect of spatial variations in age at sexual initiations after controlling for other covariates. Results are shown in (c) and (d) at the lower panel of Fig. 14.2. Evidently, significant spatial variations of state of residence of the respondents were observed. Furthermore, a clearly North – South divide was noticed with respondents in the North being

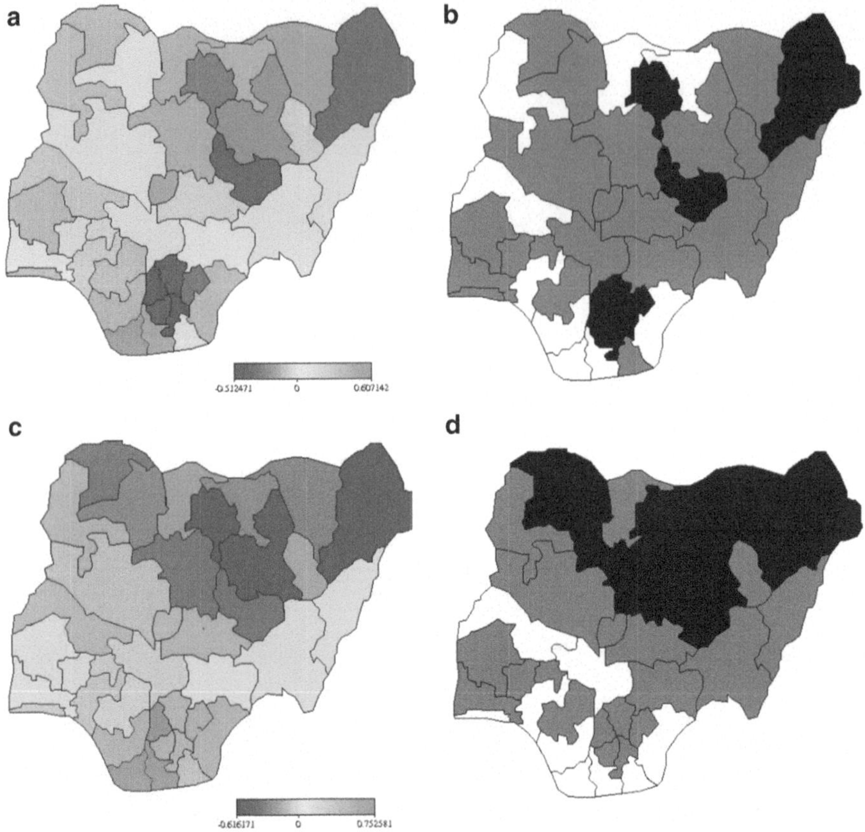

Fig. 14.2 (**a**) Spatial effects of states on age at sexual initiation and (**b**) 95% credible interval for posterior probabilities for model M_2 (*upper panels*) and (**c**) Spatial effects of states on age at sexual initiation and (**d**) 95% credible interval posterior probabilities model M_9 (*lower panels*)

associated with early initiation of sexual debut while their counterparts in the South were found to be associated with delayed sexual debut. For instance, respondents in Jigawa and Katsina states that were associated with delayed sexual initiation and respondents in Sokoto, Zamfara, Yobe and Kaduna where spatial effect were non-significant when no further covariates were adjusted (model M_2); were observed to be associated with early sexual initiation when covariates were controlled. In a similar manner, the early sexual initiation that was evident in Abia, Anambra, Ebonyi, Enugu, and Imo states when no further covariates were controlled for; disappear after controlling for other covariates.

Non-Linear Effects

Figure 14.3 shows the non-linear effects of the baseline $f_o(t)$ of age at sexual initiation (left panel) and current age of the respondents (right panel). It is clearly

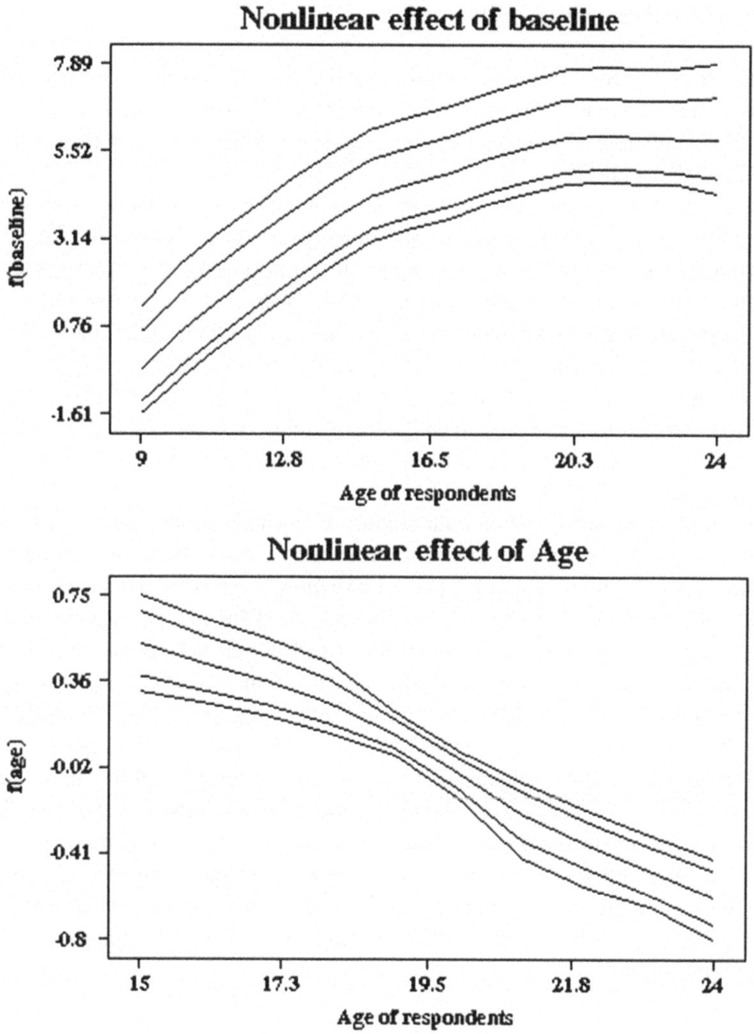

Fig. 14.3 Non-linear effects of baseline and respondents' age

observed from the Figure that the relationship between age at first sex and current age of the respondent is non-linear. This has provided us with an insight into the functional pattern of the respondent's age in relation to age at sexual debut. With this, considering age as a linear effect would have resulted in spurious and unreliable conclusion. An approximately inverse U-shape feature is evident. This implies that most of the respondents aged 20 years have had their first sexual experience.

Results of Analysis with Frailty

Prior to the inclusion of frailty components in the models, Model M_6 which included geographical information as structured spatial effects with GMRF priors in the model and with reduced set of demographic and knowledge covariates was best in terms of DIC (11758.3).

Frailty components due to census blocks, ethnic group and census blocks nested within ethnic group were included in Model M_6 to produce Models M_7, M_8 and M_9 respectively. This enables us see the impact of frailty (unobserved heterogeneity) in the data. The results are presented in Table 14.3 with their respective DIC values. It is observed that model M_7 with census blocks frailty incorporated had a better fit (DIC of 11743.4) than model M_6 which controlled for only structured spatial effects of states. However, incorporation of only random effects (frailty) due to ethnic group (M_8) did not make appreciable impact on the model fit (DIC = 11757.9 vs. 11758.3). Fitting the model with nested frailties is observed from the table to have the overall best performance with DIC of 11723.5.

The implication is that when data contain identified clusters, analyses that take clustering information into consideration through random effect, in addition to the structured spatial effect is capable of providing more robust estimates than those that ignore it. From Table 14.4, census blocks accounted for more frailty (unobserved heterogeneity) in the data than ethnic group. As observed, when only census blocks frailty was incorporated (Model M_7), the frailty variance was 0.058 (standard error 0.020). However, when only ethnic group frailty was incorporated (Model M_8), the frailty variance was 0.014 (standard error 0.015). There were slight reductions in variances of frailties when census blocks were nested within ethnic groups (Model M_9). The variances were 0.044 (standard error 0.018) and 0.014 (standard error 0.016) for census blocks and ethnic groups respectively. The implication of this is that the observations within the census blocks were more correlated than those within the ethnic groups. The between-cluster differences in these models could be due to either the observed individual or normative factors or to other unmeasured community factors.

14.6 Sensitivity Analysis

Sensitivity to the choice of hyper-parameters *a* and *b* was also investigated in this study. Various values of hyperparameters *a* and *b* were set for models with GMRF priors. These include IG(1*e*–03, 1*e*–03) (default in BayesX), IG(1*e*–05, 1*e*–05) and IG(1*e*–08, 1*e*–08). The performances were evaluated based on mixing and convergence. The results are presented in Fig. 14.4. It is observed that the models were not sensitive to the choice of priors and hyper-priors.

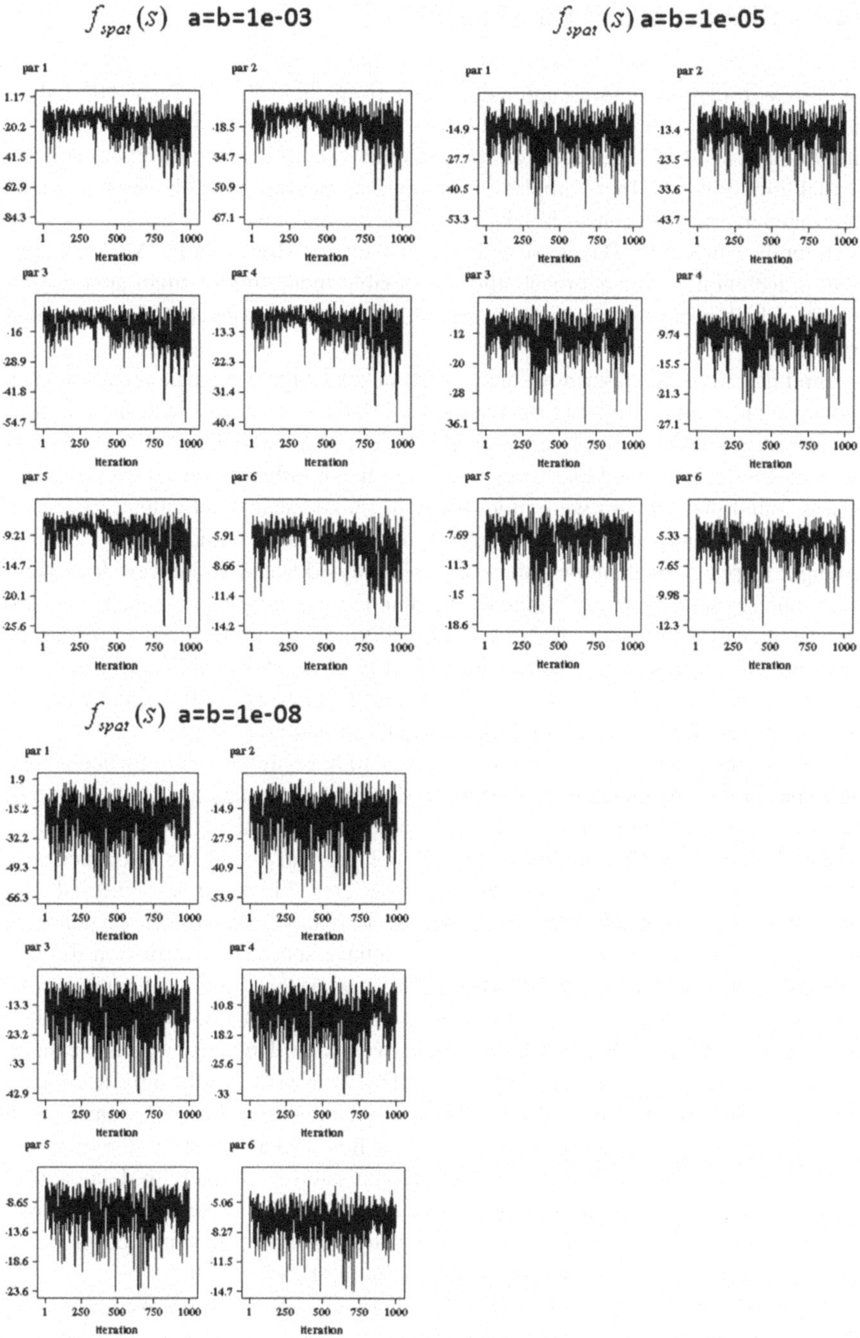

Fig. 14.4 Selected sampling paths for structured spatial effects and different choices for the parameters a and b of the IG(a, b) hyperpriors for GMRF priors

14.7 Discussion and Conclusions

A nested frailty model was applied to data from the 2005 National HIV/AIDS and Reproductive Health Survey (NARHS) on age at sexual initiation for males and females aged 15–24. This presented an extension to existing frailty models for sexual initiation data. In its simplest form, it was a two-level model, which included heterogeneity on both census blocks and ethnic groups' levels.

Inference was fully Bayesian with Markov Chain Monte Carlo (MCMC) simulation techniques. The approach allowed flexible modelling of small area district effects, which is of great advantage compared to the usual parametric and frequentist approach.

Findings from the descriptive analysis revealed a higher median age at first sex among male youth (implying delayed sexual debut) compared with their female counterparts. Furthermore, a rural-urban differential in median age at first sex was evident. Findings showed that gender had significant influence on sexual initiation. It was found that females were more likely to initiate sexual activities earlier than their male counterparts. Early sexual initiation was also found in the cohort of younger respondents than the older cohort. Highly educated youth were less likely to initiate sexual activities at younger age than the non-educated. These results are consistent with the results of Agha et al. (2006). The implication is that, policy towards 'education for all' indirectly resulted in delayed sexual debut. Therefore, policy makers should look at the issue of ensuring that every youth is empowered to be educated in that this can compliment sexual reproductive health and rights.

Though religious affiliation does not appear to have significant influence on age at sexual initiation, respondents who were Muslims, Protestant and Catholic members were observed to have reported late sexual initiation than those belonging to other religion or no religion. Respondents living in urban areas were associated with delayed sexual debut compared to the rural dwellers. This might be connected with their exposure to education relating to sexual activities. Furthermore, respondents living in urban areas were also more likely to have access to information through various media such as radio, television and newspapers on sexual reproductive health and right than those in rural areas. Such information may be through campaigns on HIV/AIDs and other reproductive health. Knowledge about sexually transmitted infection including HIV and AIDS were also significantly associated with delayed sexual debut. Correct knowledge of modes of HIV transmission were significant factors associated with age at first sexual initiation. Respondents with correct knowledge of mode of HIV transmission were likely to delay sexual initiation compared with those with incorrect knowledge. Therefore, government, policy makers and donors should strive towards ensuring universal coverage of information on sexual reproductive health including HIV and AIDS.

Regional variation was also noticed with females from North-West reporting the lowest age at first sex compared to their counterparts from other geopolitical zones. With the incorporation of spatial effects, rather than concluding that respondents from the entire South-West and South-South have delayed sexual initiation compared to those in the North-Central, which may conceal some useful information, exploration of spatial effect at a highly disaggregated level of state will avail researcher opportunity to identify states associated with early sexual initiation compared with those associated with delayed sexual debut. Through this, policy makers and donors can prioritize the use of available scarce resources in a more prudent way. Again, with findings on National Educational survey showing that states in the North are associated with lower educational attainment especially among females in the North (NPC [Nigeria] and RTI International 2011). Coupled with early sexual initiation among females in the North, this provides some explanation for the early sexual initiation in those States. Lower educational attainment that is evident among northern women is also known to be a determinant factor to early marriage (also more prevalent in the North) is also a confounder to early sexual initiation (Manda and Meyer 2005). From the analysis in this chapter, most of the states associated with early sexual initiation are in the North-East and North-West of Nigeria. This may be connected with the socio-cultural background and religious belief which encourage early marriage. The predominant religion in these parts of the country is Islam. A common view among Muslims in Nigeria is that if a female child matures under the parent's roof, there is likelihood that she will engage in premarital sexual activities and this is against Islamic doctrine. This therefore, possibly resulted in early marriage with majority having no formal education. Findings from a similar national survey on Education Data for Decision-Making (National Population Commission [Nigeria] and ORC Macro 2004) revealed that about 30 % of youth age 15–24 years have no formal education. Furthermore, more than half of the male respondents from the North-West (52.7 %) and North-East (50.7 %) had no formal education compared with their counterparts in the North-Central (22.3 %), South-East (11.5 %), South-South (7.1 %) and South-West (14.1 %). The trend is similar for females with about 78.1 % in North-West and 72.8 % in North-East without formal education. This development might possibly suggest a higher tendency for early marriage with attendant early sexual initiation in these regions.

Analyses in this Chapter have also helped to clearly discern states within a geographical region with similar socio-cultural background that are associated with early sexual initiation rather than assuming that early or delayed sexual debut is related to the whole region. Findings from the spatial analysis showed that states such as Kwara, Ondo, Kebbi were associated with delayed sexual initiation while Borno, Bauchi, Anambra states were associated with early sexual initiation. Besides the spatial effect, this analysis has allowed control for unobserved heterogeneity at cluster level. This has assisted in accounting for the effect of some unobserved covariates.

One benefit of this modelling technique is that controlling for clustering invalidates the wrong independent and identical assumption often being made regarding survival time observations that are clustered. Two levels of frailty, census blocks and ethnic groups were incorporated separately as well as census blocks nested within ethnic groups. Model that accounted for unobserved heterogeneity due to census blocks was observed to be more adequate than the ones that ignored it, while ethnic group did not seem to provide obvious frailty information in the data. The insignificant impact of the random effect of ethnic group might be due to the aggregation of ethnic groups in Nigeria into 23 in which case some differences due to ethnicity were possibly coarsened. However, model that included census blocks nested within ethnic groups was superior to all other models in terms of DIC. Promoting delayed sexual initiation among young people is an important component of the 'ABC' of HIV and AIDS prevention strategies, especially for youth in the countries with generalised epidemics of the virus as in Nigeria. Sexual abstinence serves as a protection against HIV infection as well as forestalling unwanted pregnancies among youth. The Ugandan experience (where incidence rates of HIV among youth have consistently dropped over the years) is a clear example of the success of abstinence and delayed sexual debut among youth in reducing the incidence of both unwanted pregnancies as well as HIV infections (Hogle 2002). It is, therefore, believed that if an abstinence campaign is mounted to equip young people with information, motivation and behavioural skills needed to abstain as well as social support to do so, young people will abstain or at least delay sexual debut.

It is expected that findings from this study will better assist authorities and policy makers in various states of Nigeria to have a deeper understanding of what happens in their states while planning and designing HIV prevention interventions. Based on these, appropriate policies on interventions can be formulated and strategies to address issues related to the delay of sexual debut can then be developed.

This Chapter is also expected to assist policymakers in appropriate targeting and prioritization of interventions. This will enhance an effective utilisation of scarce resources, which is predominant in developing countries like Nigeria. Furthermore, possible dialogues and consultations with parents, opinion leaders, religious leaders, community leaders as well as traditional heads/rulers will go a long way to assist in the effective and proper integration of life building and negotiation skills into the educational curriculum in states where earlier sexual debut is prevalent.

References

Adebayo, S. B., & Fahrmeir, L. (2005). Analyzing child mortality in Nigeria with Geoadditive discrete-time survival models. *Statistics in Medicine, 24*, 709–728.

Agha, S., van Rossem, R., & Ankomah, A. (2006). Community level influences on primary abstinence in Nigeria. *DHS working paper.*

Andersson-Ellstrom, A., Forssman, L., & Milsom, I. (1996). Age of sexual debut related to life-style and reproductive health factors in a group of Swedish teenage girls. *Acta Obstetricia et Gynecologica Scandinavica, 75*(5), 484–489.

Belitz, C., Brezger, A., Kneib, T., & Lang, S. (2009). *BayesX: Software for bayesian inference in structured and additive regression models. Version 2.1.* http://www.stat.uni-muenchen.de/~bayesx

Besag, J., York, Y., & Mollie, A. (1991). Bayesian Image restoration with two applications in spatial statistics (with discussion). *Annals of the Institute of Statistical Mathematics, 43*, 1–59.

Biggeri, L., Bini, M., & Grilli, L. (2001). The transition from university to work: A multilevel approach to the analysis of the time to obtain the first job. *Journal of the Royal Statistical Society A, 164*, 293–305.

Brewster, K. L. (1994). Neighborhood context and the transition to sexual activity among young Black women. *Demography, 31*, 603–614.

Brezger, A., & Lang, S. (2006). Generalized Structured Additive Regression based on Bayesian P-splines. *Computational Statistics and Data Analysis, 50*, 967–991.

Chiao,C., & Mishra,V. (2007). Trends in primary and secondary abstinence among kenyan youth. *DHS working paper* 36.

Coleman, J. (1988). Social capital in the creation of human capital. *The American Journal of Sociology, 94*(Suppl), S94–S120.

Cooper, D., Hoffman, M., Carrara, H., Rosenberg, L., Kelly, J., Stander, I., Denny, L., Williamson, A., & Shapiro, S. (2007). Determinants of sexual activity and its relation to cervical cancer risk among South African Women. *BMC Public Health, 7*, 341. doi:10.1186/1471-2458-7-341.

Cox, D. R. (1972). Regression models and life tables (with discussions). *Journal of the Royal Statistical Society, B, 34*, 187–220.

Crook, A. M., Knorr-Held, L., & Hemingway, H. (2003). Measuring spatial effects in time to event data: A case study using months from angiography to coronary artery bypass graft (CABG). *Statistics in Medicine, 22*, 2943–2961. doi:10.1002/sim.1535.

Dickson, N., Paul, C., Herbison, P., & Silva, P. (1998). First sexual intercourse: Age, coercion and later regrets reported by a birth cohort. *British Medical Journal, 316*, 29–33.

Eilers, P. H. C., & Marx, D. B. (1996). Flexible smoothing with B-Splines and penalties. *Statistical Science, 11*(2), 89–121.

Fahrmeir, L., & Lang, S. (2001a). Bayesian inference for generalized additive mixed models based on Markov Random field priors. *Applied Statistics, 50*(2), 201–220.

Fahrmeir, L., & Lang, S. (2001b). Bayesian semiparametric regression analysis of multicategorical time-space data. *Annals of the Institute of Statistical Mathematics, 52*(1), 1–18.

Fatusi, A. O., & Blum, R. W. (2008). Predictors of early sexual initiation among a nationally representative sample of Nigerian adolescents. *BMC Public Health, 8*, 136.

Federal Ministry of Health [Nigeria]. (2006). *National HIV/AIDS & Reproductive Health Survey (NARHS), 2005*. Abuja: Federal Ministry of Health.

Garcia-Calleja, J. M., Gouws, E., & Ghys, P. D. (2006). National population based HIV prevalence surveys in sub-Saharan Africa: Results and implications for HIV and AIDS estimates. *Sexually Transmitted Infections, 82*(Suppl 3), 64–70.

Goldstein, H. (1991). Multilevel modelling of survey data. *Statistician, 40*, 235–244.

Greenwood, M., & Yule, G. U. (1920). An inquiry into the nature of frequency distributions representative of multiple happenings with particular reference to the occurrence of multiple attacks of disease or of repeated accidents. *Journal of the Royal Statistical Society, 83*, 255–279.

Harrison, A., Cleland, J., Gouws, E., & Frohlich, J. (2005). Early sexual debut among young men in rural South Africa: Heightened vulnerability to sexual risk? *Sexually Transmitted Infection, 81*, 259–261.

Hastie, T., & Tibshirani, R. (1990). *Generalized additive models*. London: Chapman and Hall.

Hennerfeind, A., Brezger, A., & Fahrmeir, L. (2006). Geoadditive survival models. *Journal of the American Statistical Association, 101*, 1065–1075.

Hogle, J. M. (2002). Poliovirus cell entry: Common structural themes in viral cell entry pathways. *Annual Review of Microbiology, 56*, 677–702.

Kammann, E. E., & Wand, M. P. (2003). Geoadditive models. *Journal of the Royal Statistical Society, C, 52*, 1–18.

Kinsman, S. B., Roma, D., Furstenberg, F. F., & Schwarz, D. F. (1998). Early sexual initiation: The role of peer norms. *Paediatrics, 102*(5), 1185–1192.

Lang, S., & Brezger, A. (2004). Bayesian P-splines. *Journal of Computational and Graphical Statistics, 13*, 183–212.

Manda, S., & Meyer, R. (2005). Age at first marriage: A Bayesian multilevel analysis using a discrete time-to-event model. *Journal of the Royal Statistical Society, A, 168*(2), 439–455.

Mishra, V., Vaessen, M., Boerma, J. T., Arnold, F., Way, A., Barrère, B., Cross, A., Hong, R., & Sangha, J. (2006). HIV testing in national population-based surveys: Experience from the demographic and health surveys. *Bulletin of the World Health Organization, 84*(7), 537–545.

National Population Commission [Nigeria] and ORC Macro. (2004). *Nigeria demographic and health survey 2003*. Calverton: Maryland National Population Commission and ORC/Macro.

National Population Commission [Nigeria] and RTI International. (2011). *Nigeria Demographic and Health Survey (DHS) EdData Profile 1990, 2003 and 2008: Edication data for decision making, 2011*. Washington, DC: National Population Commission and RTI International.

Pettifor, A. E., Rees, H. V., Kleinschmidt, I., Steffenson, A. E., MacPhail, C., Hlongwa-Madikizela, L., Vermaak, K., & Padian, N. S. (2005). Young people's sexual health in South Africa: HIV prevalence and sexual behaviours from a nationally representative household survey. *AIDS, 19*, 1525–1534.

Rink, E., Tricker, R., & Harvey, S. M. (2007). Onset of sexual intercourse among female adolescents: The influence of perceptions, depression and ecological factors. *The Journal of Adolescent Health, 41*(4), 398–406.

Sargent, D. J. (1998). A general framework for random effects survival analysis in the Cox proportional hazards setting. *Biometrics, 54*, 1486–1497.

Sastry, N. (1997). A nested frailty model for survival data, with an application to the study of child survival in northeast *Brazil. Journal of the American Statistical Association, 92*, 426–435.

Spiegelhalter, D. J., Best, N. G., Carlin, B. P., & van der Linde, A. (2002). Bayesian measures of model complexity and fit (with discussion). *Journal of the Royal Statistical Society, B, 64*, 583–640.

Vaupel, J. W., Manton, K. G., & Stallard, E. (1979). The impact of heterogeneity in individual frailty on the dynamics of mortality. *Demography, 16*, 439–454.

Wienke, A. (2003). A simulation study of different correlated frailty models and estimation strategies. Max Planck Institut für demografische Forschung, *Working paper* 2003–018. www.demogr.mpg.de

Zaba, B., Pisani, E., Slaymaker, E., & Ties Boerma, J. (2004). Age at first sex: Understanding recent trends in African demographic surveys. *Sexually Transmitted Infections, 80*, 28–35.

Chapter 15
Assessing Geographic Co-morbidity Associated with Vascular Diseases in South Africa: A Joint Bayesian Modeling Approach

Ngianga-Bakwin Kandala, Samuel O.M. Manda, and William Tigbe

15.1 Introduction

The growing incidence of chronic conditions associated with changing lifestyles is creating new challenges for African countries; most of which are struggling with widespread infectious diseases. The dangers of infectious diseases such as malaria, HIV/AIDS and tuberculosis in Africa are well-known. However, the growing public health problems associated with lifestyle and chronic diseases such as heart disease, stroke, obesity, diabetes, cancer, as well as those associated with smoking, alcohol and drug abuse are not widely recognised. Changing lifestyles and dietary patterns, declining levels of physical activity and an increasingly long-lived population all play a role as African countries move through stages of nutritional and epidemiologic transitions (Mensah 2008). The shift from infectious to chronic diseases is accelerating: it's projected that by 2020, chronic diseases will account for almost three-quarters of all deaths worldwide and that 60 % of the burden of chronic diseases will occur in developing countries (WHO 2011).

In particular, stroke and high blood pressure are major causes of death and disability worldwide. Although comprehensive stroke surveillance data for Africa are lacking, the available data show that age-standardised mortality, case fatality

N.-B. Kandala (✉)
Warwick Medical School, Division of Health Sciences, University of Warwick, Coventry, UK
e-mail: n-b.kandala@warwick.ac.uk

S.O.M. Manda
Biostatistics Unit, South African Medical Research Council, Pretoria, South Africa
e-mail: Samuel.Manda@mrc.ac.za

W. Tigbe
Warwick Medical School, Division of Health Sciences, University of Warwick, Gibbet Hill Campus, CV4 7AL, Coventry, UK

N.-B. Kandala and G. Ghilagaber (eds.), *Advanced Techniques for Modelling Maternal and Child Health in Africa*, The Springer Series on Demographic Methods and Population Analysis 34, DOI 10.1007/978-94-007-6778-2_15,

and prevalence of disabling stroke in Africa are similar to or higher than in most high-income regions. In Africa, more than 90 % of patients with haemorrhagic stroke and more than half with ischaemic stroke are found to have high blood pressure (Mensah 2008). Likewise, awareness of hypertension and its prevention, treatment and control remain very low in Africa even though recent surveys show an increasing prevalence of the disease consistent with the nutritional and epidemiological transition in the region. Renewed emphasis on improved surveillance and the prevention and control of high blood pressure and stroke in Africa is needed.

However, despite the growing incidence of chronic diseases, infectious diseases show no signs of abating. Despite the success of vaccination programmes for polio among others, HIV/AIDS, tuberculosis and malaria remain prevalent and difficult to control. More than 95 % of deaths due to infectious diseases, most of which are preventable, occur in the developing world (Brenzel et al. 2006). During the next 20–30 years, these diseases will continue to burden major parts of the population, while emerging diseases such as SARS, Ebola and avian flu as well as antibiotic resistant strains of already known bacteria will also play a major role in Africa. The combined threat of chronic and infectious diseases is creating a "double burden of disease" on developing nations, which needs a joint urgent action by scientists and governments to try to tackle the burden.

The complex interactions between chronic and infectious diseases, such as the relationship between diabetes and tuberculosis, for instance, are the subject of increasing study. On the other hand the interactions between chronic diseases, such as hypertension, stroke, heart attacks and high blood cholesterol are not well documented as well as their interplay with environmental and lifestyle factors. Various ways of tackling these interactions are being identified. Preventive actions and good management are obviously major priority concerns, given the myriad health risks associated with chronic diseases. Investment in research is another priority, as are campaigns aimed at encouraging healthy and active lifestyles. Collaborations between public, private and voluntary organisations are ways forward, given the fact that most public health funds are devoted to tackling the ravages of infectious diseases. Most importantly, however, government health policy and infrastructure must ensure that all African populations enjoy sufficient nutrition and decent levels of healthcare and that all are made aware of the benefits and dangers of the populations' ever changing lifestyle choices.

Co-morbidity between vascular conditions such as hypertension, heart attacks or angina, stroke and high blood cholesterol is common in Sub-Saharan Africa. However, little is known about environmental and geographic overlaps in these illnesses. The overlapping epidemiology and aetiology of the diseases may be improved by pooling data across the diseases in a unified way using joint spatial modelling. We use recently developed multivariate spatial disease models to analyse more than one vascular disease simultaneously. These models allows for quantification of correlation structures between relative risks of related diseases as well as enabling common and disease-specific observed covariate effects and spatial patterns at the same time (Langford et al. 1999; Knorr-Held and Best 2001; Dabney and Wakefield 2005). Thus, joint spatial models have both substantive and methodological advantages over a univariate spatial model considered in Chap. 11 for an analysis of high blood pressure in South Africa. These joint mapping models have been used to model and estimate risks of related cancers (Held et al. 2005; Downing et al. 2008), childhood illnesses (Kazembe et al. 2007) and childhood cancer and diabetes (Manda et al. 2009).

In order to estimate spatial similarities and differences in the risk of four vascular diseases, high blood pressure, heart attack, stroke and high blood cholesterol in South Africa, we modelled and fitted a shared component model which jointly analyses spatial variations of two or more diseases (Knorr and Best, Dabney). The model fits common and uncommon risk factors where the risks for different diseases are described by log-odds model on binary responses pertaining to disease status at the subject level. The log odds are linearly modelled using the effects of individual confounding variables (gender, age, ethnicity, education, place of residence, co-morbidity as measure by body mass index (BMI) and lifestyle factors measured by smoking and alcohol drinking) and district-level spatial random effects. The resulting spatial residuals of risks are decomposed into shared (common to all vascular diseases) and disease-specific structured spatial random terms. Additionally, we allowed for unstructured unshared spatial terms to account for any extra binomial variation. The common and disease-specific spatially structured effects are considered as latent variables denoting common and disease-specific risk factors operating at the district level.

We present this model in the context for an analysis for co-morbidity of four vascular diseases; high blood pressure, heart attack or angina, stroke and high blood cholesterol in South Africa We considered the adult health data from the 1998 South African Health and Demographic Survey (Department of Health 2002), but aggregated to the current 52 health districts in the country. All these vascular diseases are known to share unhealthy diet as a common risk factor. Nonetheless, in this paper, we investigate the possibility of other different risk factors for these diseases, or even the presence of an interaction effect but with different spatial patterns. By applying the joint spatial modelling approach, the aims of this chapter are four-fold: (1) describing the geographic pattern of hypertension, heart attack or angina, stroke and high blood cholesterol at sub-district level in South Africa; (2) assessing the influence of vascular severity, adjusting for confounding individual-level covariates; (3) estimating the correlation between diseases at sub-district level; and (4) investigating common and disease-specific covariate effects and spatial patterns of observed and unobserved risks.

15.2 Methods

15.2.1 Individual-Level Data

South African Demographic and Health Survey (SADHS) used a stratified sample of 972 enumeration areas (EAs) at the first stage sampling. For a second stage sampling, a systematic sample of households was undertaken within each of the selected EAs, and in total 12,860 household were selected. Data collection was done using five questionnaires of which the adult health questionnaire was applied to all adults in every alternate household. The adult questionnaire collected information on adult health conditions using questions about risk factors, self-reported chronic conditions and heath service utilisation. Additionally, anthropometric and blood pressure measurements were done (Department of Health 2002). The adult health information has been instrumental in identifying new directions for the national and provincial health programmes in the country. Prevalence and treatment of chronic health conditions are crucial indicators in evaluating policies and programmes and in making projections for the future. As part of the larger international Demographic and Health Surveys programme, the health data collected contributes to a global commitment to improving lives worldwide.

We used a number of individual variables: The exposure variable investigated is the respondent geographic location (province of residence) in addition to various control variables on socio-demographic, lifestyle and co-morbidity factors known to be associated with vascular diseases. The respondent's age at the time of survey was included as an indicator of birth cohort of the participant. Other predictor variables included were socio-demographic factors such as gender, ethnicity (black/African vs. coloured, white and Asian/Indian), and education of the respondent (no education vs. Primary, secondary and higher education), and body mass index (BMI) (normal vs. underweight, overweight/obese); two lifestyle factors; smoking (non-current smoker vs. current smoker), drinking status (non-current alcohol vs. current alcohol drinker), and finally place of residence (rural vs. urban) as an environmental factor. A total of 13, 827 adults (aged 15 years or above) provided health information, of which 1,930 (13.96 %), 630 (4.56 %), 136 (0.98 %) and 173 (1.25 %) were high blood pressure, heart attack or angina, stroke and high blood cholesterol cases, respectively. The potential risk factors for these four vascular diseases available from the data are presented in Table 15.1. A majority of the sampled adult were females (58.4 %) and were, as expected of black/African origin. The mean age was 38.54 years a standard deviation of 17.90 years; about 43 % were overweight or obese. There were 25 % and 28 % current smokers and alcohol drinkers in the sample (Table 15.1).

15.2.2 Health District Level Data

An overriding objective of this study was to model jointly the prevalence rates of four vascular diseases: high blood pressure, heart attack or angina, stroke and high blood cholesterol in South Africa. In this context, we set out to explore the patterns of spatial correlation amongst them, and to estimate the relative weight of the shared risk factors for each vascular disease, both before and after adjustment for individual demographic, socioeconomic and lifestyle background. For the spatial

Table 15.1 Subject level socio-demographic, body mass index and lifestyle risk factors used in the analysis of vascular diseases in South Africa, SADHS 1998

Characteristic	Summary
Gender of subject (N (%))	
Female	8,074 (58.39)
Male	5,753 (41.61)
Age in years (Mean (SD))	38.54 (17.90)
Education (%)	
No education	1,937 (14.08)
Primary	4,030 (29.29)
Secondary	6,928 (50.35)
Higher	866 (6.29)
Population group (N (%))	
Black/African	10,457 (75.76)
Coloured	1,780 (12.90)
White	1,103 (7.99)
Indian	462 (3.35)
Residential setting (N (%))	
Rural	6,074 (43.93)
Urban	7,753 (56.07)
Body Mass Index (N (%))	
Underweight	1,323 (9.77)
Normal	6,342 (46.81)
Obese/overweight	5,850 (43.18)
Current smoker (N (%))	3,460 (25.02)
Current alcohol drinker (N (%))	3,919 (28.34)
Total (N (%))	13,827 (100)

Table 15.2 A summary of the district prevalence rates for each vascular disease

Vascular disease	Mean	Median	Minimum	Maximum
High blood pressure	15.55	15.18	3.88	50.00
Heart attack	5.66	4.89	0.00	40.00
Stroke	0.92	0.79	0.00	3.51
High blood cholesterol	1.19	0.76	0.00	9.38

analysis, we used the health district as the unit at which the residual spatial risk in the prevalence rates we estimated. The District Health System (DHS) is the basic channel through which the delivery of Primary Health Care is undertaken in South Africa (Day et al. 2010).

The minimum number of sampled adults in a health district was 10 and the maximum was 900, with mean and median number of 266 and 235. A summary of the district prevalence rates for each of the four vascular diseases is shown in Table 15.2, and the nonparametric correlations amongst the ward prevalence rates are shown in Table 15.3. Vascular disease of high blood pressure and heart attack

Table 15.3 Correlations between the standardised incidence ratios for each condition

	Blood pressure	Heart attack	Stroke	High blood cholesterol
High blood pressure	1.00	–	–	–
Heart attack	0.33	1.00	–	–
Stroke	−0.05	0.04	1.00	–
High blood cholesterol	0.17	−0.12	0.31	1.00

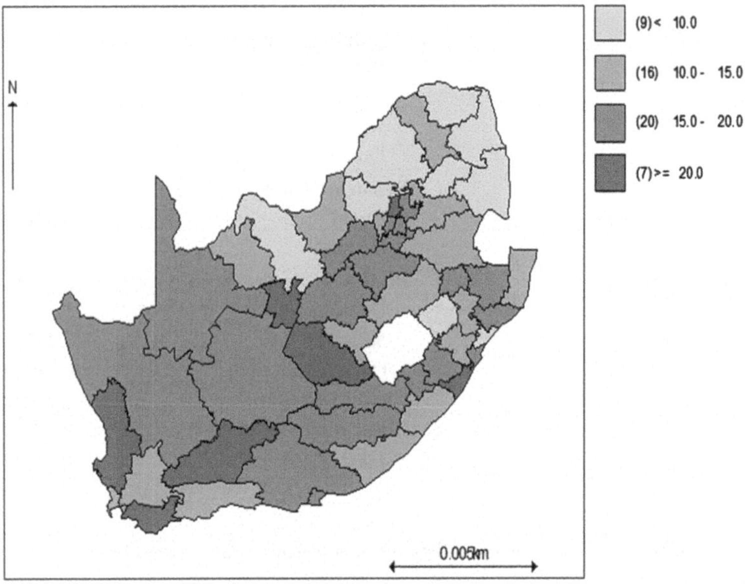

Fig. 15.1 High blood pressure prevalence by health district in South Africa

were more prevalent whilst stroke and high blood cholesterol were less prevalent. There were 15 districts out of the 52 that had a prevalence of 0 % for stroke, and 13 out of 52 had a prevalence of 0 % for high blood cholesterol. The correlation amongst the districts prevalence rates was highest for high blood pressure and heart attack (0.33), followed by stroke and high blood cholesterol (0.31). There were negative correlations between high blood pressure and stroke (−0.05) and between heart attack and blood cholesterol (−0.12); incidentally these negative correlations involve the diseases that are very rare. The disease-specific prevalence maps in Figs. 15.1, 15.2, 15.3, and 15.4 show a large amount of noise especially for the rare diseases (Figs. 15.3 and 15.4), making it difficult to discern any geographical trends in the prevalence rates. Nonetheless, some of the highest prevalence of high blood pressure and heart attacks are in the districts in the south-western parts of the country and the lowest in north-eastern parts. For stroke and high blood cholesterol, prevalence rates appear to be relatively evenly distributed across the country.

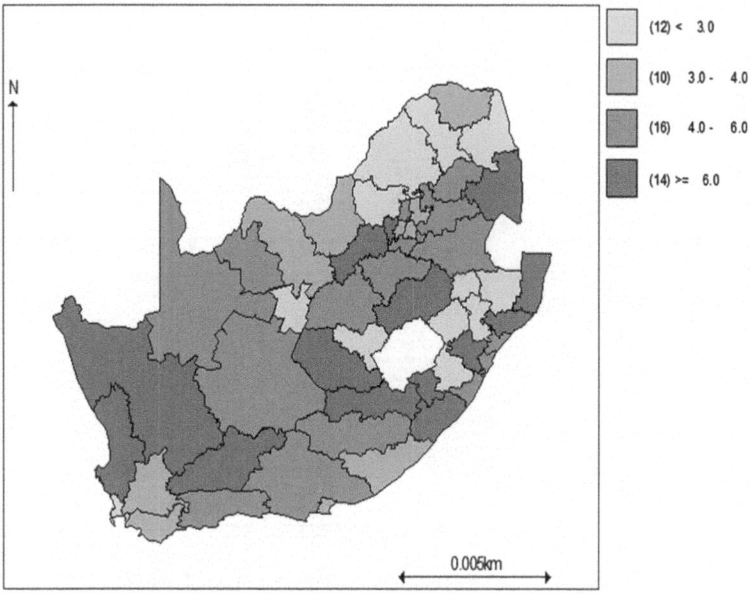

Fig. 15.2 Heart attack prevalence by health district in South Africa

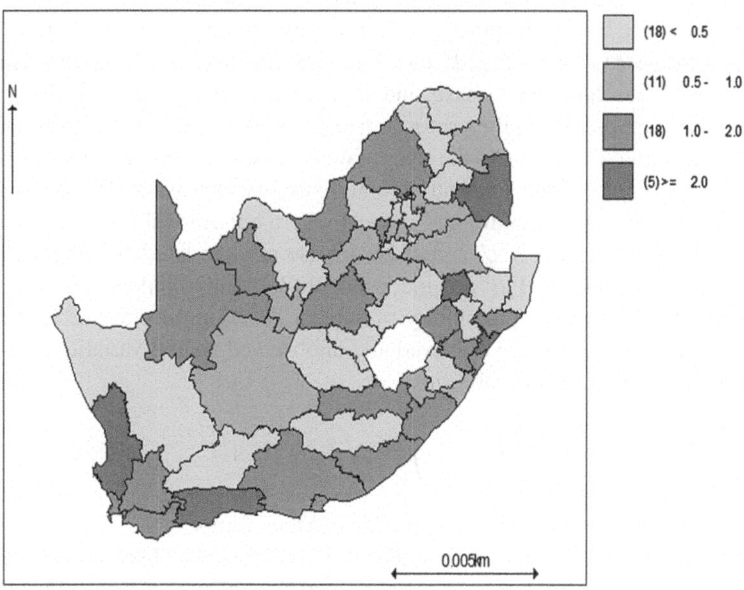

Fig. 15.3 Stroke prevalence by health district in South Africa

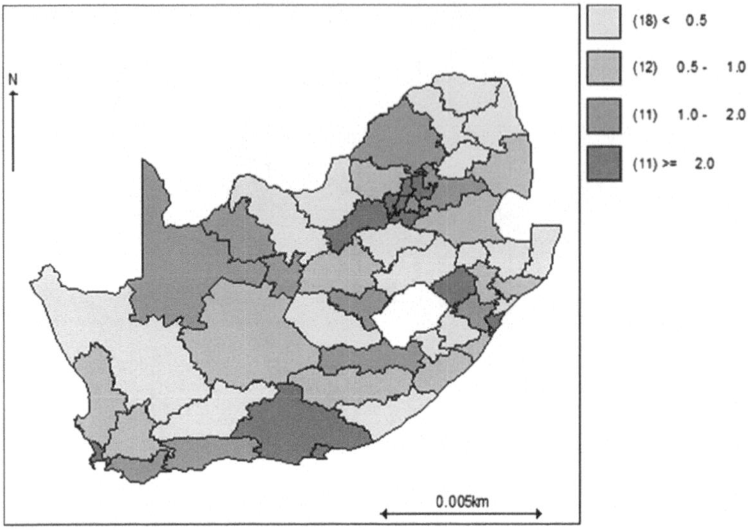

Fig. 15.4 High blood cholestroal prevalence by health district in South Africa

15.2.3 Statistical Methods

There are $J = 52$ districts, and district j has N_j adults out of the total sampled. We let Y_{ijk} be a binary response corresponding to subject i in district j for vascular disease $k(j = 1, \ldots, 52;\ i = 1, \ldots, N_j;\ k = 1, \ldots, 4)$ taking values 1 if the subject has had the disease and 0 otherwise at the time of the survey. Furthermore, suppose X_{ij} is the vector of risk covariates associated with subject ij. For the unaccounted variation in the risks of the diseases, unobserved district-spatial variation U_{jk} is introduced for district j and vascular disease k. We are working within the framework of conditional models where conditional on spatial random effects $U = (U_{j1},\ U_{j2},\ U_{j3}\ U_{j4})$ and the disease-specific fixed effects parameters β_k, the binary responses Y_{ijk} are independent Bernoulli random variables with parameters π_{ijk}, being the probability of subject ij having disease k. In order to model the probabilities of the observed and unobserved spatial variation, we use a logit link function on the probabilities:

$$log\left(\frac{\pi_{ijk}}{1-\pi_{ijk}}\right) = \alpha_k + \beta_k' X_{ij} + U_{jk}$$

where $\alpha_k{}'s$ are the disease-specific log-odds constant terms.

In order to model co-morbidity among the four vascular diseases, we can use a multivariate normal prior to assess spatial correlations amongst the four disease spatial effects U_{j1}, U_{j2}, U_{j3} and U_{j4}.As an alternative, we use a shared-component model where one shared component, relevant to all the four vascular diseases, is included. The shared spatial component could be interpreted as a proxy for variations in lifestyle and nutritional uptake choices. Within the symmetric formulations of the shared component model, we also include disease-specific spatial components for each of the four diseases (Knorr-Held and Best 2001; Held et al. 2005). Thus the mode decomposes each of the four spatial random effects U_{j1}, U_{j2}, U_{j3} and U_{j4} into a common spatial and disease specific component. The resulting model enables us to determine the extent of the variation exhibited through common as well as specific geographical patterns in the disease risks. We also allow for disease-specific unstructured heterogeneous effects ε_{jk} to account for possible extra-binomial variation that is not explained by the included fixed effect; and common and specific structured spatial terms.

Thus, the four diseases are modelled as follows on log-odds scale:

$$log\left(\frac{\pi_{ij1}}{1-\pi_{ij1}}\right) = \alpha_1 + \beta_1' X_{ij} + \gamma_1 U_j + U_{j1} + \varepsilon_{j1}$$

$$log\left(\frac{\pi_{ij2}}{1-\pi_{ij2}}\right) = \alpha_2 + \beta_2' X_{ij} + \gamma_2 U_j + U_{j2} + \varepsilon_{j2}$$

$$log\left(\frac{\pi_{ij3}}{1-\pi_{ij3}}\right) = \alpha_3 + \beta_3' X_{ij} + \gamma_3 U_j + U_{j3} + \varepsilon_{j3}$$

$$log\left(\frac{\pi_{ij4}}{1-\pi_{ij3}}\right) = \alpha_4 + \beta_4' X_{ij} + \gamma_4 U_j + U_{j4} + \varepsilon_{j4}$$

where U_{j1}, U_{j2}, U_{j3} and U_{j4} are the log odds for the risk of high blood pressure, heart attack or angina, stroke and high blood cholesterol, respectively, in health district j. The parameters $\alpha_k's$ and $\beta_k's$ are the disease-specific baseline risk and fixed effect risks associated with the risk vector X_{ij}; and U_j is the shared component common to all four vascular diseases. The unknown parameters γ allow for different risk gradients for common latent risk on the four vascular diseases.

For a Bayesian model to be completed, all unknown parameters, whether for fixed or random effects, are given prior distributions. The shared and specific spatial random effects U_j and U_{j1}, U_{j2}, U_{j3} and U_{j4} were given a prior distribution to capture local dependence in space using intrinsic conditional autoregressive (ICAR) normal models (Besag et al. 1991). We used districts sharing a common boundary with the district under investigation to define a neighbourhood set. The disease-specific heterogeneity terms were modelled to arise from a multivariate normal prior distribution with covariance matrix Σ to allow for correlations amongst the four vascular diseases. A flat prior was assigned on the overall disease-specific risk terms α_k and the fixed effects were assigned independent *Normal* $(0, 10^3)$ prior distributions. Further details about the ICAR normal prior for modelling spatially structured effects can be found in Chap. 8.

The logarithms of the scaling parameters were assigned independent *Normal* $(0, 5)$ prior distributions, and the shared and specific component precision parameters were independently assigned a conjugate hyper-prior Gamma (0.5, 0.0005) distribution (Richardson et al. 2006). The precision matrix Σ^{-1}

for the multivariate normal unstructured random effects was assigned a *Wishart* prior distribution. The shared component model for the four vascular diseases was estimated using the WinBUGS software (Spiegelhalter et al. 2004). Three independent chains were run for 40,000 iterations, using trace plots of precision parameters to assess convergence; we obtained rapid convergence by 5,000 iterations. Thus, we took the first 5,000 iterations as being in the burn-in period, and used the remaining combined 105,000 iterations from the three chains for posterior summaries.

15.3 Results

Figures 15.5, 15.6, 15.7, 15.8, and 15.9 show the covariate-adjusted smoothed estimated of the log-odds for the shared component, and for the four disease-specific components. The shared component, which can be taken to represent nutrition and lifestyle not accounted for in the model, had a larger effect on vascular disease prevalence in south-western areas of the country. Unlike the unevenness evident in the unadjusted unsmoothed (raw) prevalence maps (Figs. 15.1, 15.2, 15.3, and 15.4), now the disease-specific log-odds show clear spatial patterns. In particular, the spatial distributions of high blood pressure and stroke are concentrated highly in south-western parts of the country; the risk of heart attacks has a high concentration in the districts around the central north-eastern corridor; and high blood cholesterol is concentrated more in the top north-eastern corridor.

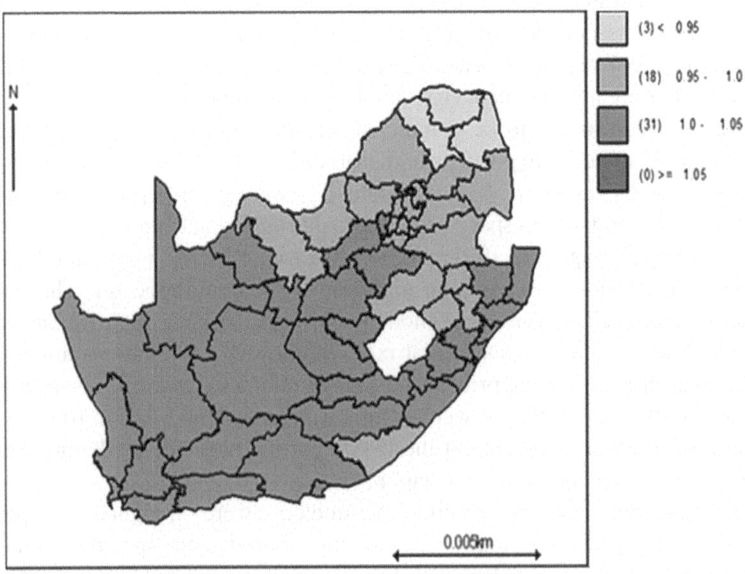

Fig. 15.5 Shared component

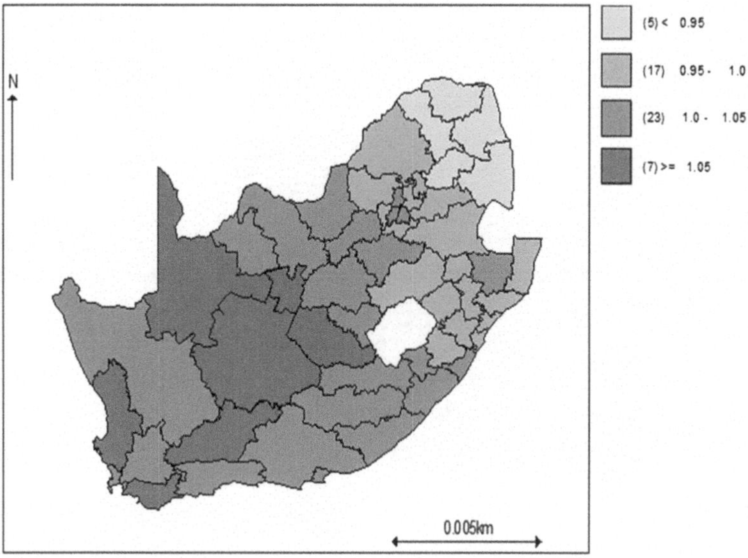

Fig. 15.6 High blood pressure specific spatial component

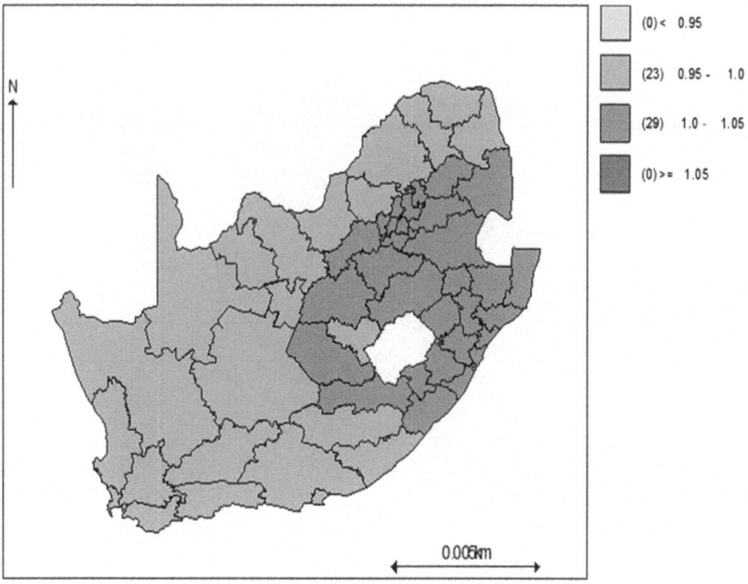

Fig. 15.7 Heart attack specific spatial component

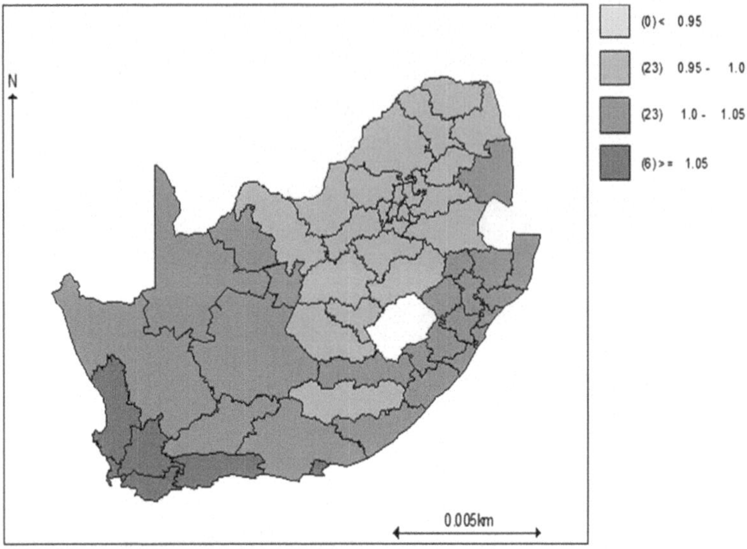

Fig. 15.8 Stroke specific spatial component

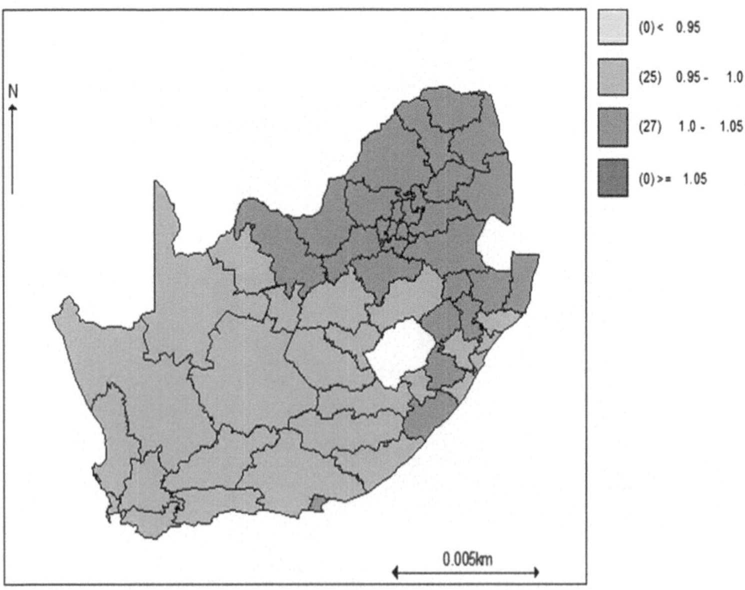

Fig. 15.9 High blood cholesterol specific spatial component

Table 15.4 Relative weights of each vascular disease for the shared component

Disease	Blood pressure	Heart attack	Stroke
Blood pressure	1.00		
Heart attack	1.071 (0.317–2.602)	1.00	
Stroke	1.070 (0.353–3.211)	1.085 (0.401–2.961)	1.00
High blood cholesterols	1.098 (0.329–3.511)	1.116 (0.345–2.870)	0.960 (0.312–3.580)

The figures represent the weight of the vascular disease listed along the top row relative to those listed along the left hand side. If the RR is >1.00 then the vascular disease along the top row has more weight

Table 15.4 shows the level of relative weight or effect that the shared component has for the different vascular diseases. The shared component, which was taken to represent nutritional and lifestyles not accounted for in the models, affected high blood pressure more slightly than the other three vascular diseases, but the relative weights were not statistically significant. The component was also slightly more important for heart attack than for stroke and high blood cholesterol and again this was not significant. However, stroke was less affected by the component relative to high blood cholesterol.

Table 15.5 shows the risks of vascular diseases on the odds ratio (OR) scale by the modelled risk factors. A male adult is associated with a reduced risk of high blood pressure and heart attack (OR = 0.45, 95 % CI 0.39–0.51, and OR = 0.57, 95 % CI 0.46–0.69), respectively, and a higher risk for high blood cholesterol (OR = 1.56, 95 % CI 1.10–1.2.26), but with equal risk for stroke (OR = 1.01, 95 % CI 0.63–1.54) compared to a female adult. Increasing age is positively associated with increased risks of all four vascular diseases (OR = 22.49 (17.58–29.23), 11.04 (7.54–16.54), 14.41 (5.21–80.40), 5.07 (2.48–11.55)), respectively, for high blood pressure, heart attack, stroke and high blood cholesterol, in the age group 65 years or above compared to 14–24 year group. There appears to be a positive association between increasing education and an increased risk of high blood cholesterol, whilst the opposite was seen for heart attack and stroke; but the relationship with high blood pressure is not systematic.

There is a statistically significant association between population groups and risk for high blood cholesterol (OR = 5.96 (3.19–11.06), 20.88 (12.26–35.33), 20.01 (10.77–44.02), respectively, in Coloureds, Whites and Indians/Asians compared to the Blacks/Africans). Ethnicity was also significantly associated with high blood pressure where Coloureds and Indians were at higher risk compared to Blacks/Africans. Whites are significantly at higher risk of heart attack that Blacks/Africans. Being White slightly increases the risk of stroke, and the risk decrease among Coloureds and Indians but the effects are not significant. Living in an urban environment impacts adversely on high blood pressure (OR = 1.36 (1.18–1.58)), whilst the opposite holds for high blood cholesterol (OR = 0.62 (0.39–0.99)). Urban residence has negative and positive effects, respectively on heart attack and stroke, but both effects are not significant. Being overweight or obese significantly decreases the risk for all of the four vascular diseases: high blood

Table 15.5 Odds ratio of vascular disease prevalence by socio-demographic, body mass and lifestyle factors

	High blood pressure	Heart attack	Stroke	High blood cholesterol
Male (Yes=1, No-0)	0.45 (0.39–0.51)	0.57 (0.46–0.69)	1.01 (0.63–1.54)	1.56 (1.10–2.26)
Age				
14–24 years	1.00	1.00	1.00	1.00
25–34 years	2.21(1.69–2.86)	2.99(2.03–4.44)	4.84(1.77–27.95)	2.70(1.35–6.10)
35–44 years	4.45(3.46–5.76)	3.55(2.44–5.38)	6.13(2.17–33.87)	2.52(1.22–5.45)
44–54 years	10.83(8.56–13.91)	5.92(4.11–9.03)	10.33(3.89–62.76)	5.36(0.19–11.54)
55–64 years	17.35 (13.5–22.4)	9.37(6.52–14.17)	13.75(4.76–70.09)	4.70(2.36–10.19)
>= 65 years	22.49(17.58–29.23)	11.04(7.54–16.54)	14.41(5.21–80.4)	5.07(2.48–11.55)
Education				
No education	1.00	1.00	1.00	1.00
Primary	1.15(0.98–1.35)	0.98(0.78–1.23)	0.67(0.39–1.12)	1.13(0.49–2.81)
Secondary	1.01(0.85–1.23)	0.70(0.53–0.91)	0.58(0.31–1.03)	1.88(0.90–4.64)
Higher	0.96(0.71–1.30)	0.35(0.19–0.61)	0.55(0.18–1.34)	2.64(1.18–7.75)
Population group				
Black/African	1.00	1.00	1.00	1.00
Coloured	1.36(1.09-1.68)	0.98(0.72–1.32)	0.86(0.43–1.57)	5.96(3.19–11.06)
White	1.07(0.86–1.34)	1.65(1.17–2.31)	1.75(0.87–3.43)	20.88(12.26–35.33)
Indian	1.49(1.07–2.06)	1.42(0.84–2.33)	0.91(0.28–2.44)	22.01(10.77–44.02)
Urban setting (Yes=1, No=0)	1.36(1.18–1.58)	0.94(0.77–1.15)	1.39(0.86–2.23)	0.62(0.39–0.99)
Body Mass Indes				
Underweight	0.77(0.58–1.01)	1.26(0.90–1.75)	1.03(0.40–2.26)	0.36(0.05–1.36)
Normal	1.00	1.00	1.00	1.00
Obese	2.18(1.93–2.46)	1.21(1.00–1.46)	1.48(0.97–2.32)	3.97(2.58–6.33)
Current smoker (Yes=1, No=0)	0.83(0.72–0.97)	0.96(0.74–1.21)	1.31(0.80–2.10)	0.95(0.64–1.41)
Current alcohol drinker (Yes=1, No=0)	1.09(0.96–1.25)	0.94(0.6–1.16)	0.66(0.40–1.03)	0.91(0.61–1.33)

pressure (OR = 2.18; 1.93–2.46); heart attack (1.21; 1.00–1.46); stroke (1.48; 0.97–2.32); and high blood cholesterol (3.97; 2.58–6.33), compared to a normal body mass index. Lifestyles such as smoking and drinking alcohol appear not to have any adverse effects on the vascular diseases; in most parts the trend seems to be negative though not statistically significant.

15.4 Discussion

We have demonstrated, by our model, the spatial distribution of vascular disease burden and influence of nutrition and lifestyle (the shared component) on vascular disease in South Africa. It appears that dietary and lifestyle factors have greater influence on vascular disease in the south-western areas of the country. This will suggest lifestyle modification will make greater impact in reducing the burden of vascular disease in these areas. Importantly, high blood pressure and stroke, which are highly related (MacMahon et al. 1990) and associated with diet (Freis 1976) and physical activity (Wareham et al. 2000), have higher concentrations in the south-western areas (Figs. 15.6, 15.7, and 15.8).

Heart attacks and angina are known to be associated with abnormal blood cholesterol (Yusuf et al. 2004). The concentration of these conditions in the north-eastern areas of South Africa reaffirms these associations and the need for a common public health approach to reduce blood cholesterol levels and risk of coronary heart disease in this specific geographical area. Low physical activity (Gill and Hardman 2003; Kraus et al. 2002), prolonged sitting (Hamilton et al. 2004) and dietary lipid (Shekelle et al. 1981) independently influence the blood cholesterol profile and vascular outcomes.

Men have reduced risk for high blood pressure and heart attack but have higher risk for high blood cholesterol. In previous studies in Europe and North America, where no spatial modelling was undertaken, the prevalence of high blood pressure was consistently higher among men compared to women in all the eight countries studied (Wolf-Maier et al. 2003). Between sexes the difference in physical activity participation and adipose tissue distribution may differ between Africa and Europe/North America. Importantly, this increased risk of high blood pressure and heart attack or angina among women poses an extra challenge for maternal health if measures are not taken to influence behaviour.

As expected, high BMI is associated with increased higher risk of vascular disease. Obesity is known to be associated with increased vascular risk (Gerber and Stern 1999; WHO 2004) and this increasing burden of chronic diseases with an increasing proportion of the population of the obese is a new challenge for African countries, most of which are struggling with more than their share of infectious diseases. The increasing burden of vascular and other non-communicable diseases associated with an increasing population of older people needs addressing. With economic growth life expectancy will continue to increase in Africa, and so is the adoption of Western lifestyle and dietary habits. These lifestyle changes, which are also associated with educational attainment, may contribute to the spatial variations in vascular disease burden in South Africa. We observed an increase in risk for high blood cholesterol associated with higher educational attainment. However, education attainment was also associated with a reduction in risk for heart attack, and probably stroke and high blood pressure (the latter two not statistically significant). This may be interpreted as interplay between diet and physical activity. It is possible that the more educated may have a high intake of dietary cholesterol but may be more physically active thereby increasing the HDL cholesterol (protective cholesterol) component. Higher physical activity is also associated with reduced blood pressure and stroke.

The adjusted odds of high blood pressure and high blood cholesterol are higher among the Coloured, White and Indian populations compared to Blacks and stroke and heart attack risk are higher among White and Indian compared to Blacks and Coloured. Therefore, aside from the spatial distribution of vascular disease in South Africa, ethnic specific measures are necessary to target high risk groups. It may also be that ethnicity is confounded by dietary and physical activities and urbanisation. Urban lifestyle in South Africa has been shown to impact negatively on the risk of high blood pressure and stroke. However, the risk of high blood cholesterol and heart attack are lower among urban dwellers. This may be due to differences in diet and/or physical activity behaviour between urban and rural dwellers.

However, smoking and alcohol consumption seem not to have negative health effects. It might be that the level and pattern of consumption of these products in South Africa are different from those observed in Western societies (Rehm et al. 2003).

We have also shown the relative weights of each vascular disease that is explained by the shared component, i.e. dietary and lifestyle factors. While these diseases are interlinked, the relative weight allows us to ascertain the relative health gain of implementing a lifestyle change in a geographic area. A combination of the disease burden and the relative weight may be used to prioritise geographically targeted public health programmes.

There are some limitations in the present study that deserve attention as those mentioned in Chap. 11. First, the cross-sectional nature of the present study does not allow establishing temporality and thus causality of the observed associations. Given the self-reporting of lifestyle factors, we cannot disregard the likelihood that health outcomes such as hypertension, stroke, high cholesterol and heart attack may influence reports of habitual smoking, drinking habits, and sleep problems and not vice versa. Second, the analysis was based on data collected in 1998, which is likely to underestimate the current prevalence of hypertension in South Africa, as reported by several recent reports. However, since 1998 there are no recent nationally representative reliable data from SA with information on hypertension. Thus, this limits our ability to apply our approach to more recent data. In addition, there was limited or lack of information for variables such as dietary habits, physical activity, and biomarker data, which are relevant to hypertension aetiology. Nevertheless, our findings corroborate the notion that high blood pressure, stroke, high cholesterol and heart attack are increasing public health issues in these settings, with evidence of considerable spatial variation in hypertension prevalence across different provinces in South Africa.

Another important issue in the use of this data is the issue of data quality because of the fact that national surveys in developing countries are prone to incomplete or partial reporting of responses. Moreover, the use of complex questionnaires inevitably allows scope for inconsistent responses to be recorded for different questions resulting in a further complication in the assessment of health outcomes.

Luckily, the MEASURE DHS program primary goals are to produce high-quality data and make it available for analysis in a coherent and consistent form. Therefore, the DHS program has a strict primary data quality policies by adopting a policy of editing and imputation which results in a data file that accurately reflects the population studied and may be readily used for analysis which ultimately reduce bias in the reporting of health outcomes including hypertension.

15.5 Conclusion

The double burden of chronic and communicable diseases in the sub-Saharan African region require rigorous public health interventions if the Millennium Development Goals (MDGs) for maternal and child health in the region are to be achieved. In Chap. 11, we highlighted the lack of appreciation of the burden of non-communicable diseases in Africa. By our novel approach, we have demonstrated in this chapter how a shared behaviour (diet, physical activity and other lifestyle variables) is distributed across South Africa. We have also shown how this behaviour may determine geographic distribution of four cardiovascular conditions – high blood pressure, heart attack/angina, stroke and high blood cholesterol. It is our firm believe that policy-makers will be able to use our maps to re-orient public health programmes on aimed at reducing chronic disease. An integrated disease management is required to address the double burden of disease in the Sub-Saharan African region.

References

Besag, J., York, J., & Mollie, A. (1991). Bayesian image restoration, with two applications in spatial statistics (with discussion). *Annals of the Institute of Statistical Mathematics, 43*, 1–59.

Brenzel, L., Wolfson, L. J., Fox–Rushby, J., Miller, M., Halsey, N. A. (2006). *Diseases control priorities project. Chapter 20: Vaccine–preventable diseases*, Washington, DC: World Bank.

Dabney, A. R., & Wakefield, J. C. (2005). Issues in the mapping of two diseases. *Statistical Methods in Medical Research, 14*, 83–112.

Day, C., Monticelli, F., Barron, P., et al. (2010). *The district health barometer 2008/09*. Durban: Health Systems Trust.

Department of Health, Medical Research Council & Measure DHS+. (2002). *South Africa demographic and health survey 1998, full report*. Pretoria: National Department of Health, South Africa.

Downing, A., Forman, D., Gilthorpe Edwards, K. L., & Manda, S. O. M. (2008). Joint disease mapping using six cancers in the Yorkshire region of England. *International Journal of Health Geographics, 7*, 41.

Freis, E. D. (1976). Salt, volume and the prevention of hypertension. *Circulation, 53*, 589–595.

Gerber, L. M., & Stern, P. M. (1999). Relationship of body size and body mass to blood pressure: Sex-specific and developmental influences. *Human Biology An International Record of Research, 71*(4), 505–528.

Gill, J. M., & Hardman, A. (2003). Exercise and postprandial lipid metabolism: An update on potential mechanisms and interactions with high-carbohydrate diets (review). *The Journal of Nutritional Biochemistry, 14*(3), 122–132.

Hamilton, M. T., Hamilton, D. G., & Zderic, T. W. (2004). Exercise physiology versus inactivity physiology: An essential concept for understanding lipoprotein lipase regulation. *Exercise and Sports Science Reviews, 32*(4), 161–166.

Held, L., Natario, I., Fenton, S. E., et al. (2005). Towards joint disease mapping. *Statistical Methods in Medical Research, 14*, 61–82.

Kazembe, L. N., Muula, A. S., Appleton, C. C., & Kleinschmidt, I. (2007). Modelling the effect of malaria endemicity on spatial variations in childhood fever, diarrhoea and pneumonia in Malawi. *International Journal of Health Geographics, 6*, 33.

Knorr-Held, L., & Best, N. G. (2001). A shared model for detecting joint and selective clustering of two diseases. *Journal of the Royal Statistical Society, Series A, 164*, 73–86.

Kraus, W. E., Houmard, J. A., Duscha, B. D., Knetzger, K. J., Wharton, M. B., McCartney, J. S., Bales, C. W., Henes, S., Samsa, G. P., Otvos, J. D., Kulkarni, K. R., & Slentz, C. A. (2002). Effects of the amount and intensity of exercise on plasma lipoproteins. *The New England Journal of Medicine, 347*(19), 1483–1492.

Langford, I. H., Leyland, A. H., Rasbash, J., et al. (1999). Multilevel modelling of geographical distributions of rare diseases. *Journal of the Royal Statistical Society, Series C, 48*, 253–269.

MacMahon, S., Peto, R., Cutler, J., et al. (1990). Blood pressure, stroke, and coronary heart disease. *Lancet, 335*, 765–774.

Manda, S. O. M., Feltbower, R. G., & Gilthorpe, M. S. (2009). Investigating spatio-temporal similarities in the epidemiology of childhood leukaemia and diabetes. *European Journal of Epidemiology, 24*(12), 743–752.

Mensah, G. A. (2008). Epidemiology of stroke and high blood pressure in Africa. *Heart, 94*, 697–705.

Rehm, J., Rehn, N., Room, R., Monteiro, M., Gmel, G., Jernigan, D., & Frick, U. (2003). The global distribution of average volume of alcohol consumption and patterns of drinking. *European Addiction Research, 9*, 147–156.

Richardson, S., Abellan, J. J., & Best, N. (2006). Bayesian spatio-temporal analysis of joint patterns of male and female lung cancer risks in Yorkshire (UK). *Statistical Methods in Medical Research, 15*, 385–407.

Shekelle, R. B., Shryock, A. M., Paul, O., et al. (1981). Diet, serum cholesterol, and death from coronary heart disease: The western electric study. *The New England Journal of Medicine, 304*, 65–70.

Spiegelhalter, D., Thomas, A., Best, N., et al. (2004). *BUGS: Bayesian Inference Using Gibbs Sampling, version 1.4*. Cambridge: MRC Biostatistics Unit.

Wareham, N. J., Wong, M. Y., Hennings, S., Mitchell, J., Rennie, K., Cruickshank, K., & Day, N. E. (2000). Quantifying the association between habitual energy expenditure and blood pressure. *International Journal of Epidemiology, 29*(4), 655–660.

WHO. (2004). *Global strategy on diet, physical activity and health*. http://www.who.int/dietphysicalactivity/strategy/eb11344/en/. Accessed 1 Feb 2011.

WHO. (2011). *World Health Organization report on nutrition*. http://www.who.int/nutrition/topics/2_background/en/index.html. Accessed 1 Feb 2011.

Wolf-Maier, K., Cooper, R. S., Banegas, J. R., et al. (2003). Hypertension prevalence and blood pressure levels in 6 European countries, Canada, and the United States. *Journal of the American Medical Association, 289*(18), 2363–2369.

Yusuf, S., Hawken, S., Ôunpuu, S., et al. (2004). Effect of potentially modifiable risk factors associated with myocardial infarction in 52 countries (the INTERHEART study): case-control study. *The Lancet, 364*, 937–952.

Chapter 16
Advances in Modelling Maternal and Child Health in Africa: What Have We Learned and What Is Next?

Gebrenegus Ghilagaber

16.1 Background

Demographic and Health Surveys (DHS) have played important role in filling the gap in the availability of survey data in developing countries. The samples drawn in the DHS use stratified multistage cluster sampling designs, and gather retrospective data on fertility history, and other background information related to maternal and child health by interviewing selected women in fertile ages. Thus, any statistical analysis of such data drawn from a complex survey needs to account for the sampling design, in addition to account for data quality. For instance, DHS datasets include geographical information that could identify spatial patterns to target health policies. Such information needs to be incorporated when the analyses of such data are undertaken.

However, the utilization of a wealth of data on maternal and child health from high quality national representative samples in the Sub Saharan region Africa (SSA), collected at comparatively enormous costs, remains sub-optimal because optimal analyses of such data demand advanced statistical techniques.

The primary aim of this volume has been to bring together such methodological advances. Thus, the volume is organized around one major (central) and two minor themes. Our central theme deals with developing or implementing new and advanced models and methods for the analysis of data collected through Demographic and Health Surveys (DHS) in African countries. Our other themes are more of substantive nature and emerge in the application of these advanced techniques to model levels, trends, and correlates of maternal and child health in the context of Africa.

G. Ghilagaber (✉)
Department of Statistics, Stockholm University, SE-106 91 Stockholm, Sweden
e-mail: Gebre@stat.su.se

N.-B. Kandala and G. Ghilagaber (eds.), *Advanced Techniques for Modelling Maternal and Child Health in Africa*, The Springer Series on Demographic Methods and Population Analysis 34, DOI 10.1007/978-94-007-6778-2_16,

16.2 Overview of the Advanced Models and Methods

To examine association between maternal and child health on one hand and individual-, family-, and community-level background variables on the other, we use various models and estimation methods. By necessity or convenience, some of the models used are static and focus on whether the event of interest (say, death of child) has occurred or not. Such models focus only on the quantum and ignore the tempo of the event by ignoring the time it takes for the event to occur. This is addressed by the dynamic survival (or event history) models used throughout the volume. The regression models fitted throughout the volume are hazard-rate regression models rather than ordinary regression. Ordinary regression models are not appropriate in the presence of censored observations as the exact event-time is unknown for the censored individuals. Hazard-rate framework, on the other hand, integrates information from censored and uncensored observations and, thus, uses the data more efficiently.

Typically, Demographic and Health Surveys (DHS) employ a nationally representative, two-stage probability sample. In the first, primary sampling units (PSUs) are selected with probability proportional to size. A complete listing of the households in the selected PSUs is carried out. The lists of households obtained are used as the frame for the second-stage sampling, which is the selection of the households to be visited by the interviewing teams during the main survey fieldwork. Women between the ages of 15 and 49 are identified in these households and interviewed.

In modeling child health, the original woman-data is converted into a child-data. In the process, children whose mother reports on their living status and other characteristics are nested within their corresponding parent (mother). Since children of the same parent are more alike than children selected at random from the population, the basic assumption of a random (independent) sample of children can't be ascertained. Further, children of the same mother are expected to be positively corrected as they share the same mother- and household characteristics (shared frailty). Thus, if this clustering (and thereby the correlation) is ignored the standard errors of covariates will be underestimated leading to spurious significance.

A sensible analytical method needs, thus, to address this issue and that is what the multi-level models in this volume do by treating children from the same parents as correlated cases (multi-levels) within the same observation (parent). Such a procedure also has the additional advantage of accounting for any parent-specific unobserved heterogeneity that may affect outcome at a child level.

We also introduce multiprocess approaches (instead of single process) to allow for interdependence among life-course processes and tackle the issue of endogeneity (reciprocal causation) and selection. Utilization of health facilities may not be uniform among potential users. Such differential utilization may lead either to underestimation or overestimation of the beneficial effects of health inputs depending on whether the selection process is adverse or favorable. The methods in this volume address this issue by making the source of selection (correlation between unobserved heterogeneity terms in various processes) part of the model. In some of the countries studied it is shown that while use of health care reduces mortality risks such beneficial effect may be underestimated if selection effects (due to more frail users of health care) is not accounted for as is done in standard modeling. In others, the effect of health care is overestimated when selection effects (due to less frail users of health care) is not accounted for.

Other features of the advanced models and methods include a more general piecewise-linear baseline hazards (rather than the restrictive piecewise constant hazards modeling), a more general Bayesian framework rather than classical approaches, and geo-additive models in order to account for geographical (area) measures.

In the two subsections below, we point out what new insights could be gained by using the advanced analytic techniques. This is done by way of summarizing the findings of relevant chapters in the themes of child and maternal health.

16.3 Child Health

In Chap. 2, children of the same mother are treated as correlated cases (multi-levels) within the same experimental unit (mother) and mother-specific unobserved heterogeneity is allowed. Further, due account is paid to selection in health care utilization by treating health care variables like prenatal care and hospital delivery as endogenous variables and modeling them simultaneously with the hazard of child mortality. The results show that standard procedures that ignore clustering and selection would underestimate or overestimate (depending on the country in question) the beneficial effects of health inputs on child survival.

In Chap. 3, spatial effect is interpreted as representing the cumulative effect of unidentified or unmeasured additional covariates that may reflect impacts of environmental and socio-cultural factors. As a result, it is shown that failure to take into consideration the spatial dimension would invariably lead to an overestimation of the precision in predicting childhood mortality risks in un-sampled districts.

The geoadditive latent variable models in Chap. 4 offer possibilities to jointly analyze child morbidity and malnutrition. One of the outcomes is the possibility to measure the degree of spatial correlation between the indicators of diseases and those of malnutrition.

In Chap. 5, pathway in the association between wealth and child health is investigated. It is shown that wealth is an indirect factor seen as an enabling factor in health seeking behavior.

Chapter 6 synthesizes various traditions and shows that multiplicative hazard model is (1) a model-based alternative to the problem of standardization and (2) a discrete-data version of the common proportional hazards model. Further, its log-linear parameterization enables investigators to estimate its parameters using commonly available software that are developed for other purposes such as contingency table analysis.

Chapter 7 uses spatial models to identify geographic variations in level of immunization coverage across Nigeria, thereby providing policy-makers with tools to enhance appropriate policy formulation on improving access to and coverage of immunization.

The methods used in Chap. 8 offer valuable tools for producing robust and flexible covariate-adjusted maps of under-five morality that may indicate underlying latent risk profiles. The authors also indicated how the otherwise limited information in most survey data can be enriched with external sources using the geographical information system tools.

Results in Chap. 9 confirm findings in previous chapters that failure to account for hierarchical nature of data leads to underestimation of standard errors of some factors resulting in spurious significance.

16.4 Maternal Health

Chapter 10 presents a flexible family of parametric distributions for modeling the tempo of fertility by embedding a number of commonly known distributions as special cases of a more general extended generalized gamma model. As a number of common distributions like exponential, Weibull, and lognormal are nested within the more general model, the relative merit of each can be tested through standard likelihood ratio test. This provides a statistically well grounded, theoretically appropriate, and empirically evident procedure on how to identify the most appropriate distribution for a given dataset.

Among the many and novel findings in Chap. 11 are the maps generated as tools to help policy-makers re-evaluate the lack of focus on non-communicable diseases (chronic diseases) in Sub-Saharan Africa and focus on integrated diseases management approach, which will accelerate the achievement of the Millennium Development Goals (MDGs) for maternal and child health in the region.

The mixture of triangular distributions proposed in Chap. 12 has the ability to detect peaks, periods of increase and decrease, multi-modal, giving a much more detailed picture than traditional distributions like the Weibull. Application of such model to the timing of first birth in South Africa yields expected estimates of birth cohort effects, in line with the suggested increased access to birth control and abortion over the years. A contradicting picture emerges from using the other models. Based on such appropriate model, it is shown that South Africa has made positive steps in improving maternal health among teenagers and in combating the adverse effects of early childbearing on both the mother and child.

The use of Bayesian variable selection procedure for fitting a parsimonious model to fertility data in Nigeria is demonstrated in Chap. 13. The approach permits automatic identification of variables to be included in the model and also specify the form in which a continuous covariate enters the model (linearly or nonlinearly). Use of such model on fertility data reveals that woman's educational attainment is a major proximate determinant of fertility in Nigeria.

A nested frailty model which included heterogeneity on both census blocks and ethnic groups' levels was implemented on age at sexual initiation for males and females aged 15–24 in Chap. 14. Such an approach allowed flexible modeling of small area district effects which is of great advantage compared to the usual parametric and frequentist approach. Findings from the descriptive analysis revealed, among others, a higher median age at first sex among male youth (implying delayed sexual debut) compared with their female counterparts. One benefit of such modeling technique is that controlling for clustering invalidates the wrong independence and identical-distribution-assumption often made regarding survival time observations that are clustered.

Lastly, in Chap. 15, a novel approach demonstrates how a shared behavior such as diet, physical activity and other lifestyle variables is distributed across South Africa and how such behavior may determine geographic distribution of four cardiovascular conditions – high blood pressure, heart attack/angina, stroke and high blood cholesterol. The maps produced are expected to enable policy-makers to re-orient public health programmes aimed at reducing chronic disease. Thus, the double burden of chronic and communicable diseases in the sub-Saharan African region require rigorous public health interventions if the Millennium Development Goals (MDGs) for maternal and child health in the region are to be achieved.

16.5 Some Potential Extensions for the Future

Since every chapter in this volume is designed to be as self-contained as possible, most of the methods and examples are treated independently, leaving little room for the inter-method, inter-chapter, or inter-data comparisons. This may be one of the limitations of the volume.

Except for death, the other events studied in this volume are not a certain event to all individuals. In other words, there may be long-term survivors – individuals who may never experience the event irrespective of the length of exposure time. Accordingly, alternative models that allow for this feature (partition the censored observations among real censoring and long-term survivors) could be appropriate.

The multiprocess procedure used in one of the chapters estimates two or more equations jointly and allows investigators to model the correlation (source of selection bias) directly, thereby mitigating the bias due to selection. The tradeoff in the procedure is that we have to assume that the mother specific heterogeneity terms in the two equations are jointly normally distributed. If the true model is known, then a proper model will eliminate selection bias. In real life, we don't know what the true model is, however. We may theorize that there is an unobserved mother effect which is normally distributed. If the distribution of that effect is in fact something other than normal, the selection bias will be reduced but not necessarily eliminated. Thus, while the modeling approach we used is designed to certainly mitigate selection biases, it may not be taken for granted that such biases are fully eliminated. A possible area for future studies would, therefore, be a deeper examination on the validity of the distributional assumptions (and proposal of alternative distributions) as well as investigation of the robustness to violations of distributional assumptions of the procedure used here.

Index

N.-B. Kandala and G. Ghilagaber (eds.), *Advanced Techniques for Modelling Maternal and Child Health in Africa*, The Springer Series on Demographic Methods and Population Analysis 34, DOI 10.1007/978-94-007-6778-2,

The manufacturer's authorised representative in the EU is Springer Nature Customer Service Centre GmbH, Europaplatz 3, 69115 Heidelberg, Germany. If you have any concerns regarding our products, please contact ProductSafety@springernature.com

Printed and bound by CPI Group (UK) Ltd, Croydon, CR0 4YY
25/09/2026
02222869-0015